Cardiomyopathy: An Issue of Cardiology Clinics

Cardiomyopathy: An Issue of Cardiology Clinics

Edited by Sasha Luther

hayle
medical

New York

Hayle Medical,
750 Third Avenue, 9th Floor,
New York, NY 10017, USA

Visit us on the World Wide Web at:
www.haylemedical.com

ISBN: 978-1-63241-921-7

Cataloging-in-publication Data

Cardiomyopathy : an issue of cardiology clinics / edited by Sasha Luther.
    p. cm.
Includes bibliographical references and index.
ISBN 978-1-63241-921-7
1. Myocardium--Diseases. 2. Heart--Diseases. 3. Cardiology. I. Luther, Sasha.
RC685.M9 C37 2020
616.124--dc23

Table of Contents

Preface

The main aim of this book is to educate learners and enhance their research focus by presenting diverse topics covering this vast field. This is an advanced book which compiles significant studies by distinguished experts in the area of analysis. This book addresses successive solutions to the challenges arising in the area of application, along with it; the book provides scope for future developments.

Cardiomyopathy is a set of diseases which affect the muscles of the heart. It is of various types - dilated cardiomyopathy, hypertrophic cardiomyopathy, restricted cardiomyopathy, takotsubo cardiomyopathy and arrhythmogenic right ventricular dysplasia. Each of these affects the cardiac muscle in a different way. The heart muscle enlarges and thickens in hypertrophic cardiomyopathy, while ventricles enlarge and weaken in dilated cardiomyopathy. Early on in the development of the disease, there are few or no symptoms. Gradual fatigue, chest pain, arrhythmias, and swelling of the feet or abdomen can be observed. Cardiomyopathies often lead to progressive heart failure-related disability or cardiovascular death. A cardiomyopathy can be detected through a physical exam, ECG, stress test, blood test or echocardiogram. Treatment differs for different cardiac conditions. To manage fatal heart rhythms defibrillators may be used, while for severe heart failure ventricular assist devices (VADs) can be used. Medications and implanted pacemakers are used to manage slow heart rates. This book is a valuable compilation of topics, ranging from the basic to the most complex advancements in the diagnosis and treatment of cardiomyopathy. It presents this complex subject in the most comprehensible and easy to understand language. This book will help new researchers by foregrounding their knowledge in this condition.

It was a great honour to edit this book, though there were challenges, as it involved a lot of communication and networking between me and the editorial team. However, the end result was this all-inclusive book covering diverse themes in the field.

Finally, it is important to acknowledge the efforts of the contributors for their excellent chapters, through which a wide variety of issues have been addressed. I would also like to thank my colleagues for their valuable feedback during the making of this book.

Editor

Clinical predictors of a positive genetic test in hypertrophic cardiomyopathy in the Brazilian population

Julia Daher Carneiro Marsiglia[1*], Flávia Laghi Credidio[1], Théo Gremen Mimary de Oliveira[1], Rafael Ferreira Reis[1], Murillo de Oliveira Antunes[2], Aloir Queiroz de Araujo[3], Rodrigo Pinto Pedrosa[4], João Marcos Bemfica Barbosa-Ferreira[5], Charles Mady[2], José Eduardo Krieger[1], Edmundo Arteaga-Fernandez[2] and Alexandre Costa Pereira[1]

Abstract

Background: Hypertrophic cardiomyopathy is a genetic autosomal dominant disease characterized by left ventricular hypertrophy. The molecular diagnosis is important but still expensive. This work aimed to find clinical predictors of a positive genetic test in a Brazilian tertiary centre cohort of index cases with HCM.

Methods: In the study were included patients with HCM clinical diagnosis. For genotype x phenotype comparison we have evaluated echocardiographic, electrocardiographic, and nuclear magnetic resonance measures. All patients answered a questionnaire about familial history of HCM and/or sudden death. β-myosin heavy chain, myosin binding protein C, and troponin T genes were sequenced for genetic diagnosis.

Results: The variables related to a higher probability of a positive genetic test were familial history of HCM, higher mean heart frequency, presence of NSVT and lower age. Probabilities of having a positive molecular genetic test were calculated from the final multivariate logistic regression model and were used to identify those with a higher probability of a positive molecular diagnosis.

Conclusions: We developed an easy and fast screening method that takes into account only clinical data that can help to select the patients with a high probability of positive genetic results from molecular sequencing of Brazilian HCM patients.

Keywords: Genetics, *MYH7*, *MYBPC3*, *TNNT2*, Molecular, Screening

Background

Hypertrophic cardiomyopathy (HCM) is a genetic autosomal dominant disease characterized by left ventricular (LV) hypertrophy, without dilatation, usually asymmetric and mainly septal in the absence of any other cardiac or systemic disease that can lead to secondary hypertrophy [1,2]. The main symptoms, when present, are dyspnea on exercise, angina, heart palpitations, pre-syncope or syncope, but many patients may remain asymptomatic and some may have sudden death (SD) as the first manifestation of the disease. The estimated prevalence is 0.2% (1:500), corresponding to 0.5% of all cardiomyopathies [3].

The disease is caused by a mutation in sarcomere, disc-Z, or calcium handling genes. So far, over 20 genes have been associated with the disease, and over 1,000 different mutations have been described. However, the most common genes causing the disease are β-myosin heavy chain (*MYH7*), myosin binding protein C (*MYBPC3*), and troponin T (*TNNT2*) [4].

Molecular diagnosis is very important for several reasons. When the clinical diagnosis is a certainty, establishment of the molecular defect is a diagnostic confirmation, because HCM is a genetic disease. On the other hand, a genetic diagnosis can help in uncertain cases, such as when this is little hypertrophy, hypertrophy in athletes, or hypertensive patients are being screened [2]. In addition, genetic diagnosis allows the identification of children and

* Correspondence: julia.marsiglia@usp.br
[1]Laboratory of Genetics and Molecular Cardiology, Heart Institute (InCor), University of São Paulo, São Paulo, Brazil
Full list of author information is available at the end of the article

adults with subclinical manifestations of the disease, especially in the familial context.

Although genetic testing is important, and it is recommended by the European Cardiology Society, it is not yet a reality in most clinical settings, mainly due to its high cost and the lack of well-established genotypic and phenotypic correlations. Some authors previously reported the use of clinical features to predict a positive genetic test [5,6], as this can help to optimize genetic testing by prioritizing patients with a high chance of a positive genetic test.

Thus, this work aimed to find clinical predictors of a positive genetic test in a Brazilian tertiary centre cohort of index cases with HCM.

Methods

Patients

All the subjects included in the study are HCM index patients clinically diagnosed by expert cardiologists. All of them are patients treated in the respective hospitals the researchers are affiliated and were invited to participate of the research during the periodic consultation. The assistant physician explained about the research and referred them to the Molecular genetics Analysis Laboratory. A septum thickness above 15 mm in the absence of any other disease that could lead to secondary hypertrophy was the criterion used. It included patients from the Heart Institute, a tertiary centre at the University of São Paulo Medical School, but also patients from other cities in Brazil, namely Vitória, Manaus, and Recife. All participants signed the informed consent, and the University of São Paulo Hospital's Research Ethics Committee (CAPPesq) approved the project. Only one patient per family was included in the present analysis.

Examinations

For genotype x phenotype comparison, clinical data were obtained from the patients' medical records. We have evaluated echocardiographic, electrocardiographic, and nuclear magnetic resonance measures, when available. All patients answered a questionnaire about familial history of HCM and sudden death. The presence of a familial history was divided in three categories: absent, when there was no history, present, when at least one relative had a confirmed diagnosis for HCM and unsure, when the patient mentions that there is a history of cardiac disease in the family but without an established HCM diagnosis.

Electrocardiography

Tracings were analysed for the presence or absence of atrial fibrillation, LV hypertrophy, left bundle branch block, left atrial enlargement, delta waves and abnormal Q waves.

Ambulatory ECG monitoring

Tracings were recorded with 3 bipolar leads for 24 hours using commercially available equipment and analysed by an experienced reader. Complex ventricular arrhythmia was defined as the presence of non-sustained ventricular tachycardia (NSVT) defined as >3 consecutive ventricular ectopic complexes occurring at a rate of >100 beats/min.

Echocardiography

Two-dimensional echocardiography with M-mode recording was obtained following the recommendations of the American Society of Echocardiography (ASE) [7]. The resting systolic gradients were measured with colour-guided continuous-wave Doppler (CWD) across LV cavity and outflow tract, avoiding the effect of mitral regurgitation when present. The examinations were performed using standard equipment with 2.5 and 3.5 MHz transducers.

Genetic testing

The polymerase chain reaction (PCR) was performed from DNA using primers that cover the entire coding region from β-myosin heavy chain (*MYH7*), myosin binding protein C (*MYBPC3*), and troponin T (*TNNT2*) genes (primer sequences available upon request). After PCR, the fragments were purified with the ExoSAP-IT® enzyme (GE Healthcare). The sequencing reaction was performed with BigDye Terminator V3.1 Cycle sequencing Kit® (Life Technologies) and EDTA/ethanol precipitation protocol. The samples were sequenced in an automatic sequencer ABI3500xl (Life Technologies).

The sequences were evaluated with the SeqMan program (DNASTAR Lasergene, Madison, WI) and compared with the reference sequence in the NCBI database. For *MYH7*, *MYBPC3*, and *TNNT2*, the references were, respectively, NM_000257.2, NM_000256.3, and NM_000364.2 [8]. When an undescribed mutation was found, we used bioinformatics algorithms to evaluate the pathogenic potential of the alteration. The SIFT [9] and *Polyphen* [10] programs were used only for substitutions, and the *MutationTaster* [11] was used to analyze deletions, insertions, and intron alterations. A mutation was labeled as pathogenic if (1) it had been previously described as causing disease; (2) it generated an aminoacid change and was considered pathogenic by all 3 programs above or in 2 programs but the aminoacid was conserved.

Statistical analysis

Statistical analyses were performed with the SPSS program 15.0. The ANOVA test was used to compare means, Fisher's exact test for frequencies comparison, and uni- and multivariate logistic regression for constructing the prediction model. The variables with a statistical difference in the ANOVA test were tested in the univariate logistic regression and independent variables with a p value < 0.1 were included in the multivariate logistic regression. We did not use any hierarchical or stepwise approach in the multivariate logistic regression model.

Accuracy of the final prediction model was explored through ROC analysis. Sensitivity, specificity, positive and negative predictive values according to model cut offs were determined. The prediction model was generated with the probability of a positive genetic test derived from the regression model (where (β) are the regression coefficients of variables in the final model). These probabilities were imputed in a ROC analysis and a cut-off maximizing specificity and sensitivity was chosen.

$$p = \frac{e^{\beta_0 + \beta_1 x}}{1 + e^{\beta_0 + \beta_1 x}}$$

Results

This study analysed 268 patients, 58% males and 42% females with a median age of 46 years (SD = 15.6). The youngest was 13 years old and the oldest 90. We obtained the data from ECG and echocardiogram from all the patients and data from holter and resonance were obtained respectively from 176 and 116 patients. The variable used for the analysis were obtained as followed: presence or absence of atrial fibrillation, obtained from

ECG, septal and posterior wall thickness, left atrium size and ejection fraction, obtained from echocardiogram, medium heart rate and presence of NSVT from Holter and presence or absence of fibrosis from cardiac resonance.

The median septal thickness was 20 mm (SD = 6), posterior wall thickness (PW) was 12 mm (SD = 5), left atrium size (LA) was 42 mm (SD = 8), and ejection fraction (EF) was 71% (SD = 9). There were no statistical differences in these criteria regarding sex.

Among the patients, we found a pathogenic mutation in 131 of them (48.8%). Seventy-eight (59.5%) of the mutations were in the *MYH7* gene, 50 (38.2%) in the *MYBPC3* gene, and 3 (2.3%) in the *TNNT2* gene. All variant used for this analysis were considered pathogenic according to our criteria described on Methods section. The full variant list can be found a previous article from our group [12]. The comparison between clinical features and presence or absence of an identified mutation has shown that patients with a mutation are, on average, younger in age, younger in age at diagnosis, have higher average cardiac frequency, and higher frequency of patients with NSVT (Table 1).

Familial history of HCM was also correlated with the presence or absence of an identified mutation (Table 2), and it was found that when there is a proven familial history, the chance of finding a mutation is significantly higher than when there is no familial history. When the familial history was unsure, as in the cases when the

Table 1 Clinical features with absence or presence of a mutation in one of the studied genes

		Mutation				
		Absence		Presence		
		Mean	SD	Mean	SD	p value
Age at diagnosis (years)		38	16	33	13	**0.026**
Current age (years)		48	17	43	13	**0.028**
MCF (bpm)		67	9	71	11	**0.006**
Septum (mm)		20	6	21	5	0.179
PW (mm)		12	3	12	6	0.581
LA (mm)		42	8	43	8	0.164
EF (%)		71	9	71	9	0.638
		Count	Frequency (%)	Count	Frequency (%)	
Sex	M	79	57.2	76	58.3	0.902
	F	59	42.8	54	58.5	
AF	No	91	93.8	90	87.4	0.150
	Yes	6	6.2	13	12.6	
Obstructive	No	73	64.6	81	70.4	0.397
	Yes	40	54.1	34	29.6	
NSVT	No	63	75.9	50	54.9	**0.004**
	Yes	20	24.1	41	45.1	

SD Standard deviation, *MCF* medium cardiac frequency, *PW* posterior wall thickness, *LA* left atrium size, *EF* ejection fraction, *AF* atrial fibrillation, *obstructive* ventricular gradient above 30 mmHg, *NSVT* non-sustained ventricular tachycardia. p-values < 0.05 are marked in bold.

Table 2 Comparison of positive, negative and unsure HC familiar history and mutation identification

| | | HC familial history | | | | | |
| | | Absent | | Present | | Unsure | |
		Count	Frequency	Count	Frequency	Count	Frequency
Mutation	Absent	16	69.6%	23	37.1%	33	50%
	Present	7	30.4%	35	62.9%	33	50%

patient mentioned relatives with cardiac disease, but without a clinical diagnosis of HCM, the odds of identifying a mutation were higher than in those with a negative family history and statistical similarity to those with a confirmed familial history.

The variables with a statistical difference in the ANOVA test were tested in the univariate logistic regression and independent variables with a p value < 0.05 were included in the multivariate logistic regression: familial history of HCM, average heart frequency, NSTV and age (Table 3). Probabilities of having a positive molecular genetic test were calculated from the final multivariate logistic regression model and were used to identify those with a higher probability of a positive molecular diagnosis. The predicted probabilities distribution and ROC curve are shown respectively in Figures 1 and 2. The AUC is 0.775 and 0.55 was used as the cut-off value for the ROC curve.

Discussion
Genetic test positivity prediction model
The genetic test positivity prediction model developed in this study is useful to analyse *a priori* a patient's chance of finding a mutation when ordering genetic testing. In the clinical practice scenario, cardiologists can give a more accurate estimate to patients regarding the molecular test. In the large scale screening scenario, such as in national cascade screening projects, only patients with a greater chance of having a positive genetic test would be analysed, which could optimize the use of reagents and analysis time. This model is particularly important in centres with fewer resources, because the genetic test

is still very expensive. Especially in the Brazilian scenario, where few academic centres have the structure and budget to perform the test, this method can serve as a cost-effective tool. Our main focus with this model is the cascade screening. Patients with borderline hypertrophy or with uncertain diagnosis were not included in this study, so such predictor may not be accurate for this group.

The sensitivity and specificity values can be adjusted according to a particular interest. For example, if one wants to maximize the number of positive patients included, the sensitivity and specificity can be modulated by changing cut-off values. In the simulations for the studied population, adjusting the predicted probability cutoff for 0.34, which represents an approximate 90% sensitivity, from the 122 included in the analysis, 91 would be tested. Of those, 60 patients would be positive. From the 31 patients not tested, only 7 would have a positive result, so we would not be testing 24 patients predicted as negative. These savings, in a national screening program, can signify an important economic resource.

To applied this model, one can use the values from Table 3 to calculate the predicted probability of a positive genetic test. P is equal the predicted probability, β_0 is the constant value, β_1 is the variable constant and x is the variable value if continuous or 0 and 1 if the variable is categorical.

In this work, we are using predicted probability, thus what we can conclude is regarding higher or lower probabilities, not certainties. For example, we saw in the logistic regression model that each patient's year addition

Table 3 Variables included in the multivariate logistic regression

| | B | S.E. | Wald | df | Sig. | Exp(B) | 95.0% C.I. for EXP(B) | |
							Lower	Upper
HCFH			7.222	2	0.027			
HCFH (1)	1.767	0.661	7.152	1	0.007	5.856	1.603	21.387
HCFH (2)	1.261	0.665	3.594	1	0.058	3.53	0.958	13.004
AHF	0.044	0.021	4.471	1	0.034	1.045	1.003	1.089
NSVT	1.603	0.479	11.193	1	0.001	4.969	1.943	12.709
Age	−0.053	0.018	9.211	1	0.002	0.948	0.916	0.981
Constant	−2.507	1.718	2.13	1	0.144	0.081		

HCFH Familial history of HC, *HCFH (1)* familial history of cardiac disease with confirmed HC diagnosis, *HCFH (2)* familial history of cardiac disease without HC diagnosis, *AHF* average heart frequency, *NSVT* non-sustained ventricular tachycardia.

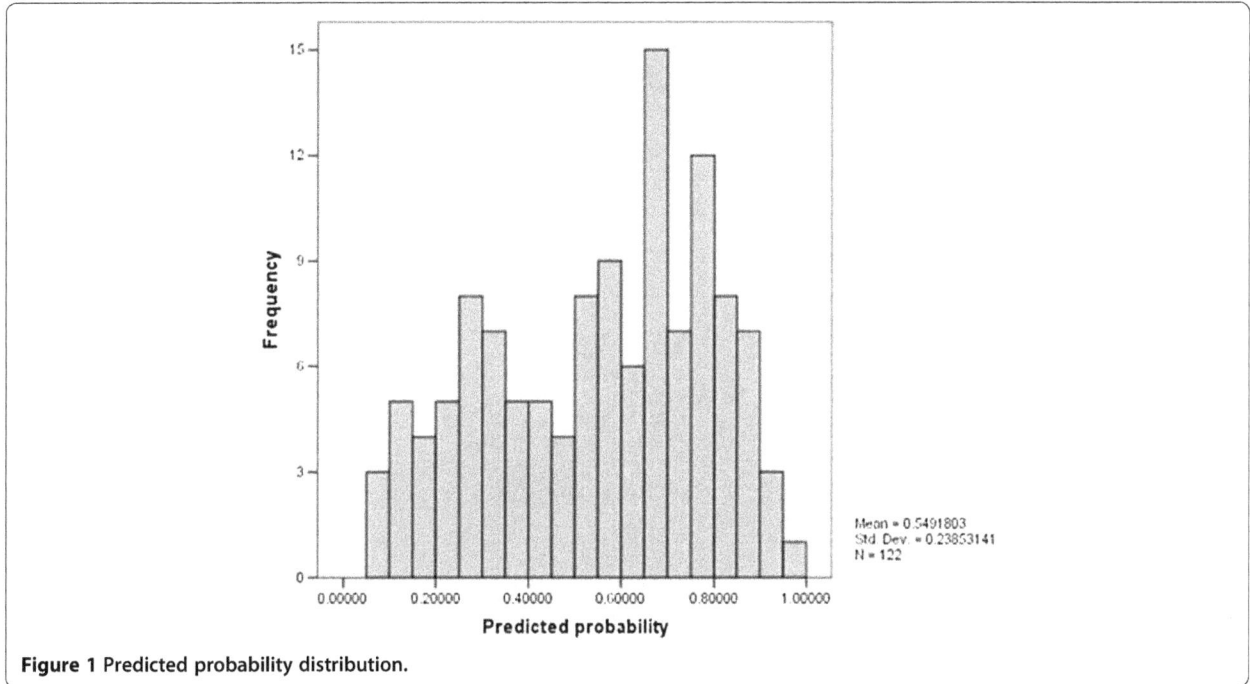

Figure 1 Predicted probability distribution.

decreases the chance of finding a mutation in the genetic test. We did not define a cutoff for this measure, meaning that one can find the mutation in any age, but the older the patient is, the lower is the probability of finding a mutation. On the other hand, the presence of a confirmed HCM family history increases the chance of finding a mutation almost 6 times when compared to patients who don't have a positive HCM family history.

Ingles et al. [5] also used this approach to identify positivity predictors for genetic testing in an Australian HCM population. The multivariate analysis of this population identified female sex, LV thickness, HCM familial history, and SD familial history as associated with a higher chance of mutation identification. The authors considered familial history as a key predictor of a positive genetic test in their population, with a 3 times higher chance of a positive result compared to patients without a familial history, which was similar to what we found in this study. In their study, this detection rate was even higher when the patient also had an SD familial history. Differently from what was found in this study, age at diagnosis was not significant in the Australian population, although the p value was 0.052.

Another study performed by Gruner et al. [6] in a Toronto HCM population showed that in these patients age at diagnosis, female sex, HCM familial history, and SD familial history were also correlated with a higher probability of a mutation identification. In addition, the study correlated hypertension and dyslipidaemia as negative predictive factors, with a higher frequency of both in

genetically negative patients. Other strong predictors identified were morphology subtype, as previously described [13] and maximal wall LV thickness and LW thickness.

The identification of NSVT as one of the predictors for a positive genetic test is a very interesting observation, since this is one risk factor for sudden death in HCM patients. In a previous work, Olivotto et al. [14]

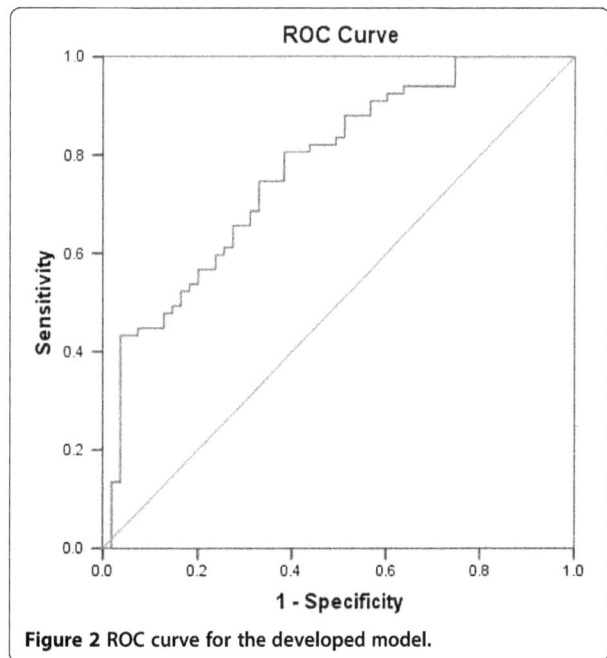

Figure 2 ROC curve for the developed model.

compared patients with and without an identified sarcomeric mutation and found that there was a difference regarding those, with patients with a positive genetic test being related to a less favourable clinical outcome, especially regarding end stage heart failure, but not sudden death. This finding in our study may show that the presence of a mutation can indeed be related with a higher risk of sudden death related risk factors.

Study limitations

The limitations of this study are the lack of patients with hypertension, since it was an exclusion criterion for HCM diagnosis in the participating centres; therefore, we could not test it as a negative predictor. Also, we only studied the three most important genes (*MYH7*, *MYBPC3*, and *TNNT2*), thus patients with mutations in other sarcomeric genes may be wrongly labelled as mutation negative. But the frequency of these genes in HCM is very low, so we believe that the lack of these data does not change the results found.

These finding may be limited to the Brazilian population. Replication studies in other populations should be made to confirm these results.

As new technology becomes available, such as next generation sequencing screening techniques, this reality may change and screening programs will have to constantly adapt to new molecular data.

Conclusion

In conclusion, we developed an easy and fast screening method that takes into account only clinical data that can help to select the patients with a high probability of positive genetic results for molecular sequencing of Brazilian HCM patients. This method can be applied in centres with limited resources to save time and money.

Competing interest

No competing financial interests exist. None of the authors had any funding by commercial agencies. Júlia Marsiglia, Flávia Laghi Credidio, Théo Gremen Mimary de Oliveira and Rafael Ferreira Reis had scholarships from national Science funding agencies (CNPq and CAPES). The other researchers are employees from the respective institutes and didn't receive any extra funding for developing this work and writing or publishing this article.

Authors' contribution

JDCM - acquisition of data, analysis and interpretation of the data, Statistical analysis, Drafting of the manuscript. FLC - acquisition of data, analysis and interpretation of the data, critical revision of the manuscript for important intellectual content. TGMO - acquisition of data, analysis and interpretation of the data, critical revision of the manuscript for important intellectual content. RFR - acquisition of data, analysis and interpretation of the data, critical revision of the manuscript for important intellectual content. MOA - acquisition of data, critical revision of the manuscript for important intellectual content. AQA - acquisition of data, analysis and interpretation of the data, critical revision of the manuscript for important intellectual content. RPP - acquisition of data, analysis and interpretation of the data, critical revision of the manuscript for important intellectual content. JMBBF - acquisition of data, analysis and interpretation of the data, critical revision of the manuscript for important intellectual content. CM - acquisition of data, critical revision of the manuscript

for important intellectual content. JEK - obtaining funding, critical revision of the manuscript for important intellectual content. EAF - conception and design of the research, acquisition of data, analysis and interpretation of the data, critical revision of the manuscript for important intellectual content. ACP - Conception and design of the research, analysis and interpretation of the data, statistical analysis, obtaining funding, critical revision of the manuscript for important intellectual content, Supervision. All authors read and approved the final manuscript.

Acknowledgments

We would like to thank to Luciana Turolla Wanderley for all the help in the experiments and interpretation of results.

Author details

[1]Laboratory of Genetics and Molecular Cardiology, Heart Institute (InCor), University of São Paulo, São Paulo, Brazil. [2]Clinical Unit of Cardiomyopathies, Heart Institute (InCor), University of São Paulo, São Paulo, Brazil. [3]Federal University of Espírito Santo, Vitória, Brazil. [4]Chagas Disease and Heart Failure Outpatient Service, PROCAPE-University of Pernambuco/UPE, Recife, Brazil. [5]Federal University of Amazonas, Manaus, Brazil.

References

1. Maron BJ: Hypertrophic cardiomyopathy. *Lancet* 1997, **350**(9071):127–133.
2. Richard P, Villard E, Charron P, Isnard R: **The Genetic Bases of Cardiomyopathies.** *J Am Coll Cardiol* 2006, **48**(9_Suppl_A):A79–A89.
3. Maron BJ, Gardin JM, Flack JM, Gidding SS, Kurosaki TT, Bild DE: **Prevalence of hypertrophic cardiomyopathy in a general population of young adults. Echocardiographic analysis of 4111 subjects in the CARDIA Study. Coronary Artery Risk Development in (Young) Adults.** *Circulation* 1995, **92**(4):785–789.
4. Bos JM, Towbin JA, Ackerman MJ: **Diagnostic, prognostic, and therapeutic implications of genetic testing for hypertrophic cardiomyopathy.** *J Am Coll Cardiol* 2009, **54**(3):201–211.
5. Ingles J, Sarina T, Yeates L, Hunt L, Macciocca I, McCormack L, Winship I, McGaughran J, Atherton J, Semsarian C: **Clinical predictors of genetic testing outcomes in hypertrophic cardiomyopathy.** *Genet Med* 2013, **15**(12):972–977.
6. Gruner C, Ivanov J, Care M, Williams L, Moravsky G, Yang H, Laczay B, Siminovitch K, Woo A, Rakowski H: **Toronto hypertrophic cardiomyopathy genotype score for prediction of a positive genotype in hypertrophic cardiomyopathy.** *Circ Cardiovasc Genet* 2012, **6**(1):19–26.
7. Henry WL, DeMaria A, Gramiak R, King DL, Kisslo JA, Popp RL, Sahn DJ, Schiller NB, Tajik A, Teichholz LE, Weyman AE: **Report of the American Society of Echocardiography Committee on Nomenclature and Standards in Two-dimensional Echocardiography.** *Circulation* 1980, **62**(2):212–217.
8. *The National Center for Biotechnology Available from.* http://www.ncbi.nlm.nih.gov/.
9. Kumar P, Henikoff S, Ng PC: **Predicting the effects of coding non-synonymous variants on protein function using the SIFT algorithm.** *Nat Protoc* 2009, **4**(7):1073–1081.
10. Adzhubei IA, Schmidt S, Peshkin L, Ramensky VE, Gerasimova A, Bork P, Kondrashov AS, Sunyaev SR: **A method and server for predicting damaging missense mutations.** *Nat Methods* 2010, **7**(4):248–249.
11. Schwarz JM, Rodelsperger C, Schuelke M, Seelow D: **MutationTaster evaluates disease-causing potential of sequence alterations.** *Nat Methods* 2010, **7**(8):575–576.
12. Marsiglia JD, Credidio FL, de Oliveira TG, Reis RF, Antunes Mde O, de Araujo AQ, Pedrosa RP, Barbosa-Ferreira JM, Mady C, Krieger JE, Arteaga-Fernandez E, Pereira AC: **Screening of MYH7, MYBPC3, and TNNT2 genes in Brazilian patients with hypertrophic cardiomyopathy.** *Am Heart J* 2012, **166**(4):775–782.
13. Binder J, Ommen SR, Gersh BJ, Van Driest SL, Tajik AJ, Nishimura RA, Ackerman MJ: **Echocardiography-guided genetic testing in hypertrophic cardiomyopathy: septal morphological features predict the presence of myofilament mutations.** *Mayo Clin Proc* 2006, **81**(4):459–467.
14. Olivotto I, Girolami F, Ackerman MJ, Nistri S, Bos JM, Zachara E, Ommen SR, Theis JL, Vaubel RA, Re F, Armentano C, Poggesi C, Torricelli F, Cecchi F: **Myofilament protein gene mutation screening and outcome of patients with hypertrophic cardiomyopathy.** *Mayo Clin Proc* 2008, **83**(6):630–638.

2

Right ventricular systolic dysfunction and remodelling in Nigerians with peripartum cardiomyopathy

Kamilu Musa Karaye[1,2]*, Krister Lindmark[2,3] and Michael Henein[2,3]

Abstract

Background: The literature on right ventricular systolic dysfunction (RVSD) in peripartum cardiomyopathy (PPCM) patients is scanty, and it appears that RV reverse remodelling in PPCM has not been previously described. This study thus aimed to assess RVSD and remodelling in a cohort of PPCM patients in Kano, Nigeria.

Methods: A longitudinal study carried out in 3 referral hospitals in Kano, Nigeria. Consecutive PPCM patients who had satisfied the inclusion criteria were recruited and followed up for 12 months. RVSD was defined as the presence of either tricuspid annular plane systolic excursion (TAPSE) <16 mm or peak systolic wave (S') tissue Doppler velocity of RV free wall <10 cm/s. For the purpose of this study, recovery of RV systolic function was defined as an improvement of reduced TAPSE to ≥16 mm or S' to ≥10 cm/s, without falling to reduced levels again, during follow-up.

Results: A total of 45 patients were recruited over 6 months with a mean age of 26.6 ± 7.0 years. RV systolic function recovery occurred in a total of 8 patients (8/45; 17.8 %), of whom 6 (75.0 %) recovered in 6 months after diagnosis. The prevalence of RVSD fell from 71.1 % at baseline to 36.4 % at 6 months ($p = 0.007$) and 18.8 % at 1 year ($p = 0.0008$ vs baseline; $p = 0.41$ vs 6 month). Patients with RVSD had higher serum creatinine, and TAPSE accounted for 19.2 % ($p = 0.008$) of the variability of serum creatinine at 6 months. Although 83.3 % of the deceased had RVSD, it didn't predict mortality in the regression models ($p > 0.05$).

Conclusion: RVSD and reverse remodelling were common in Nigerians with PPCM, in whom the first 6 months after diagnosis seem to be critical for RV recovery and survival.

Keywords: Peripartum cardiomyopathy, Right ventricular dysfunction, RV remodelling

Background

Peripartum cardiomyopathy (PPCM) is an important cause of heart failure (HF) in many parts of the world including Northern Nigeria, and is associated with significant morbidity and mortality [1, 2]. We previously described right ventricular (RV) systolic dysfunction in PPCM patients using tricuspid annular plane systolic excursion (TAPSE), and reported RV systolic dysfunction (RVSD) in 54.6 % of the patients [3]. It is believed that left ventricular (LV) function recovers in 23–41 % of

PPCM patients over time, but the literature on RVSD in PPCM is still scanty and to the best of our knowledge, RV reverse remodelling in PPCM has not been previously described [2]. We hypothesised that many PPCM patients would also experience RV reverse remodelling over time. The present study thus aimed to assess RVSD and reverse remodelling over 1 year in a cohort of PPCM patients in Kano, Nigeria.

Methods

This is a longitudinal study carried out in Murtala Mohammed Specialist Hospital (MMSH), Aminu Kano Teaching Hospital (AKTH) and a private cardiology clinic in Kano, Nigeria.

* Correspondence: kkaraye@yahoo.co.uk
[1]Department of Medicine, Bayero University and Aminu Kano Teaching Hospital, 3 New Hospital Road, Kano, Nigeria
[2]Department of Public Health and Clinical Medicine, Umea University, SE-901 87 Umea, Sweden
Full list of author information is available at the end of the article

Clinical evaluation

The study conformed to the ethical guidelines of the Declaration of Helsinki, on the principles for medical research involving human subjects [4]. The research protocol was approved by the Research Ethics Committees of AKTH and Kano State Hospitals Management Board before the study started. Inclusion criteria were: (i) new diagnosis of PPCM before commencement of medical treatment; (ii) onset of HF symptoms between last few months of pregnancy and first 5 months postpartum, (iii) at least 18 years of age; (iv) contact telephone number, except patients who gave reassurance that they were willing to attend the follow-up, and (v) giving written informed consent. We excluded PPCM patients who were on HF treatment, as well as those who presented more than 5 months since delivery. PPCM was defined according to the recommendations of the HF Association of the European Society of Cardiology Working Group on PPCM, and LV systolic dysfunction was defined as LV ejection fraction (LVEF) <45 % [2].

At the study sites, physicians and obstetricians were invited to refer all patients with suspected PPCM to the principal investigator (PI) for further evaluation. Patients were then interviewed, clinically evaluated and recruited consecutively. For each subject, a 12-lead electrocardiogram (ECG) at rest and trans-thoracic echocardiogram were carried out by the PI at the study centres according to standard recommendations [5]. The echocardiographic examination was carried out using Sonoscape S8 Doppler Ultrasound System (Shenzhen, China, 2010). Plasma hemoglobin and serum urea, electrolytes and creatinine were measured at the laboratories of AKTH according to standard protocols.

The PI re-evaluated the patients at 6 and 12 months follow-up, using the same protocol as at recruitment including ECG and echocardiographic examinations, but blood tests were not repeated.

Cardiac function assessment

Echocardiography was performed according to standard recommendations [5, 6]. RV basal diameter (RVb), Right atrial longitudinal dimension (RAL) and RA end-systolic area (RAA) were measured in each patient. Tricuspid annular plane systolic excursion (TAPSE) was recorded from the apical four-chamber view with the M-mode cursor positioned at the free wall angle of the tricuspid valve (TV) annulus [7]. RV long axis amplitude of motion (i.e. TAPSE) was measured from end-systolic to end-diastolic points [7], and its peak systolic velocity (S') was measured from myocardial tissue Doppler imaging (TDI). All recordings of TAPSE and S' were obtained during held end-expiration. Care was taken to align M-mode or TDI beam along the direction of tricuspid annulus motion, with the minimum

angle in between. TDI sample volume was positioned at 10 mm from the insertion site of the tricuspid leaflets or 10 mm away within RV lateral wall and adjusted to cover the longitudinal excursion of the tricuspid annulus both in systole and diastole [5]. RVSD was defined as the presence of either TAPSE <16 mm or S' of RV lateral tricuspid annulus <10 cm/s [6]. For the purpose of this study, recovery of RV systolic function was defined as an improvement of reduced TAPSE to ≥16 mm or S' to ≥10 cm/s, without falling to reduced levels again, during follow-up.

Pulmonary artery systolic pressure (PASP) was estimated using continuous wave Doppler of the maximum velocity of the tricuspid regurgitant jet (v), from which the retrograde pressure drop was calculated using the modified Bernoulli equation ($4 V^2$), and adding to it the estimated right atrial pressure (RAP) [8]. RAP was estimated using the diameter and collapse of the inferior vena cava during spontaneous respiration, as previously described [9]. Pulmonary hypertension (PHT) was defined as mean pulmonary arterial pressure (mPAP) of ≥25 mmHg at rest [10]. mPAP was estimated from PASP using the Chemla formula as: mPAP = (0.61 × PASP) +2 (mmHg) [11].

Statistical analysis

Continuous variables were explored for the presence of skewness, which was corrected with logarithmic ($\log_{10}$) transformation. Patients' baseline characteristics were described using frequencies and mean, while time period between patients' delivery and recruitment was described using the median and inter-quartile range (IQR). Chi-square, Fisher's exact probability and Student t-tests were used to compare categorical and continuous variables as appropriate. Spearman correlation coefficient (ρ_s) was used to assess the association between TAPSE and mPAP and serum creatinine, while logistic regression models were used to assess the associations between RVSD or mortality and variables of interest. Linear regression was also used to assess the relationship between TAPSE and mPAP. Estimates for regression analyses were expressed as Odds Ratios (OR) and 95 % Confidence Intervals (CI). The regression results were tested with Hosmer and Lemeshow's goodness of fit test, and a p-value ≥0.05 implied that the model's estimates fit the data at an acceptable level. The statistical analysis was carried out using SPSS version 16.0 software. Two-sided p-value <0.05 was considered as minimum level of statistical significance.

Results

The study flow is shown in Fig. 1. A total of 71 patients suspected to have PPCM were referred to the PI for possible inclusion, but only 51 (71.8 %) satisfied the diagnostic criteria, and all of them developed the disease

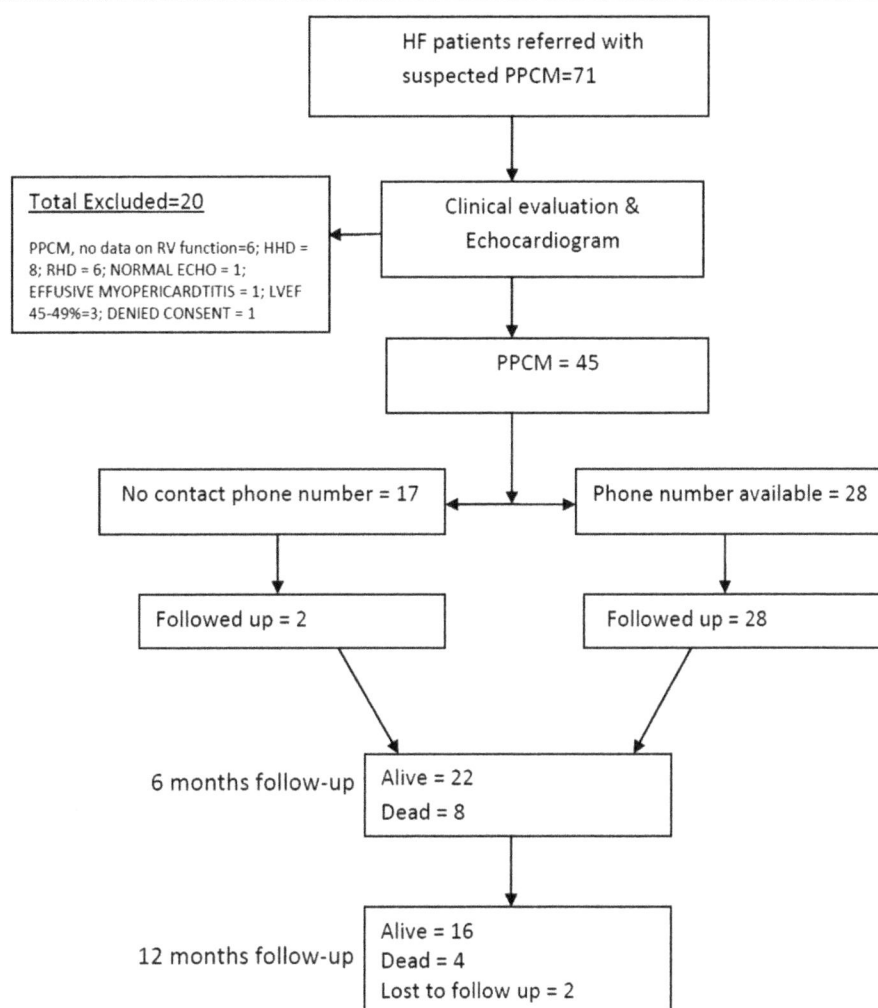

Fig. 1 Flow chart of recruitment and follow-up of patients

postpartum. Of the 51 PPCM patients, 45 (88.2 %) had complete data for RVSD assessment at baseline, and of these 22 (48.9 %) were reviewed at 6 months, 8 (17.8 %) had died, while the remaining 15 (33.3 %) were lost to follow-up. At 1 year, 16/45 (35.6 %) patients were alive, 12 (26.7 %) had died and 17 (37.8 %) were lost to follow-up. The median time from delivery to recruitment for the patients was 6.0 (IQR: 3–15) weeks, and they were recruited in July to December 2013.

Baseline clinical characteristics of patients with and without RVSD (Table 1)

Of the 45 recruited patients, 32 (71.1 %) had RVSD while the remaining 13 (28.9 %) had normal RV systolic function. When these 2 groups were compared, the differences were not statistically significant except for higher serum creatinine among those with RVSD ($p = 0.02$), who also tended to have lower diastolic blood pressure (DBP) ($p = 0.05$).

RV remodelling

Baseline echocardiographic variables were compared between patients with and without RVSD in Table 2. Those with RVSD had significantly lower mean TAPSE and S' ($p < 0.001$), but RV basal diameter, RAA, RAL, mPAP, and prevalence of PHT was not significantly different ($p > 0.05$) between the groups. Mean PAP was 29.3 ± 12.1 mmHg among all subjects respectively, out of whom a total of 30 (66.7 %) had PHT.

The pattern of RV reverse remodelling is presented in Fig. 2, which shows increased TAPSE ($p = 0.049$) at 6 months, but RAL ($p = 0.04$) reduced at 12 months and mPAP fell at both 6 ($p = 0.008$) and 12 months ($p = 0.020$) follow up. The prevalence of RVSD reduced from 71.1 % at baseline to 36.4 % (8/22 patients) at 6 months ($p = 0.007$) and to 18.8 % (3/16 patients) at 12 months ($p = 0.001$ vs baseline and $p = 0.41$ vs 6 month). In addition, the prevalence of PHT fell to 36.4 % ($p = 0.019$) at 6 months and 31.3 % ($p = 0.03$)

Table 1 Baseline clinical characteristics of patients with and without RVSD

Variables	Patients with RVSD $N = 32$ (71.1 %)	Patients without RVSD $N = 13$ (28.9 %)	p-value
Age (years)	26.1 ± 7.5	27.7 ± 5.4	0.500
NYHA class:			0.809
II	13 (40.6 %)	6 (46.2 %)	
III	12 (37.5 %)	5 (38.5 %)	
IV	7 (21.9 %)	1 (7.7 %)	
Parity ≥ 2	25 (78.9 %)	10 (76.9 %)	0.758
Breastfeeding	30 (93.8 %)	13 (100 %)	–
BMI (Kg/m^2)	21.4 ± 4.6	21.9 ± 3.9	0.704
Systolic BP (mmHg)	116 ± 23	128 ± 26	0.172
Diastolic BP (mmHg)	83 ± 18	94 ± 16	0.051
Heart rate/min	111 ± 16	104 ± 21	0.302
Pedal oedema	26 (81.3 %)	8 (61.5 %)	0.312
Hepatomegaly	19 (59.4 %)	6 (46.2 %)	0.515
Pregnancy associated hypertension	13 (40.6 %)	9 (69.2 %)	0.158
Haemoglobin (g/dL)	12.2 ± 1.8	12.9 ± 1.3	0.202
Log$_{10}$ Creatinine	2.0 ± 0.2	1.9 ± 0.1	0.020*
Sodium (mmol/L)	136.3 ± 6.3	135.5 ± 5.2	0.655
Treatment:			
ACEI/ARB	15 (46.9 %)	7 (53.9 %)	0.749
Frusemide	32 (100 %)	13 (100 %)	–
Spironolactone	31 (96.9 %)	11 (84.6 %)	0.196
Digoxin	28 (87.57 %)	12 (92.3 %)	>0.999
Beta blockers	2 (6.3 %)	1 (7.7 %)	>0.999
Warfarin	1 (3.1 %)	1 (7.7 %)	0.499
α-Methyl Dopa	4 (12.5 %)	2 (15.4 %)	>0.999

Key: *NYHA* New York Heart Association functional classification, *BMI* body mass index, *ACEI* angiotensin concerting enzyme inhibitors, *ARB* angiotensin receptor blockers. Results are presented as means ± standard deviations, or as numbers with percentages in parentheses. * p-vlaue is statistically significant

at 12 months. RV systolic function recovery occurred in a total of 8 patients (8/45; 17.8 %), of whom 6 (75.0 %) recovered in 6 months. Improvement in TAPSE alone was observed in 2 patients; in S' alone in another 2 patients, while both TAPSE and S' improved in 4 other patients.

Further analysis showed that although baseline TAPSE was significantly associated with mPAP at 6 months follow-up ($\rho_s = -0.531$; $p = 0.023$), it did not predict its variability ($R^2 = 0.217$; $p = 0.051$). Baseline TAPSE correlated with $\log_{10}$ creatinine ($\rho_s = +0.332$; $p = 0.048$), and accounted for 19.2 % ($p = 0.008$) of the variability of serum creatinine (Fig. 3). In addition, RVSD significantly increased the odds for $\log_{10}$ creatinine >1.95 (equivalent to serum creatinine 89.1 μmol/l) by 5.8 fold (OR = 5.83; CI = 1.263–26.944; $p = 0.024$).

When the baseline characteristics of subjects followed up were compared with those who were lost, differences between the groups were not statistically significant.

RVSD and mortality

Of the 30 patients followed-up, 2 (6.7 %) were lost to follow-up and 12 died (40.0 %), of whom 8 (66.7 %) did so within the first 6 months. The deceased had a median survival time of 19.5 weeks. Of the 12 deceased patients, 10 (83.3 %) had RVSD while the remaining 2 (16.7 %) had normal RV systolic function ($p = 0.47$). Variables assessed in Tables 1 and 2 were compared between the deceased (12 subjects) and the survivors (16 subjects) at 1 year follow up, and the only significant difference between the groups was a lower serum haemoglobin level in the former (12.1 ± 1.3 g/dl) as compared to the latter (13.5 ± 1.4 g/dl) ($p = 0.012$). Step wise univariate regression analyses were then carried out in which the serum haemoglobin and the other variables in the Tables were assessed for possible association with 1 year mortality. However, the one year mortality wasn't predicted by any variable in the univariate regression models, including RVSD ($p = 0.284$), serum creatinine ($p = 0.441$)

Table 2 Baseline echocardiographic characteristics of patients with and without RVSD

Variables	Patients with RVSD ($N = 32$)	Patients without RVSD ($N = 13$)	p-value
Right atrial end-systolic area, cm^2	19.7 ± 7.6	15.8 ± 8.1	0.149
Right atrial length, mm	42.9 ± 10.2	42.5 ± 11.1	0.916
Right ventricular basal diameter, mm	49.6 ± 9.3	47.7 ± 10.7	0.583
TAPSE, mm	13.1 ± 2.6	20.3 ± 2.2	<0.001*
Right ventricular S', cm/s	10.6 ± 3.2	15.3 ± 3.9	<0.001*
RIMP	1.09 ± 0.60	1.76 ± 1.30	0.032*
RV wall thickness, mm	3.6 ± 1.2	3.5 ± 0.8	0.952
Tricuspid Valve E:A ratio	1.21 ± 0.44	0.90 ± 0.35	0.019*
Tricuspid Valve E/e'	5.08 ± 2.73	3.46 ± 1.45	0.023*
Left atrial diameter, mm	43.2 ± 6.4	41.9 ± 6.2	0.548
LV end-diastolic diameter, mm	62.0 ± 7.5	62.4 ± 11.7	0.910
LV ejection fraction, %	32.4 ± 9.3	36.6 ± 7.7	0.127
LV stroke volume index, L/m^2	39.9 ± 12.3	51.4 ± 17.9	0.017
Anti-log$_{10}$ mitral valve E:A	1.50 ± 0.62	1.31 ± 0.25	0.154
Mitral valve E/e'	15.96 ± 7.13	15.61 ± 7.06	0.882
PA acceleration time, ms	61.8 ± 22.4	78.9 ± 28.0	0.037*
PA systolic pressure, mmHg	47.4 ± 19.4	39.2 ± 21.5	0.246
Mean PAP, mmHg	30.6 ± 11.6	25.9 ± 13.1	0.273
Pulmonary hypertension	23 (71.9 %)	7 (53.9 %)	0.304

Key: *TAPSE* Tricuspid annular plane systolic excursion, *LV* left ventricle, *E:A* transvalvular filling velocities ratio, *E/e'* ratio of early filling to averaged early diastolic tissue Doppler velocities of mitral or tricuspid valves, *PAP* pulmonary artery pressure, *RIMP* right ventricular (RV) index of myocardial performance. Results are presented as means ± standard deviations, or as numbers with percentages in parentheses. *p-vlaue is statistically significant

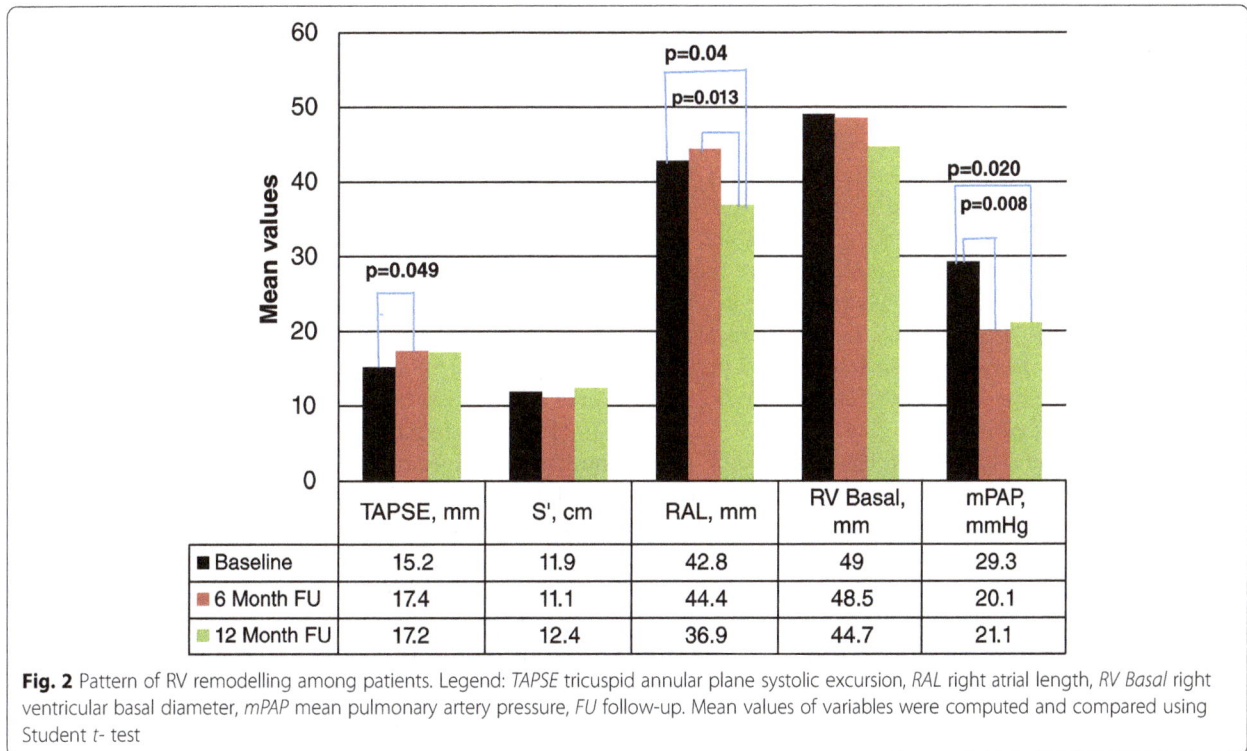

Fig. 2 Pattern of RV remodelling among patients. Legend: *TAPSE* tricuspid annular plane systolic excursion, *RAL* right atrial length, *RV Basal* right ventricular basal diameter, *mPAP* mean pulmonary artery pressure, *FU* follow-up. Mean values of variables were computed and compared using Student *t*- test

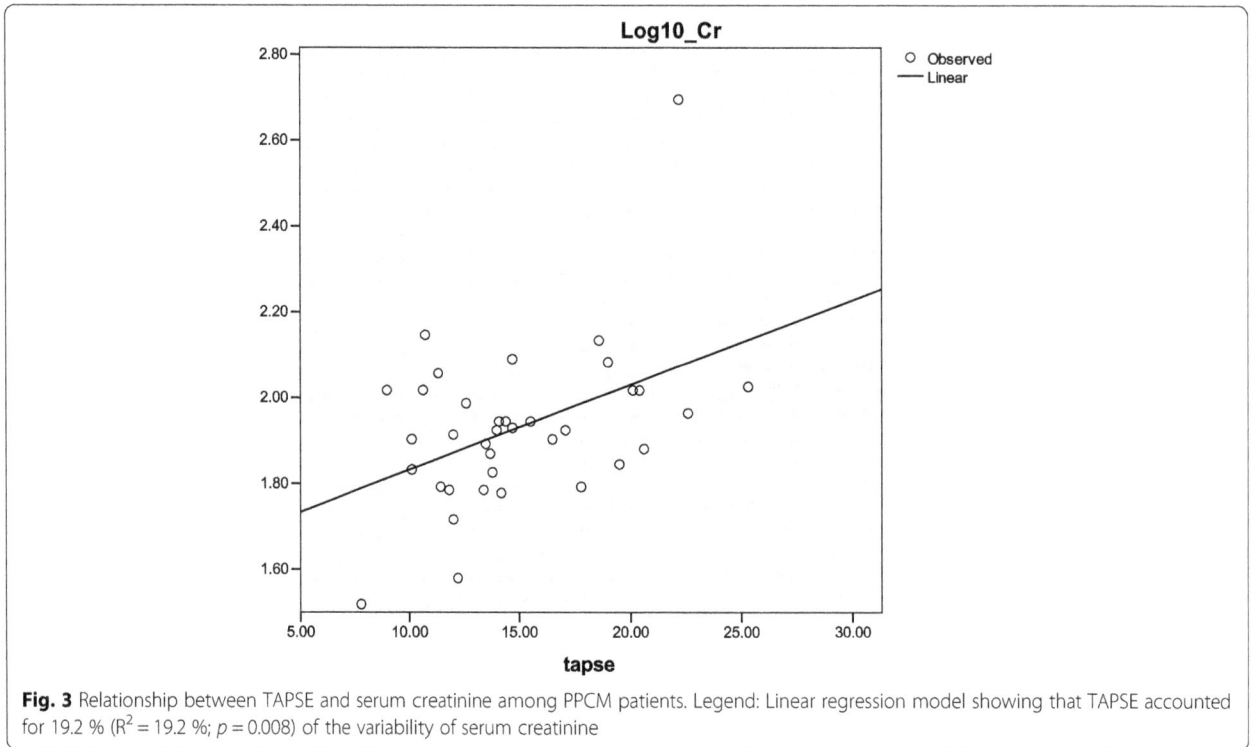

Fig. 3 Relationship between TAPSE and serum creatinine among PPCM patients. Legend: Linear regression model showing that TAPSE accounted for 19.2 % (R^2 = 19.2 %; p = 0.008) of the variability of serum creatinine

and haemoglobin (p = 0.053) (Hosmer & Lemeshow test X^2 = 9.69; p = 0.288).

Discussion

The present longitudinal study assessed RVSD and RV remodelling and its response to treatment and potential recovery in a group of PPCM patients from Kano, Nigeria. The prevalence of RVSD, in the form of reduced TAPSE and RV free wall S' velocity was evident in 71.1 % of the patients at baseline, and fell to 36.4 % at 6 months and to 18.8 % at 12 months follow-up. Likewise, PHT was found in 66.7 % of patients at baseline, and persisted in 36.4 % at 6 months, and to 31.3 % at 12 months follow up. RV systolic function recovery occurred in a total of 8 patients (8/45; 17.8 %), of whom 6 (75.0 %) recovered in 6 months. Forty percent of the followed-up patients died within 1 year; two-thirds of them within the first 6 months after diagnosis.

RVSD, its recovery and potential relationship with mortality are not well studied in PPCM. Based on reduced TAPSE, we have previously reported a prevalence of RVSD of 54.6 % in PPCM patients [3]. Adding RV reduced myocardial velocity (S') raised the prevalence of patients with RVSD in this study to 71.1 %, suggesting a more accurate means for identifying such patients. The second important observation in the current study is the significant recovery of RVSD along with its pressure afterload in the form of PHT. Indeed, 6 months from

the time of presentation, the prevalence of RVSD, PHT fell by more than 50 % despite poor adherence to heart failure conventional medications. Thus, the observed RV reverse remodelling seems to be related to the recovery of the pulmonary circulation status rather than to the effect of medications as has been previously observed in the LV [12]. This claim is supported by the modest relationship we found between TAPSE and mPAP at 6 months follow-up. Our finding might be explained by the significant RV function recovery in more than 50 % of patients at 6 months, thus suggesting a different pathophysiologic mechanism to right ventricular - pulmonary circulation coupling in PPCM compared with DCM, which has a more chronic course of disturbances of ventricular function [13]. In addition, TAPSE was linearly related to serum creatinine, confirming the adverse relationship between RVSD and renal impairment [14, 15]. Whether this reflects the aggressive nature of cardiac decompensation in PPCM, since all the patients developed LV systolic dysfunction with LVEF <45 % within a few postpartum days, remains to be verified in a larger group of patients.

Thus, our findings show that the first 6 months of PPCM diagnosis seem to be crucial for RV function recovery as well as survival. These findings are supported by Whitehead et al. who reported 87 % of PPCM deaths occurring within the first 6 months of diagnosis, and Elkayam who observed that LV function normalises in approximately 50 % of women with PPCM within the same period [12, 16]. These findings urge intensive medical treatment for such young patients within the first few days and weeks of their presentation. Finally, our mortality rate of 40 % in the present study seems high compared to 13 % over 6 months in South Africa [17]. This could be partly explained by the high maternal mortality in Nigeria in general, which was as high as 496.4 per 100,000 live births in 2013 [18].

Clinical implications

In the absence of magnetic resonance imaging, which is known for its superior accuracy in assessing RV structure and function, bedside echocardiography has an acceptable accuracy for diagnosing and monitoring RV function in PPCM patients, and it is widely available and affordable, particularly in countries where PPCM is relatively more prevalent [19]. With the high mortality recorded in the present study, PPCM patients should receive intensive care in the acute phase, with thorough assessment and follow up of LV as well as RV function in an attempt to identify the vulnerable ones who need closer follow up.

Study limitations

Although important, B-type natriuretic peptide (BNP) or N-terminal pro-BNP and other biomarkers could not be assessed because the tests were not readily available at the study centres. Secondly, it is important to point out that 15 of the 45 patients could not be followed-up because they were not contactable in spite of adequate counselling. Their inability to come for follow-up isn't unrelated to the significant security challenges being faced by northern Nigeria including Kano, making movements and keeping to appointments extremely difficult. Thirdly, cardiac magnetic resonance imaging could have shed more light on the nature of the myocardial pathology in PPCM, but this facility was not available at the study centres [19].

Conclusion

The present study assessed RVSD and pulmonary circulation disturbances in a group of PPCM patients in Kano, Nigeria. These were prevalent in over two-thirds of the patients at presentation and improved by more than 50 % at 6 months despite the lack of adherence to medical therapy. However, the studied cohort suffered a relatively high mortality which was not predicted by RVSD or other variables, in keeping with the overall high maternal mortality in Nigeria. These findings urge intensive care for such young patients during the acute phase of the disease to support cardiac function recovery and reduce mortality.

Abbreviations

PPCM: peripartum cardiomyopathy; HF: heart failure; RV: right ventricle; TAPSE: tricuspid annular plane systolic excursion; RVSD: right ventricular systolic dysfunction; LV: left ventricle; MMSH: Murtala Mohammed specialist hospital; AKTH: Aminu Kano teaching hospital; LVEF: LV ejection fraction; PI: principal investigator; ECG: electrocardiogram; RAA: right atrial area; RVb: RV basal dimension; RAL: RA length; TV: tricuspid valve; TDI: tissue Doppler imaging; PASP: pulmonary artery systolic pressure; RAP: RA pressure; PHT: pulmonary hypertension; mPAP: mean pulmonary artery pressure; RIMP: right ventricular index of myocardial performance; ρ_s: Spearman correlation coefficient; OR: odds ratio; CI: confidence interval; DBP: diastolic blood pressure; BNP: B-type natriuretic peptide.

Competing interest

The authors hereby declare that we have no competing interests regarding this manuscript.

Authors' contributions

KMK conceptualised and designed the study, and acquired, analysed and interpreted data, drafted the article and revised it critically for important intellectual content, and approved the final submitted version. KL analysed and interpreted data, revised the article critically for important intellectual content, and approved the final submitted version. MYH designed the study, analysed and interpreted data, revised the article critically for important intellectual content, and approved the final submitted version.

Author details

[1]Department of Medicine, Bayero University and Aminu Kano Teaching Hospital, 3 New Hospital Road, Kano, Nigeria. [2]Department of Public Health and Clinical Medicine, Umea University, SE-901 87 Umea, Sweden. [3]Department of Cardiology, Umea Heart Centre, SE-901 87 Umea, Sweden.

References

1. Karaye KM, Sani MU. Factors associated with poor prognosis among patients admitted with heart failure in a Nigerian tertiary medical centre: a cross-sectional study. BMC Cardiovasc Disord. 2008;8(1):16.
2. Sliwa K, Hilfiker-Kleiner D, Petrie MC, Mebazaa A, Pieske B, Buchmann E, et al. Heart Failure Association of the European Society of Cardiology Working Group on Peripartum Cardiomyopathy. Current state of knowledge on aetiology, diagnosis, management and therapy of peripartum cardiomyopathy: a position statement from the Heart Failure Association of the European Society of Cardiology Working Group on peripartum cardiomyopathy. Eur J Heart Fail. 2010;12(8):767–78.
3. Karaye KM. Right ventricular systolic function in peripartum and dilated cardiomyopathies. Eur J Echocardiogr. 2011;12(5):372–4.
4. World Medical Association Declaration of Helsinki. Ethical Principles for Medical Research Involving Human Subjects. J Postgrad Med. 2002;48:206–8.
5. Lang RM, Badano LP, Mor-Avi V, Afilalo J, Armstrong A, Ernande L, et al. Recommendations for cardiac chamber quantification by echocardiography in adults: an update from the American Society of Echocardiography and the European Association of Cardiovascular Imaging. J Am Soc Echocardiogr. 2015;28(1):1–39.
6. Rudski LG, Lai WW, Afilalo J, Hua L, Handschumacher MD, Chandrasekaran K, et al. Guidelines for the echocardiographic assessment of the right heart in adults: a report from the American Society of echocardiography. Endorsed by the European Society of Cardiology, and the Canadian Society of echocardiography. J Am Soc Echocardiogr. 2010;23:685–713.
7. Lindqvist P, Henein M, Kazzam E. Right ventricular outflow tract fractional shortening: an applicable measure of right ventricular systolic function. Eur J Echocardiogr. 2003;4:29–35.
8. Sciomer S, Magri D, Badagliacca R. Non-invasive assessment of pulmonary hypertension: Doppler echocardiography. Pulm Pharmacol Ther. 2007;20:135–40.
9. Posteraro A, Salustri A, Trambaiolo P, Amici E, Gambelli G. Echocardiographic estimation of pulmonary pressures. J Cardiovasc Med. 2006;7:545–54.
10. Galie' N, Hoeper MM, Humbert M, Torbicki A, Vachiery JL, Barbera JA, et al. Guidelines for the diagnosis and treatment of pulmonary hypertension. The

Task Force for the Diagnosis and Treatment of Pulmonary Hypertension of the European Society of Cardiology (ESC) and the European Respiratory Society (ERS), endorsed by the International Society of Heart and Lung Transplantation (ISHLT). Eur Heart J. 2009;30:2493–537.

11. Chemla D, Castelain V, Humbert M, Hébert JL, Simonneau G, Lecarpentier Y, et al. New Formula for Predicting Mean Pulmonary Artery Pressure Using Systolic Pulmonary Artery Pressure. Chest. 2004;126:1313–7.

12. Elkayam U. Clinical characteristics of peripartum cardiomyopathy in the United States: diagnosis, prognosis, and management. J Am Coll Cardiol. 2011;58(7):659–70.

13. Di Mauro M, Calafiore AM, Penco M, Romano S, Di Giammarco G, Gallina S. Mitral valve repair for dilated cardiomyopathy: predictive role of right ventricular dysfunction. Eur Heart J. 2007;28(20):2510–6.

14. Mullens W, Abrahams Z, Francis GS, Sokos G, Taylor DO, Starling RC, et al. Importance of venous congestion for worsening of renal function in advanced decompensated heart failure. J Am Coll Cardiol. 2009;53(7):589–96.

15. Guinot PG, Arab OA, Longrois D, Dupont H. Right ventricular systolic dysfunction and vena cava dilatation precede alteration of renal function in adult patients undergoing cardiac surgery: an observational study. Eur J Anaesthesiol. 2014;31:1–8.

16. Whitehead SJ, Berg CJ, Chang J. Pregnancy-related mortality due to cardiomyopathy: United States, 1991–1997. Obstet Gynecol. 2003;102:1326–31.

17. Blauwet LA, Libhaber E, Forster O, Tibazarwa K, Mebazaa A, Hilfiker-Kleiner D, et al. Predictors of outcome in 176 South African patients with peripartum cardiomyopathy. Heart. 2013;99(5):308–13.

18. Kassebaum NJ, Bertozzi-Villa A, Coggeshall MS, Shackelford KA, Steiner C, Heuton KR, et al. Global, regional and national levels and causes of maternal mortality during 1990–2013: a systematic analysis for the Global Burden of Disease Study 2013. Lancet. 2014;384(9947):980–1004.

19. Blecker GB, Steendijk P, Holman ER, Yu C-M, Breithardt OA, Kaandorp TAM, et al. Assessing right ventricular function: the role of echocardiography and complementary technologies. Heart. 2006;2(Suppl I):i19–26.

3

Molecular mechanisms behind progressing chronic inflammatory dilated cardiomyopathy

Daiva Bironaite[1]*, Dainius Daunoravicius[2], Julius Bogomolovas[3], Sigitas Cibiras[2,5], Dalius Vitkus[4], Edvardas Zurauskas[2], Ieva Zasytyte[5], Kestutis Rucinskas[5], Siegfried Labeit[3], Algirdas Venalis[1] and Virginija Grabauskiene[2,5]

Abstract

Background: Inflammatory dilated cardiomyopathy (iDCM) is a common debilitating disease with poor prognosis that often leads to heart failure and may require heart transplantation. The aim of this study was to evaluate sera and biopsy samples from chronic iDCM patients, and to investigate molecular mechanism associated with left ventricular remodeling and disease progression in order to improve therapeutic intervention.

Methods: Patients were divided into inflammatory and non-inflammatory DCM groups according to the immunohistochemical expression of inflammatory infiltrates markers: T-lymphocytes (CD3), active-memory T lymphocyte (CD45Ro) and macrophages (CD68). The inflammation, apoptosis, necrosis and fibrosis were investigated by ELISA, chemiluminescent, immunohistochemical and histological assays.

Results: The pro-inflammatory cytokine IL-6 was significantly elevated in iDCM sera (3.3 vs. 10.98 μg/ml; $P < 0.05$). Sera levels of caspase-9, −8 and −3 had increased 6.24-, 3.1- and 3.62-fold, ($P < 0.05$) and only slightly (1.3-, 1.22- and 1.03-fold) in biopsies. Significant release of Hsp60 in sera (0.0419 vs. 0.36 ng/mg protein; $P < 0.05$) suggested a mechanistic involvement of mitochondria in cardiomyocyte apoptosis. The significant MMP9/TIMP1 upregulation in biopsies (0.1931 - 0.476, $P < 0.05$) and correlation with apoptosis markers show its involvement in initiation of cell death and ECM degradation. A slight activation of the extrinsic apoptotic pathway and the release of hsTnT might support the progression of chronic iDCM.

Conclusions: Data of this study show that significant increase of IL-6, MMP9/TIMP1 and caspases-9, −8, −3 in sera corresponds to molecular mechanisms dominating in chronic iDCM myocardium. The initial apoptotic pathway was more activated by the intramyocardial inflammation and might be associated with extrinsic apoptotic pathway through the pro-apoptotic Bax. The activated intrinsic form of myocardial apoptosis, absence of necrosis and decreased fibrosis are most typical characteristics of chronic iDCM. Clinical use of anti-inflammatory drugs together with specific anti-apoptotic treatment might improve the efficiency of therapies against chronic iDCM before heart failure occurs.

Keywords: Apoptosis, Dilated cardiomyopathy, Heart, Inflammation, Necrosis

Background

Inflammatory processes usually characterize myocarditis, the progression of which leads to development of dilated cardiomyopathy (DCM) causing heart failure and finally to heart tissue destruction [1,2]. Dilated cardiomyopathy (DCM) is a heart muscle disease which leads to the enlargement of one or both ventricles and consequent systolic dysfunction. DCM is a consequence of persistent exposure to various cellular stress signals, including pro-inflammatory, viral, oxidative, neuro-hormonal, and other micro- or macro environmental factors [3]. Accumulating data showed an importance of inflammatory component in the development of DCM, indicating a relation between myocarditis, autoimmunity and DCM even if immunosuppressive therapy is not always effective [4,5]. Therefore, a better understanding of the molecular mechanisms dominating in inflammatory DCM (iDCM) is needed in order to improve treatment and prevent further heart destruction.

* Correspondence: d.bironaite@imcentras.lt
[1]Dept. of Stem Cell Biology, State Research Institute, Center for Innovative Medicine, Zygimantu 9, LT01102 Vilnius, Lithuania
Full list of author information is available at the end of the article

Pro-inflammatory cytokines are not constitutively expressed in the heart but are rapidly expressed in response to cardiac injury [6]. In most cases increased inflammation is in most cases a natural response to injury, helping to heal and recover damaged tissues, whereas overwhelming inflammation aggravates the disease [7]. High levels of accumulated pro-inflammatory factors induce various pathogenic effects, such as improper functioning of the left ventricle, cardiomyocyte death and/or fibrosis [8-10]. It was shown that inflammatory mediators, such as IL-6 and tumor necrosis factor - alpha (TNF-α) can activate apoptotic Fas-Fas ligand pathway in chronic heart failure [11]. Additionally, inflammatory cytokines activate members of the matrix metalloproteinase (MMP) family, zinc-depended endopeptidases, which participate in remodeling of ECM and fibrotic processes [12]. It is agreed, that likewise to heart failure, the main processes characterizing DCM are hypertrophy or loss/death of myocytes and interstitial fibrosis [13]. Despite of that, not all previously mentioned features fit to various forms of DCM. Therefore, in the present study, we have investigated the level of inflammation and subsequent induction of apoptosis, necrosis and fibrosis in sera and biopsies of chronic iDCM patients with purpose to estimate which of previously mentioned processes are mostly and firstly activated. A more detailed estimation of molecular mechanisms will allow more efficient use of therapeutic means to treat chronic iDCM and thereby prevent further myocardium destruction.

Methods

Inclusion and exclusion criteria

Study subjects were 32 consecutive patients (25 males, 7 females, mean age 43.14 ± 11.86 years), admitted to a tertiary referral Centre with clinically diagnosed DCM. All patients showed enlarged LV associated with significantly impaired systolic function (LVEF less 45%) on echocardiography in association with long duration of heart failure symptoms. At enrolment, the average duration of observed symptoms was 24–30 month. In addition to clinical severity of heart failure according to the New York Heart Association classification, heart failure was also identified by determination of concentration of brain natriuretic peptide (BNP) in sera.

Exclusion criteria: 1) Known causes of heart failure, such as hypertension, significant coronary artery disease, valvular heart diseases, although not relative mitral regurgitation, endocrine diseases, significant renal diseases or drug or alcohol abuse; 2) Acute myocarditis suspected by clinical presentation and diagnostic tests (signs or symptoms of systemic infections; elevated erythrocyte sedimentation rate, reactive C protein level and TnT/TnI, acute chest pain with ST/T wave changes such as:

ST-segment elevation or depression and T-wave inversions; new onset of non-specific ECG signs like: bundle branch block, AV-block and/or ventricular arrhythmias; regional wall motion abnormalities on echocardiography; edema and/or LGE on CMR).

All patients signed written informed consent for cardiac catheterization and endomyocardial biopsies (EMB), which includes resulting analysis to elucidate a possible origin of the myocardial and coronary artery diseases. Inflammatory cardiomyopathy was defined as a cardiomyopathy with decreased LVEF, increased LVEDD, and a positive myocardial inflammation score according to the Dallas criteria as well as criteria of the ESC/WHO [14-16]. All patients were subdivided into two groups: inflammation-positive (n = 22) and inflammation-negative (n = 10) according to immunohistochemically proven upregulation of inflammatory infiltrate markers. CD3 (T lymphocyte), CD45Ro (active-memory T lymphocyte) and CD68 (macrophage) were determined immunohistochemicaly by counting positively stained cells per mm^2. Immunohistochemical stainings (IHC) of collected samples revealed the significant amounts of inflammatory cellular infiltrates (≥ 14 leucocytes/mm^2 including up to 4 monocytes/macrophages/mm^2 with the presence of CD3 positive T-lymphocytes ≥ 7 cells/mm^2) in the biopsy samples (Figure 1). A cut off for inflammation samples (diffuse, focal or confluent) and the presence or the absence of necrosis and fibrosis were determined as earlier described [15].

Additional medical examinations

All patients were interviewed about their medical history and underwent a careful physical examination, as well as laboratory studies, including test of thyroid function, serum electrolytes (sodium, potassium), hsCRP, glucose, HbA1c, cholesterol, triglyceride, HDL, LDL, cardiac enzymes (CK, CK-MB, AST), hsTnT, urea, creatinine, uric acid, coagulation tests (PT, aPTT), blood count (hemoglobin, haematocrit, RBC, WBC and platelet count). Each patient underwent investigations such as blood pressure on admission, ECG, echocardiography, Holter monitoring and spiroergometry. The same basic medical treatment scheme was applied to all patients. Essential physical and laboratory data are shown in Table 1.

Cardiac catheterization and endomyocardial biopsies

Before EMB, each patient underwent coronary angiography to exclude coronary artery disease as well as right heart catheterization to assess haemodynamic parameters: mean pulmonary artery (PA) pressure, pulmonary capillary wedge pressure (PCWP) and pulmonary vascular resistance (PVR). Right ventricular EMB was obtained using a flexible bioptome via the right

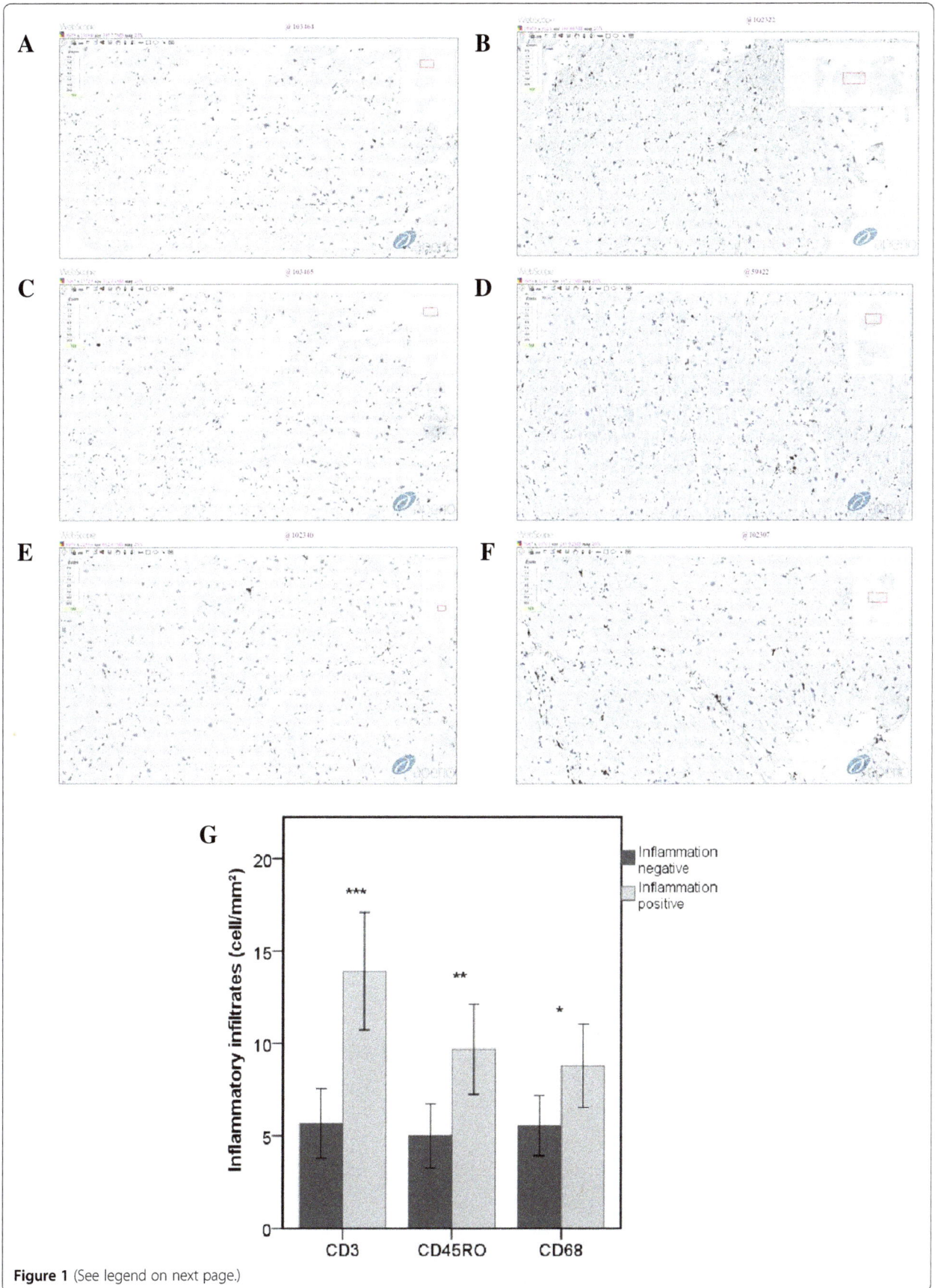

Figure 1 (See legend on next page.)

femoral vein [17]. Myocardial dilatation was assessed by ultrasound. Biopsies were taken from the right inter-ventricular septum from patients with confirmed absence of ischemia and cardiovascular pathology (stenosis and occlusion). Biopsy specimens were immediately placed at –80°C and later processed for appropriate studies. At least three EMBs samples were subjected to the conventional histological and immunohistochemical evaluation, while two EMBs were stored in a biobank as retained biosamples. Blood collection tubes (8.5 ml) were used for serum sampling of each patient at the same time as EMB.

Preparation of blood samples
Collected blood samples were placed in vacutainer tubes without anticoagulants and kept at room temperature for 30–45 min to allow clotting. Samples were centrifuged for 15 min at the manufacturer's recommended speed (1,000 - 2,000 RCF). The upper layer was carefully

aspired, checked for turbidity, aliquated into cryovials, labeled and stored at –80°C. Before measurement, all serum samples were thawed on ice, centrifuged at 12,000 g for 5 min and, if necessary, appropriately diluted.

Biochemical assays of inflammatory infiltrates and cytokines
Inflammatory infiltrates were estimated on fixed, paraffin-embedded material. For classification of biopsies, the previously mentioned markers (Santa Cruz Biotechnology, Inc.), CD3 (T lymphocytes), CD45Ro (active-memory T lymphocytes) and CD68 (macrophages) were applied. Positive cells were registered by an experienced pathologist and expressed as number of cells per mm^2.

The pro-inflammatory cytokines TNF-α, IL-6 and IL-1β in serum samples were assayed by solid-phase, chemoluminescent immunometric assays using IMMULITE/Immulite 1000 systems (Immulite, Siemens)

Table 1 Baseline characteristics of patients

Variable	Inflammation negative group		Inflammation positive group		
	Total No. of pts.	Value	Total No. of pts.	Value	p Value
Sex (male/female)	10	8 (80%) / 2 (20%)	22	17 (77%)/5 (33%)	0.863¿
Age (years)	10	46.7 ± 5.87	22	42.36 ± 2.07	0.389
NYHA					
II	10	1 (10%)	22	0 (0%)	0.132¿
III	10	7 (70%)	22	15 (68%)	0.918¿
IV	10	2 (20%)	22	7 (32%)	0.491¿
Cardiac parameters					
LBBB (%)	10	3 (30%)	22	5 (22.7%)	0.659¿
Permanent AF (%)	10	2 (20%)	22	0 (0%)	0.000¿*
LVEF (%)	10	24.10 ± 2.28	22	23.05 ± 1.35	0.678
LVEDD (cm)	10	6.89 ± 0.17	22	6.89 ± 0.19	0.998
LVEDDI (cm/m2)	10	3.68 ± 0.21	22	3.71 ± 0.09	0.847
Mean Ao (mmHg)	10	92.00 ± 3.95	22	86.06 ± 2.71	0.291
Mean RAP (mmHg)	10	16.22 ± 3.19	22	11.44 ± 1.74	0.164
Mean PCWP (mmHg)	10	25.00 ± 2.79	22	23.45 ± 2.70	0.731
Mean PAP (mmHg)	10	34.89 ± 4.33	22	32.95 ± 3.24	0.734
CI (L/min/m2)	10	2.38 ± 0.33	22	2.2 ± 0.14	0.573

Data are presented as the means ± SE. *Significant at 0.05 level. ¿Chi- square test. *Abbreviations:* NYHA – New York Heart Association functional class; LBBB – left bundle branch block; AF – atrial fibrillation; LVEF - left ventricular ejection fraction; LVEDD – left ventricular end-diastolic diameter; LVEDDI – left ventricular end-diastolic diameter index; Ao – aortic; RAP – right atrial pressure; PCWP – pulmonary capillary wedge pressure; PAP – pulmonary artery pressure; CI – cardiac index.

according to the manufactures' instructions: TNF-α (Catalog No: LKNFZ (50 tests), LKNF1 (100 tests); IL-6 (Catalog No: LK6PZ (50 tests), IL-1β (Catalog No: LKL1Z (50 tests)).

Biochemical assays for apoptosis and necrosis

ELISA was used to assay endomyocardial biopsies and serum samples. The following biomarkers were analyzed: Bcl-2, caspase-9, caspase-8 (Novus Biologicals Europe, Cambridge, UK); Bax (Elabscience Biotechnology Co., Ltd, China); caspase 3, MMP9, TIMP1, APO1/Fas/CD95, FasL (Invitrogen, Paisley, UK) and HSP60 (AssayPro, Saint Charles, Missouri, USA).

All collected serum samples were centrifuged at 12,000 g for 5 min, aliquated in 50 μl portions and stored at −80°C. Before measurement, serum samples were thawed on ice, appropriately diluted and analyzed by ELISA.

Collected heart tissue biopsies were immediately inserted into clean tubes and kept at −80°C. Before measurement, tissue samples were lysed in 100 μl of RIPA lysis buffer (Thermo Scientific Inc., USA), supplemented with protease- and phosphatase mini-inhibitor tablets, 1 mM PMSF, 1 mM Na2VO4 and 25 mM NaF according to the manufacturer's suggestion (Thermo Scientific Inc., USA). Biopsy samples were sonicated at 10 mV for 2 × 5 s on ice by a Bandelin Sonopuls sonicator, kept for 30 min on ice, centrifuged at 12,000 g for 15 min, aliquoted and stored at −80°C.

Amount of protein in serum and biopsy samples were measured using a modified Lowry Protein Assay kit according to the manufacturer's recommendations (Thermo scientific Inc., USA). Absorbance was measured with a spectrophotometer (Asys UVM 340 Microplate Reader UK - Biochrom Ltd.) set to 750 nm. The exact protein concentration of each unknown sample was estimated using bovine serum albumin (BSA) as a standard. Total protein concentrations were expressed as μg/ml. Final concentration of biomarkers was expressed as ng/mg of protein or pg/mg protein.

The myocardial injury marker, high-sensitivity troponin T (hsTnT), was measured in serum using an Elecsys 2010 analyzer (Roche Diagnostics, Indianapolis, Indiana) and expressed as pg/ml. Myocardial necrosis was estimated and scored by a competent pathologist on at least three independent routinely stained (Haematoxylin and Eosin (H&E)) sections. Normal myofibres had peripheral nuclei, intact sarcolema and non-fragmented nuclei. Pyknosis of muscle fiber nuclei, edema, and beginning of leuco-diapedesis from the capillaries suggested that the myocardial cells had reached the stage of necrosis.

Histochemical measurement of fibrosis in endomyocardial biopsies

Tissues collected for histological analyzes were fixed in 10% neutral buffered formalin, and then paraffin-embedded in a tissue processor. Total cardiac fibrosis (including interstitial and perivascular forms) was assessed. Specimens were stained with Masson's trichrome connective tissue stain according to a standard protocol. Keratin and normal muscle fibers stained red, whereas fibrotic areas stained blue. Digital images from the experimental glass slides were obtained using ScanScope Digital Slide Scanner (Aperio, Vista, CA) at a 20× magnification and archived on a devoted Spectrum Server 11.1.0.751 (Aperio). Quality control of the scanned images and all further analysis were performed using ImageScope V11.1.2.760 (Aperio) and WebScope V11.1.0.756 (Aperio).

Digital analysis of the slides was done using a Colocalization V9 algorithm that was run for the whole slides, ignoring the number of tissue cross sections on it – making the process fully automated. A colocalization algorithm uses the deconvolution method to separate the stains and classifies each pixel according to the number of stains present. For colocalization, the threshold for each stained sample is specified for a required stain (e.g. Masson's trichrome) and the algorithm reports the percentage of areas for each stain combination is detected: 1, 2, 3, 1 + 2, 1 + 3, 2 + 3, 1 + 2 + 3 or none (up to 3 areas were analyzed). The algorithm also provides an eight-color mark-up image for visualization of colocalized stains. Summing up the stain combinations 3, 2 + 3 and 1 + 3 calculated the total percentage of cardiac fibrosis.

PCR assay

Intramyocardial viruses were estimated by PCR assay [18]. Briefly, genomic DNA and total RNA were extracted simultaneously using ZR-Duet™ DNA/RNA Miniprep kit (Zymo Research, Irvine, CA, USA). RNA (1 μg) was reversely transcribed in 20 μl reaction volumes using random hexamers and First Strand cDNA Synthesis Kit (Thermo Fisher, Vilnius, Lithuania) according to the vendor's recommendations. Forward primers for the second round of PCR were labeled with 6-carboxyfluorescein (FAM) at the 5′ end. Final PCR products were 10-fold diluted and analyzed by capillary electrophoresis on a Genetic Analyzer 3130*xl*, using GeneScan™ 600 LIZ™ Size Standard and Gene Mapper Software v4.1 (Applied Biosystems, Foster City, CA, USA) for sizing PCR fragments. The following virus species were detected in the biopsies of 16 patients: parvo virus B19 (n = 11), human herpes virus type 6 (n = 4), hepatitis C virus (n = 1), Eppstein-Barr virus (n = 1), entero virus (n = 1), and varicella zoster virus (n = 1). The frequencies of detected viral genomes were equal in each tested group (50%) and, therefore, it did not influence the results.

Statistical analysis

All statistical analyses were performed using the SPSS package (version 19.0 for Windows; SPSS Inc., Chicago, IL, USA) at not higher than 5% significance level. The normality of the data distribution was tested by the Shapiro-Wilk test. Significance of measurements was tested by Student's t test or the Wilcoxon–Mann–Whitney rank sum non-parametric test. For comparative purposes Pearson's correlation coefficient was used.

Ethical approval

The study was approved by the local Lithuanian Bioethics Committee (license No. 158200-09-382-l03; No. 158200-382-PP1-23). All patients signed written informed consent to include their data in the study for each investigational procedure. The investigation conforms to the principles outlined in the *Declaration of Helsinki*.

Results

Inflammatory markers in dilated cardiomyopathy

Here, we monitored the inflammatory process by detecting expression of CD3, CD45Ro and CD68 in inflammatory infiltrates by immunohistochemistry (Figure 1). In addition, we determined levels of inflammatory cytokines TNF-α, IL-6 and IL-1β in sera. Representative immunohistochemical micrographs show the increased and diffused expression of CD3, CD45Ro and CD68 (Figure 1A, B, C, D, E and F). Total expression of cytokines in infiltrates from inflammatory-negative and -positive groups is shown in Figure 1G. T-lymphocyte receptors (CD3) and active memory T-lymphocytes (CD45Ro) were significantly upregulated 2.38-fold ($P < 0.001$) and 2.1-fold ($P < 0.01$), respectively (Figure 1G). Significant accession of CD3 and CD45Ro in iDCM myocardium also suggests increased myocardial micro-vascular permeability.

Our data showed upregulation of the specific and general inflammatory markers interleukin-6 (IL-6) and C-reactive protein (hsCRP), respectively, in iDCM serum samples (3.45-fold, $P < 0.05$ and 2.76-fold) (Table 2). Changes of tumor necrosis factor alpha (TNF-α) and interleukin-1beta (IL-1β), also known as catabolin, were not significant in the iDCM sera.

Changes of apoptotic and necrotic biomarkers in iDCM samples

Data presented in Figure 2A show significant correlation between CD3 and IL-6. Significant correlation of IL-6 and hsCRP with the mitochondrial chaperonic protein Hsp60 and pro-apoptotic Bax in sera, respectively, suggests that myocardial inflammation mostly affected the integrity of mitochondrial membranes (Figure 2B and C). Levels of the mitochondrial membrane stabilizing protein Hsp60 in inflammation-positive sera were 8.97-fold higher ($P < 0.05$). Changes of APO1/Fas/CD95

(FasR), the main receptor of extrinsic apoptotic pathway, and its ligand (FasL) in sera and biopsies were not significant (Table 2).

Data presented in Figure 3A demonstrate statistically significant ($P < 0.05$) increase of caspase-9, –8 and –3 in sera with the most prominent expression of caspase-9. Enhanced expression of the same caspases in endomyocardial biopsy samples (Figure 3B) was, however, slight and insignificant. The upregulation of high sensitivity troponin T (hsTnT), a major structural sarcomeric protein of the heart and a marker of necrosis and/or cardiomyocyte injury, in sera was not significant (Table 2). However, the sarcomeric protein hsTnT in iDCM sera strongly correlated with the levels of caspases-8, Bax and caspase-3 in biopsies, suggesting cardiomyocyte injury and caspase-regulated release of hsTnT (Table 3).

The correlation analysis of apoptotic biomarkers in iDCM sera and biopsies

Data in Figure 4A demonstrate that caspase-9, a serum cysteine-aspartic acid specific protease, also named apoptosis-initiating caspase, significantly correlated with the general inflammatory marker C-reactive protein (hsCRP) confirming the sensitivity of the intrinsic apoptotic pathway to inflammation. In parallel, the significant correlation between caspase-9 and MMP9 tells us that caspase-9 might be either directly activated by the MMP9 or, alternatively, through the other mediators of the intrinsic apoptotic pathways, such as Bcl-2 and Bax (Figure 4C and D; $P < 0.05$). Results presented in Figure 4E and F show that levels of caspase-9 are strongly correlated ($P < 0.05$) with the executing caspase-3 and extrinsic apoptotic pathway-initiating caspase-8, suggesting the interaction between the intrinsic and extrinsic apoptotic pathways. Furthermore, a significant correlation was observed between caspase-8 and the APO1/Fas/CD95 levels in iDCM sera (Figure 5A). Caspase-8 also significantly correlated with the pro-apoptotic Bax and MMP9 confirming the intersection of extrinsic and intrinsic pathways at mitochondrial level and caspase-8 activation by MMP9 (Figure 5B and C).

Next, we have investigated correlation of apoptotic biomarkers in iDCM myocardium. Caspase-9 in heart tissues, similarly to that in sera, significantly correlated with pro-inflammatory cytokine IL-6, and caspase-8 in myocardium correlated with Bax and caspase-3 (Table 3). The executing caspase-3 also demonstrated significant correlation with both the intrinsic (Bax, Bcl-2) and extrinsic (APO1/Fas/CD95 and FasL) apoptotic pathways (Table 3). Similarly to that in sera, members of both apoptotic pathways (Bcl-2, APO1/Fas/CD95 and FasL) in biopsies significantly correlated with MMP9 and its inhibitor TIMP1 (Table 3).

Table 2 Summarized data of measured biomarkers

Variable	Inflammation negative group		Inflammation positive group		
	Total No. of pts.	Value	Total No. of pts.	Value	p Value
Markers of inflammation in serum					
TNF-α (pg/mL)	8	7.9313 ± 0.5106	21	14.2819 ± 5.0280	0.223
IL-6 (pg/mL)	8	3.3938 ± 0.8554	21	11.4038 ± 3.3614	0.031*
IL-1β (pg/mL)	8	5.0000 ± 0.0000	21	4.7619 ± 0.2381	0.329
CRP (μg/mL)	8	7.6875 ± 5.0460	19	21.5563 ± 6.9633	0.066¡
Markers of apoptosis in serum					
Bcl2 (ng/mg protein)	10	0.0288 ± 0.0288	22	0.0536 ± 0.0455	0.889¡
Bax (ng/mg protein)	10	2.152717 ± 0.24	22	2.3354 ± 0.1606	0.535
Caspase-9 (ng/mg protein)	10	0.012955 ± 0.0013	22	0.0808 ± 0.0283	0.038*
Caspase-8 (ng/mg protein)	10	0.001 ± 0.0001	22	0.0031 ± 0.0009	0.043*¡
Caspase-3 (ng/mg protein)	10	0.0029 ± 0.0022	22	0.0105 ± 0.0023	0.025*
APO1/Fas/CD95 (ng/mg protein)	10	0.0000 ± 0.0000	22	0.00004 ± 0.00004	0.857¡
FasL (ng/mg protein)	10	0.0000 ± 0.0000	22	0.0000 ± 0.0000	N.A.
HSP60 (ng/mg protein)	10	0.0419 ± 0.0253	22	0.3760 ± 0.1468	0.035*
Markers of apoptosis in biopsy					
Bcl2 (ng/mg protein)	10	83.5523 ± 26.2936	21	63.8790 ± 17.2137	0.540
Bax (ng/mg protein)	10	5.6452 ± 2.6905	21	6.8873 ± 3.7924	0.724¡
Caspase-9 (ng/mg protein)	10	29.6575 ± 12.5969	21	38.7122 ± 9.6108	0.950¡
Caspase-8 (ng/mg protein)	10	0.9483 ± 0.1640	21	1.1611 ± 0.1962	0.413
Caspase-3 (ng/mg protein)	10	0.2503 ± 0.0773	21	0.2586 ± 0.0649	0.935
APO1/Fas/CD95 (ng/mg protein)	10	3.4651 ± 0.6568	21	4.1921 ± 0.6607	0.443
FasL (ng/mg protein)	10	4.5550 ± 1.3594	21	4.0588 ± 1.1083	0.780
HSP-60 (ng/mg protein)	10	24.1262 ± 6.9102	21	19.2656 ± 4.5617	0.565
Marker of heart tissue contraction in serum					
hsTnT (pg/mL)	8	35.4988 ± 9.0908	20	66.4145 ± 26.9755	0.289
Markers of extracellular matrix degradation in serum					
MMP9 (ng/mg protein)	10	1.3867 ± 0.0674	22	1.5261 ± 0.0508	0.115
TIMP1 (ng/mg protein)	10	5.9610 ± 0.3597	22	6.1223 ± 0.1497	0.686
MMP9/TIMP1	10	0.2355 ± 0.0090	22	0.2511 ± 0.0086	0.223
Markers of extracellular matrix degradation in biopsy					
MMP9 (ng/mg protein)	10	2.3698 ± 1.1931	21	2.7630 ± 0.9394	0.798
TIMP1 (ng/mg protein)	10	9.4917 ± 1.7605	21	7.8056 ± 1.4029	0.462
MMP9/TIMP1	10	0.1931 ± 0.0729	21	0.4760 ± 0.1048	0.035*
Frequency of viral genome	5	50%	11	50%	
BNP (pg/mL)	10	1277.8500 ± 428.5054	22	1603.2591 ± 276.3777	0.532

Data are presented as the means ± SE. *Significant at 0.05 level. ¡ Wilcoxon–Mann–Whitney rank sum nonparametric test. *Abbreviations:* TNF-α - tumor necrosis factor α; IL-6 – interleukin-6; IL-1β – interleukin 1β; Bcl-2 – B-cell lymphoma 2 protein; Bax – Bcl-2–associated X protein; Hsp60 – heat shock protein 60; MMP9 – matrix metalloproteinase 9; TIMP1 – tissue inhibitor of matrix metalloproteinase 1; TNF-a – tumor necrosis factor-alfa; IL-1β – interleukin 1 beta; IL-6 – interleukin 6; hs TnT – high sensitivity troponin T; CRP – C-reactive protein, BNP- B-type natriuretic protein; N.A. – not available.

Estimation of fibrosis in iDCM biopsies

The final experimental part was dedicated to investigate the level of fibrosis in the EMB samples. Data in Figure 6A and B show that the level of fibrosis (blue stain) in inflammatory-positive biopsies was slightly lower compared to the inflammatory-negative ones. The quantitative expression of fibrosis staining confirmed our observation (Figure 6C). The exact roles of collagen I

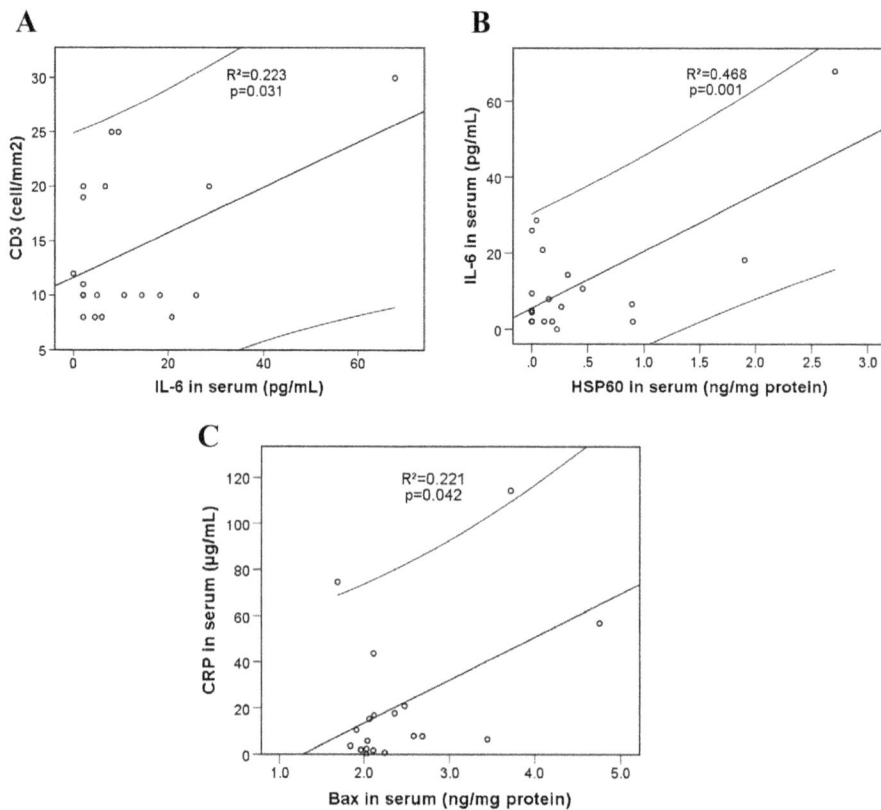

Figure 2 Correlation between inflammatory and mitochondrial membrane destabilization markers. (A). Correlation between serum inflammatory cytokine IL-6 and CD3. **(B)**. Correlation between IL-6 and mitochondrial membrane stabilizing chaperone Hsp60 in serums. **(C)**. Correlation between C-reactive protein (CRP) and Bax in serums. Correlation analysis was done by the statistical SPPS programme. Correlation was significant at a level of $P <0.05$. Linear regression line is presented within 95% confidence interval. Regression coefficients (R^2) are shown in the graphs.

and III in fibrosis were impossible to evaluate due to the absence of collagen I and III quantification algorithm under polarized light. This part needs additional investigations.

Discussion

Inflammatory cardiomyopathy is often defined by myocarditis in association with cardiac dysfunction and inflammation as a main factor of interconnection [15,19]. Long-term studies have shown that less than 15% of patients with acute myocarditis developed dilated cardiomyopathy [20]. It was also demonstrated that patients with proved active myocarditis in biopsies and idiopathic DCM had the same long-term outcome (56% vs. 54%, respectively) [21]. Therefore, investigation of underlying basic molecular mechanisms and their possible pharmacological modulation could improve treatment of chronic iDCM.

Formerly the inflammatory markers were thought to be only indicators of risk but not causal factors [22]. However, it was shown that the pro-inflammatory

cytokines, such as TNF-α, IL-6 and IL-1β, might act synergistically at both mRNR and protein levels by impairing cardiac contraction [23,24]. Pro-inflammatory IL-6 has been reported to be involved in the remodeling of left ventricle after myocardial infarction and induced heart failure leading to skeletal muscle atrophy and heart disorders [25,26]. The molecular mechanisms by which IL-6 affect myocardium can be related to a negative ionotropic effect and upregulation of nitric oxide synthase, downregulation of SERCA2, stimulation of collagen synthesis to name a few [27-29]. The activation of molecular mechanism in heart usually depends on the origin, duration and intensity of toxic stimuli.

Recently, a strong and direct influence of IL-6 was shown on mitochondrial function: IL-6 inhibited adipocyte mitochondrial membrane potential, ATP production and increased intracellular ROS levels [30,31]. Similar to IL-6, a general inflammatory biomarker C-reactive protein (hsCRP) also correlated with poor DCM prognosis, heart failure and mitochondrion-mediated

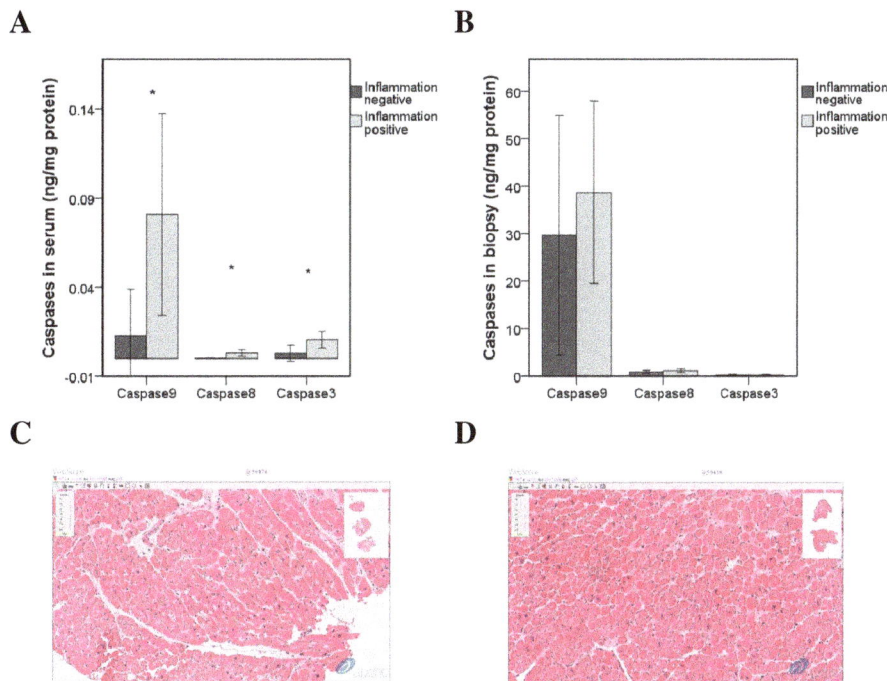

Figure 3 Levels of pro-caspases-9, −8, and −3 in iDCM samples. (A). Levels of caspases in iDCM serum samples. **(B).** Levels of caspases in iDCM biopsies. **(C).** Histological estimation of necrosis in inflammation-negative EMB. **(D).** Histological estimation of necrosis in inflammation-positive EMB. Images are representative from one EMB of each group. Data are presented as means ± SE from at least three independent measurements. Data were considered significant at *$P < 0.05$.

myocyte apoptosis [32-34]. It was also shown that, CRP contributes to IL-6 expression which is a stronger prognostic predictor of heart failure than CRP [35,36]. In agreement with previous observations, our data show significant upregulation of IL-6 in chronic iDCM sera and its significant correlation with numbers of infiltrated T-lymphocytes (CD3) and secreted intra-mitochondrial Hsp60 protein

levels. The significant correlation of CRP with pro-apoptotic Bax and strong upregulation of caspase-9 in sera confirmed that inner apoptotic pathway is more sensitive to inflammation compared to the extrinsic one. Additionally, the absence of necrosis and insignificant upregulation of apoptosis markers in biopsies suggest the beginning of cell death in chronic iDCM myocardium.

Table 3 Correlation of apoptotic, necrotic and inflammatory biomarkers in EMB

	Casp-9 in biopsy	Casp-8 in biopsy	Casp-3 in biopsy	Bcl2 in biopsy	FasR in biopsy	FasL in biopsy	MMP9 in biopsy	TIMP1 in biopsy	Bax in biopsy	IL-6 in serum
Casp-8 in biopsy	0.303									
Casp-3 in biopsy	0.063	**0.436***								
Bcl2 in biopsy	−0.202	0.175	**0.486***							
FasR in biopsy	−0.097	−0.074	**0.526***	**0.739****						
FasL in biopsy	−0.046	0.007	**0.442***	**0.835****	**0.907****					
MMP9 in biopsy	−0.229	0.024	0.419	**0.764****	**0.730****	**0.824****				
TIMP1 in biopsy	−0.012	−0.205	0.213	**0.517***	**0.795****	**0.722****	0.401			
Bax in biopsy	0.283	**0.584****	**0.678****	0.056	0.139	0.053	0.128	−0.127		
IL-6 in serum	**0.518***	−0.016	−0.011	−0.262	−0.202	−0.154	−0.041	−0.227	0.131	
hs TNT in serum	0.434	**0.598****	**0.563***	−0.125	−0.067	−0.165	−0.120	−0.249	**0.954****	0.231

Two tailed significance: *$P < 0.05$; **$P < 0.01$. Significant correlations are in bold type.
Abbreviations: Casp-3 – Caspase-3; Casp-8 – Caspase-8; Casp-9 – Caspase-9; IL-6 – Interleukin-6; Bcl-2 – B-cell lymphoma 2 protein; FasR—Fas receptor; FasL – Fas ligand; MMP9 – matrix metalloproteinase 9; TIMP1 – tissue inhibitor of matrix metalloproteinase 1; Bax – Bcl-2–associated X protein; Hsp60 – heat shock protein 60; hsTnT – high sensitivity Troponin T.

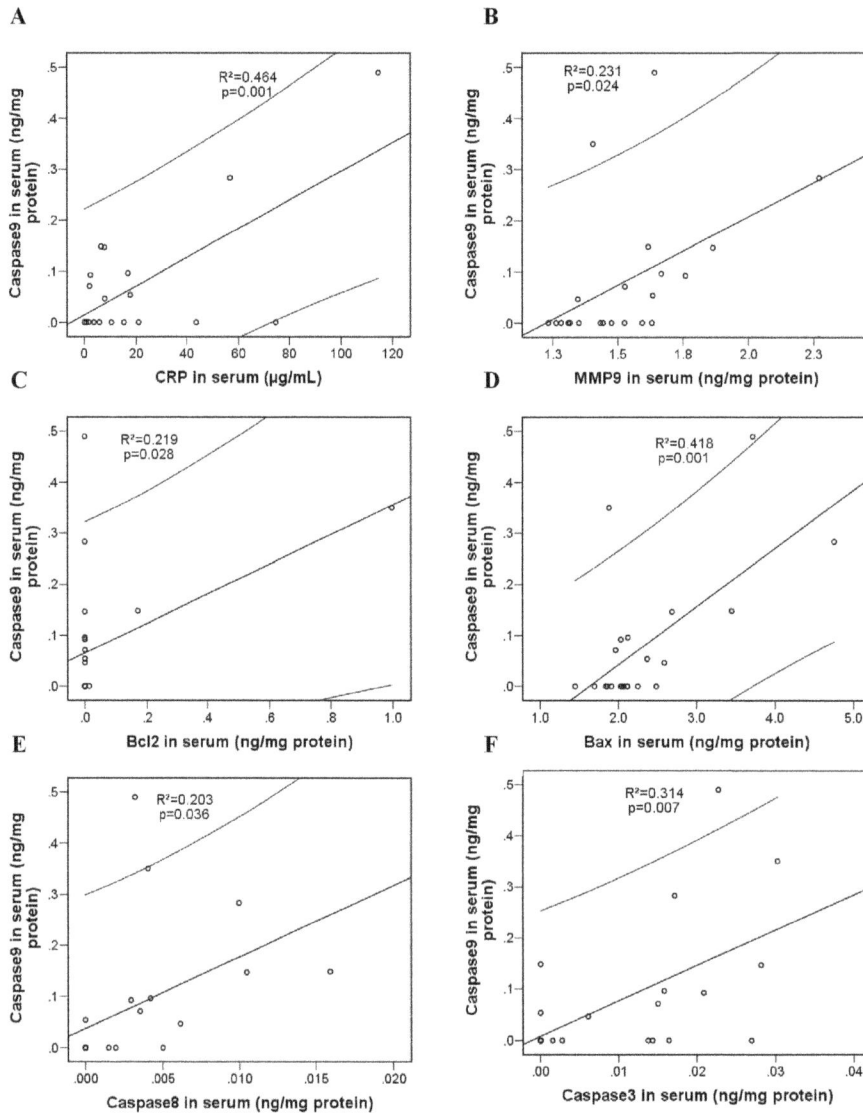

Figure 4 Correlation of caspase-9 with biomolecules in serum samples. Caspase-9 correlated with: **(A)**. C-reactive protein (CRP). **(B)**. matrix metalloproteinase-9 (MMP-9). **(C)**. B-cell lymphoma 2 protein (Bcl-2). **(D)**. Bcl-2–associated X protein (Bax). **(E)**. Caspase-8. **(F)**. Caspase-3. Correlation analysis was done by the statistical SPPS programme. Linear regression line is presented within 95% confidence interval. Regression coefficients (R^2) and statistical significance ($P < 0.05$) are shown in the graphs.

Many recent findings demonstrate interaction between both apoptotic pathways strengthening toxic effects in heart [37]. It was shown that the member of the extrinsic apoptotic pathway pro-caspase-8 cleaves the BH3 domain-only protein Bid, which in turn, activates Bax, stimulates its integration into mitochondrial membranes and release of cytochrome c [38,39]. In agreement with previous observations, data of the present study show a significant correlation between caspase-8 and Bax levels in iDCM sera, suggesting that Bax can be one of the most important intersection points between the intrinsic and extrinsic apoptotic pathways. However, the mediators of extrinsic apoptotic pathway in iDCM samples had low initial level and intensity of activation suggesting this pathway being a supporter but not a main leader of heart cell death. The other authors' observations confirmed that the extrinsic apoptotic pathway might have low impact on cardiomyocyte death in left ventricular tissue [40].

The ECM is an important mediator between different cell types within the myocardium supporting its structural network which can be degraded by proteolytic enzymes matrix metalloproteinases (MMPs). In animal

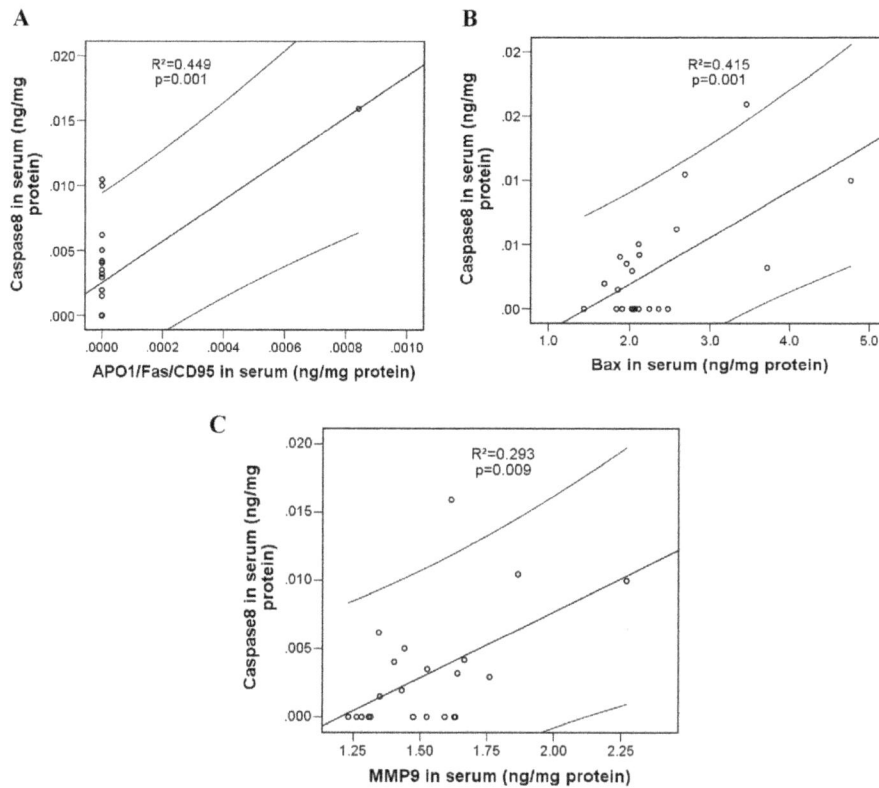

Figure 5 Correlation between caspase-8 and biomolecules in serum samples. Correlation of caspase-8 with: **(A)**. Fas receptor (APO1/Fas/CD95). **(B)**. Bcl-2–associated X protein (Bax). **(C)**. Matrix metalloproteinase-9 (MMP-9). Correlation analysis was done using SPPS program. Linear regression line is presented within 95% confidence interval. Coefficients of regression (R^2) and statistical significance ($P < 0.05$) are shown in the graphs.

model, a time-dependent increase of myocardial MMPs levels were related to the progression of left ventricular dilation and dysfunction [41]. Similar to the intrinsic apoptotic pathway, MMP-9 was also found to be sensitive to inflammation and to participate in the pathogenesis of cardiomyopathy [42]. Additionally, it was shown that chronic heart failure involves endothelial apoptosis in response to MMP-9 activation [43]. Data of this study showed that the MMP-9/TIMP1 ratio in iDCM biopsies was significantly upregulated and significantly correlated with the markers of both apoptotic pathways (Bcl-2, Fas receptor and Fas ligand). These observations suggest that upregulation of MMP-9/TIMP1 are more related to the activation of apoptotic pathways than to the stimulation of fibrosis. Parallelly, the significant correlation between hsTnT and apoptotic proteins caspases-8, Bax and caspase-3 also reveals hsTnT contribution to the impairment of cardiomyocyte and/or contraction ability by activation of pro-apoptotic signaling cascades.

Conclusions

The present study demonstrates that persistent myocardial stressors increase T-lymphocytes in myocardium

of iDCM patients which correlates with the augmented secretion of inflammatory cytokines, such as IL-6. Chronic myocardial inflammation subsequently affects mitochondria and induces significant release of Hsp60 and caspase-9, −8 and −3, suggesting activation of both apoptotic pathways with stronger implication on the intrinsic pathway. The pro-apoptotic Bax is an important intersection point for the extrinsic- and intrinsic apoptotic pathways, blockage of which might improve iDCM treatment. The significant activation of MMP-9/TIMP1 was enough to support apoptosis but not fibrosis.

Taken together, our study suggests that biomarkers secreted to the serum parallels intramyocardial processes and, therefore, might be useful not only for the diagnosis but also for detailed studies of the molecular mechanism behind chronic iDCM. The observed absence of necrosis and fibrosis in chronic iDCM shows that disease had still not reached an end-stage and might be controlled by anti-inflammatory and specific anti-apoptotic drugs.

Limitations

The main limitation of this study is that it contains a relatively low number of iDCM patients. The study also

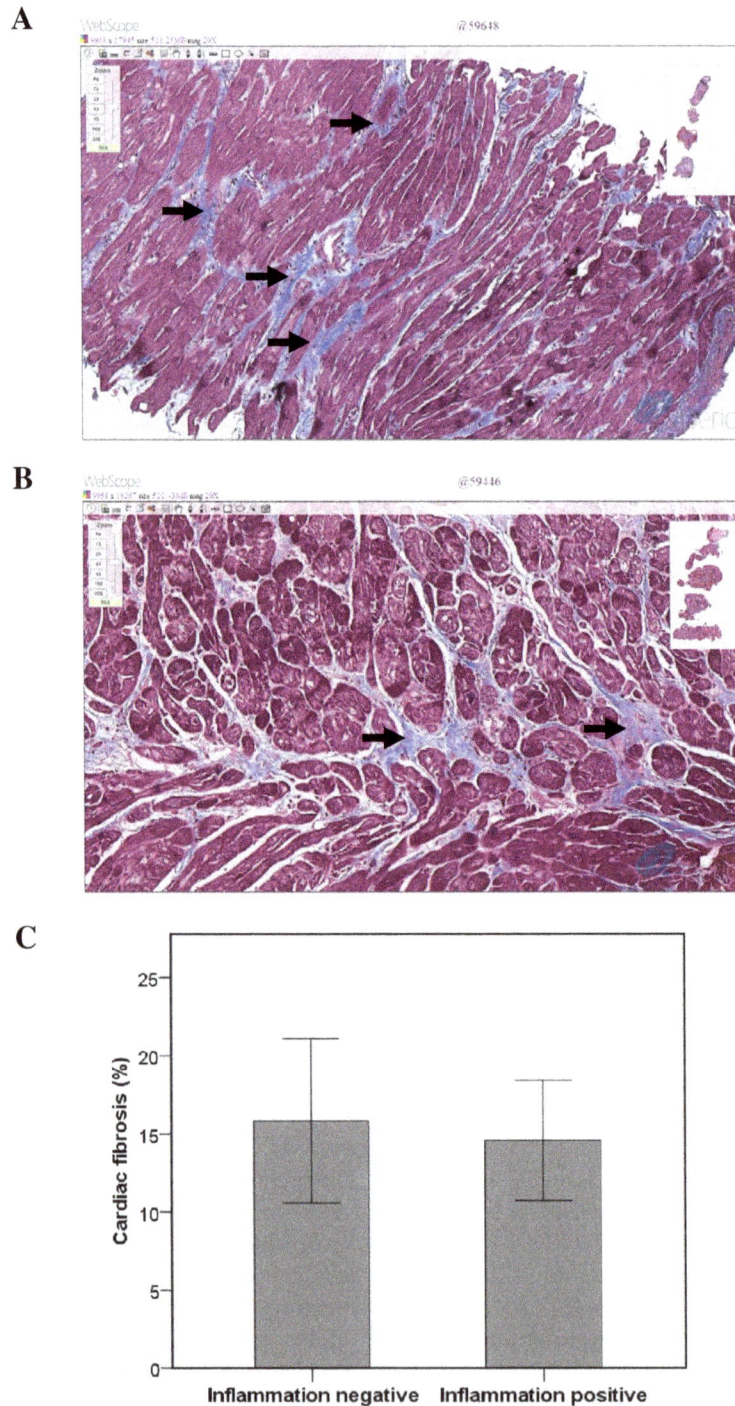

Figure 6 **Histopathological findings of fibrosis in right ventricular EMB. (A)**. Inflammation-negative EMB. **(B)**. Inflammation-positive EMB. **(C)**. Quantitative expression of fibrosis. Micrographs show one representative picture from one patient of each group. Fibrosis is colored blue. Magnification × 10.

lacks normal heart biopsies because of ethical reasons. However, the main goal of this study was to investigate the main processes, molecular mechanism and signaling pathways dominating in chronic iDCM of unknown origin. The collection of additional iDCM samples continues and, hopefully, in the future we will be able to understand more about iDCM diagnosis and its treatment.

Competing interests
The authors declare that they have no competing interests.

Authors' contributions
DB and DD drafted the manuscript. DD performed statistical analysis. SC, KR and DV performed cardiac catheterization and collection of sera and EMB samples. DB performed serum- and EMB ELISA analyses. EZ performed microscope evaluation of the samples. DD designed and performed the digital analyses. IZ - selected patients. JB and SL - participated in the consideration of results. AV - provided with laboratory equipment. AG - manager of study. All authors have participated in conception and design of the study, reviewed the analysis of results as well as read and approved the final manuscript.

Acknowledgements
This work was supported by the Research Council of Lithuania (grant number: MIP-086/2012 and MIP-011/2014) and European Union, EU-FP7, SarcoSi project (number: 291834) for support.

Author details
[1]Dept. of Stem Cell Biology, State Research Institute, Center for Innovative Medicine, Zygimantu 9, LT01102 Vilnius, Lithuania. [2]Department of Pathology, Forensic Medicine and Pharmacology, Vilnius University, Faculty of Medicine, Vilnius, Lithuania. [3]Department of Integrative Pathophysiology, Universitätsmedizin Mannheim, Mannheim, Germany. [4]Department of Physiology, Biochemistry, Microbiology and Laboratory Medicine, Vilnius University, Faculty of Medicine, Vilnius, Lithuania. [5]Vilnius University, Faculty of Medicine, Clinic of Cardiovascular Diseases, Vilnius, Lithuania.

References
1. Mason JW. Myocarditis and dilated cardiomyopathy: an inflammatory link. Cardiovasc Res. 2003;60:5–10.
2. Gopal DM, Sam F. New and emerging biomarkers in left ventricular systolic dysfunction-insight into dilated cardiomyopathy. J Cardiovasc Transl Res. 2013;6:516–27.
3. Maisch B, Noutsias M, Ruppert V, Richter A, Pankuweit S. Cardiomyopathies: classification, diagnosis, and treatment. Heart Fail Clin. 2012;8:53–78.
4. Kawai C. From myocarditis to cardiomyopathy: mechanisms of inflammation and cell death: learning from the past for the future. Circulation. 1999;99:1091–100.
5. Mason JW, O'Connell JB, Herskowitz A, Rose NR, McManus BM, Billingham ME, et al. A clinical trial of immunosuppressive therapy for myocarditis. The Myocarditis Treatment Trial Investigators. N Engl J Med. 1995;333:269–75.
6. Kapadia S, Lee JR, Torre-Amione G, Birdsall HH, Ma TS, Mann DL. Tumor necrosis factor gene and protein expression in adult feline myocardium after endotoxin administration. J Clin Invest. 1995;96:1042–52.
7. Eddy LJ, Goeddel DV, Wong GHW. Tumor necrosis factor-® pretreatment is protective in a rat model of myocardial ischemia-reperfusion injury. Biochem Biophys Res Commun. 1992;184:1056–9.
8. Schwimmbeck PL, Badorff C, Rohn G, Schulze K, Schultheiss HP. The role of sensitized T-cells in myocarditis and dilated cardiomyopathy. Int J Cardiol. 1996;54:117–25.
9. Yamaji K, Fujimoto S, Ikeda Y, Masuda K, Nakamura S, Saito Y, et al. Apoptotic myocardial cell death in the setting of arrhythmogenic right ventricular cardiomyopathy. Acta Cardiol. 2005;60:440–65.
10. Leslie KO, Schwarz J, Simpson K, Huber SA. Progressive interstitial collagen deposition in Coxsackievirus B3-induced murine myocarditis. Am J Pathol. 1990;136:683–93.
11. Kinugawa T, Kato M, Yamamoto K, Hisatome I, Nohara R. Proinflammatory cytokine activation is linked to apoptotic mediator, soluble fas level in patients with chronic heart failure. Int Heart J. 2012;53:182–6.
12. Toprak G, Yüksel H, Demirpençe Ö, Islamoglu Y, Evliyaoglu O, Mete N. Fibrosis in heart failure subtypes. Eur Rev Med Pharmacol Sci. 2013;17:2302–9.
13. Davies MJ, McKenna WJ. Dilated cardiomyopathy: an introduction to pathology and pathogenesis. Br Heart J. 1994;72:S24.
14. Caforio AL, Pankuweit S, Arbustini E, Basso C, Gimeno-Blanes J, Felix SB, et al. European Society of Cardiology Working Group on Myocardial and Pericardial Diseases. Current state of knowledge on aetiology, diagnosis, management, and therapy of myocarditis: a position statement of the European Society of Cardiology Working Group on Myocardial and Pericardial Diseases. Eur Heart J. 2013;34:2636–48. 2648a-2648d.
15. Karatolios K, Pankuweit S, Kisselbach C, Maisch B, Hellenic J. Inflammatory cardiomyopathy. Hellenic J Cardiol. 2006;47:54–65.
16. Richardson P, McKenna W, Bristow M, Maisch B, Mautner B, O'Connell J, et al. Report of the 1995 World Health Organization/International Society and Federation of Cardiology Task Force on the Definition and Classification of cardiomyopathies. Circulation. 1996;93:841–2.
17. Cooper LT, Baughman KL, Feldman AM, Frustaci A, Jessup M, Kuhl U, et al. The role of endomyocardial biopsy in the management of cardiovascular disease: a scientific statement from the American Heart Association, the American College of Cardiology, and the European Society of Cardiology. Circulation. 2007;116:2216–33.
18. Allard A, Albinsson B, Wadell G. Rapid typing of human adenoviruses by a general PCR combined with restriction endonuclease analysis. J Clin Microbiol. 2001;39:498–505.
19. Maisch B, Portig I, Ristic AD, Hufnagel G, Pankuweit S. Definition of inflammatory cardiomyopathy myocarditis: on the way to consensus – a status report. Herz. 2000;25:200–9.
20. D'Ambrosio A, Patti G, Manzoli A, Sinagra G, Di Lenarda A, Silvestri F, et al. The fate of acute myocarditis between spontaneous improvement and evolution to dilated cardiomyopathy: a review. Heart. 2001;85:499–504.
21. Grogan M, Redfield MM, Bailey KR, Reeder GS, Gersh BJ, Edwards WD, et al. Long-term outcome of patients with biopsy-proved myocarditis: comparison with idiopathic dilated cardiomyopathy. J Am Coll Cardiol. 1995;26:80–4.
22. Rao M, Jaber BL, Balakrishnan VS. Inflammatory biomarkers and cardiovascular risk: association or cause and effect? Semin Dial. 2006;19:129–35.
23. Carty CL, Heagerty P, Heckbert SR, Enquobahrie DA, Jarvik GP, Davis S, et al. Association of genetic variation in serum amyloid-A with cardiovascular disease and interactions with IL6, IL1RN, IL1beta and TNF genes in the Cardiovascular Health Study. J Atheroscler Thromb. 2009;16:419–30.
24. Yamagishi S, Inagaki Y, Nakamura K, Abe R, Shimizu T, Yoshimura A, et al. Pigment epithelium-derived factor inhibits TNF-alpha-induced interleukin-6 expression in endothelial cells by suppressing NADPH oxidase-mediated reactive oxygen species generation. J Mol Cell Cardiol. 2004;37:497–506.
25. Kobara M, Noda K, Kitamura M, Okamoto A, Shiraishi T, Toba H, et al. Antibody against interleukin-6 receptor attenuates left ventricular remodelling after myocardial infarction in mice. Cardiovasc Res. 2010;87:424–30.
26. Janssen SP, Gayan-Ramirez G, Van den Bergh A, Herijgers P, Maes K, Verbeken E, et al. Interleukin-6 causes myocardial failure and skeletal muscle atrophy in rats. Circulation. 2005;111:996–1005.
27. Finkel MS, Oddis CV, Jacob TD, Watkins SC, Hattler BG, Simmons RL. Negative inotropic effects of cytokines on the heart mediated by nitric oxide. Science. 1992;257:387–9.
28. Villegas S, Villarreal FJ, Dillmann WH. Leukemia inhibitory factor and interleukin-6 downregulate sarcoplasmic reticulum Ca^{2+} ATPase (SERCA2) in cardiac myocytes. Basic Res Cardiol. 2000;95:47–54.
29. Mir SA, Chatterjee A, Mitra A, Pathak K, Mahata SK, Sarkar S. Inhibition of signal transducer and activator of transcription 3 (STAT3) attenuates interleukin-6 (IL-6)-induced collagen synthesis and resultant hypertrophy in rat heart. J Biol Chem. 2012;287:2666–77.
30. Ji C, Chen X, Gao C, Jiao L, Wang J, Xu G, et al. IL-6 induces lipolysis and mitochondrial dysfunction, but does not affect insulin-mediated glucose transport in 3 T3-L1 adipocytes. J Bioenerg Biomembr. 2011;43:367–75.
31. White J, Dawson B, Landers G, Croft K, Peeling P. Effect of supplemental oxygen on post-exercise inflammatory response and oxidative stress. Eur J Appl Physiol. 2013;113:1059–67.
32. Kaneko K, Kanda T, Yamauchi Y, Hasegawa A, Iwasaki T, Arai M, et al. C-Reactive protein in dilated cardiomyopathy. Cardiology. 1999;91:215–9.
33. Yang J, Wang J, Zhu S, Chen X, Wu H, Yang D, et al. C-reactive protein augments hypoxia-induced apoptosis through mitochondrion-dependent pathway in cardiac myocytes. Mol Cell Biochem. 2008;310:215–26.
34. Yin WH, Chen JW, Jen HL, Chiang MC, Huang WP, Feng AN, et al. Independent prognostic value of elevated high-sensitivity C-reactive protein in chronic heart failure. Am Heart J. 2004;147:931–8.
35. Nakagomi A, Seino Y, Endoh Y, Kusama Y, Atarashi H, Mizuno K. Upregulation of monocyte proinflammatory cytokine production by C-reactive protein is significantly related to ongoing myocardial damage and future cardiac events in patients with chronic heart failure. J Card Fail. 2010;16:562–71.

36. Jug B, Salobir BG, Vene N, Sebestjen M, Sabovic M, Keber I. Interleukin-6 is a stronger prognostic predictor than highsensitive C-reactive protein in patients with chronic stable heart failure. Heart Vessels. 2009;24:271–6.

37. Konstantinidis K, Whelan RS, Kitsis RN. Mechanisms of cell death in heart disease. Arterioscler Thromb Vasc Biol. 2012;32:1552–62.

38. Chou JJ, Li H, Salvesen GS, Yuan J, Wagner G. Solution structure of BID, an intracellular amplifier of apoptotic signaling. Cell. 1999;96:615–24.

39. Roucou X, Montessuit S, Antonsson B, Martinou JC. Bax oligomerization in mitochondrial membranes requires tBid (caspase-8-cleaved Bid) and a mitochondrial protein. Biochem J. 2002;368:915–21.

40. Wollert KC, Heineke J, Westermann J, Ludde M, Fiedler B, Zierhut W, et al. The cardiac Fas (APO-1/CD95) Receptor/Fas ligand system: relation to diastolic wall stress in volume-overload hypertrophy in vivo and activation of the transcription factor AP-1 in cardiac myocytes. Circulation. 2000;101:1172–8.

41. Spinale FG, Coker ML, Thomas CV, Walker JD, Mukherjee R, Hebbar L. Time-dependent changes in matrix metalloproteinase activity and expression during the progression of congestive heart failure: relation to ventricular and myocyte function. Circ Res. 1998;82:482–95.

42. Fares RC, Gomes Jde A, Garzoni LR, Waghabi MC, Saraiva RM, Medeiros NI, et al. Matrix metalloproteinases 2 and 9 are differentially expressed in patients with indeterminate and cardiac clinical forms of Chagas disease. Infect Immun. 2013;81:3600–8.

43. Ovechkin AV, Tyagi N, Rodriguez WE, Hayden MR, Moshal KS, Tyagi SC. Role of matrix metalloproteinase-9 in endothelial apoptosis in chronic heart failure in mice. J Appl Physiol (1985). 2005;99:2398–405.

4

Microarray profiling of long non-coding RNA (lncRNA) associated with hypertrophic cardiomyopathy

Wei Yang, Yuan Li, Fawei He and Haixiang Wu[*]

Abstract

Background: Hypertrophic cardiomyopathy (HCM) is an inherited disorder with around 1400 known mutations; however the molecular pathways leading from genotype to phenotype are not fully understood. LncRNAs, which account for approximately 98 % of human genome, are becoming increasingly interesting with regard to various diseases. However, changes in the expression of regulatory lncRNAs in HCM have not yet been reported. To identify myocardial lncRNAs involved in HCM and characterize their roles in HCM pathogenesis.

Methods: Myocardial tissues were obtained from 7 HCM patients and 5 healthy individuals, and lncRNA and mRNA expression profiles were analyzed using the Arraystar human lncRNA microarray. Real-time PCR was conducted to validate the expression pattern of lncRNA and mRNA. Gene ontology (GO) enrichment and KEGG analysis of mRNAs was conducted to identify the related biological modules and pathologic pathways.

Results: Approximately 1426 lncRNAs (965 up-regulated and 461 down-regulated) and 1715 mRNAs (896 up-regulated and 819 down-regulated) were aberrantly expressed in HCM patients with fold change > 2.0. GO analysis indicated that these lncRNAs–coexpressed mRNAs were targeted to translational process. Pathway analysis indicated that lncRNAs–coexpressed mRNAs were mostly enriched in ribosome and oxidative phosphorylation.

Conclusion: LncRNAs are involved in the pathogenesis of HCM through the modulation of multiple pathogenetic pathways.

Keywords: Hypertrophic cardiomyopathy, LncRNA, Gene ontology, KEGG pathway

Background

Hypertrophic cardiomyopathy (HCM) represents the most common inherited cardiac disease with an estimated prevalence of 0.2 % in the general population [1, 2]. Classically, HCM is morphologically characterized by varying degrees of myocardial hypertrophy, myocyte disarray and interstitial fibrosis [3, 4]. It is also a leading cause of sudden cardiac death in young people, including athletes [5]. Approximately 25 % of individuals with HCM demonstrate left ventricular outflow tract (LVOT) obstruction [6]. It has been accepted that HCM is caused predominately by genetic variants. To date, around 1400 mutations have been identified as being responsible for HCM pathology and more than 60 % of

genetic variants occurred in 9 sarcomeric genes, including *MYH7*, *MYL2* and *MYBPC3* [7–10]. However, the molecular mechanisms that underlie the pathogenesis of HCM remain largely unknown.

Long non-coding RNAs (lncRNAs) are defined as the transcripts of more than 200 nucleotides that structurally resemble mRNAs but do not encode proteins [11]. The Encyclopedia of DNA Elements (ENCODE) project has reported that >90 % of the genome can be transcribed and the non-coding transcripts account for approximately 98 % [12]. Normally, lncRNAs are involved in a variety of biological processes, such as cell-cycle control, differentiation, apoptosis, chromatin remodeling as well as epigenetic regulation [13, 14]. Dysregulation of lncRNAs has been reported in numerous human diseases, including cancer [15] and neurological diseases [16]. However, dysregulation of lncRNAs in patients with

* Correspondence: HXW_1971@163.com
Department of Ultrasonics, The Second Hospital of Sichuan, No. 55, People's South Road, Wuhou District, 610041 Chengdu, Sichuan, China

HCM has never been reported. In the present study, we hypothesized that lncRNAs were dysregulated in hypertrophied myocardial tissues.

In order to reveal the potential roles of lncRNAs in the pathogenesis of HCM, we performed microarray analysis to identify dysregulated lncRNAs and mRNAs in HCM patients, compared to control subjects.

Methods

Ethical statement

All subjects provided written informed consent prior to participation and all procedures in the present study were approved by the Ethics Committee of the second people's hospital of Sichuan.

Tissues from patients with HCM and healthy individuals

Hypertrophied myocardial tissues used in this study were obtained from 7 HCM patients (4 males and 3 females) with severe symptoms (New York Heart Association functional classes III or IV) who underwent septal myectomy at outpatient department of Chengdu first people's hospital (from May 2013 to December 2013). All patients were diagnosed by two experienced clinicians, based on two-dimensional echocardiography demonstrating an unexplained left ventricular hypertrophy (diastolic interventricular septal thickness ≥ 15 mm and the ratio of septal to posterior wall thickness ≥1.3) in the absence of another cardiac or systemic disease capable of producing a similar magnitude of hypertrophy. Besides, 5 normal myocardial tissues, excised from 5 healthy individuals (3 males and 2 females) at autopsy who voluntarily donated their body for research to the Center of Forensic Medicine in West China, were used as a control group. It is worth noting that we didn't perform genetic scanning of 1400 known candidate genes in patients.

The following data was collected for all subjects: gender, age at diagnosis or death, heart rate, family history of hypertrophic cardiomyopathy, previous angina pectoris, systolic blood pressure (SBP) and diastolic blood pressure (DBP) (Table 1). Diseases that would affect cardiac structures and functions were absent in any individual. These diseases included, but not limited to, primary hypertension with duration of more than 10 years, secondary hypertension, ischemic heart disease, congenital heart disease, rheumatic heart disease, aortic stenosis and other similar diseases.

RNA extraction

Myocardial specimens were quickly excised and snap-frozen in liquid nitrogen. Tissues were homogenized in TRIZOL reagent (Invitrogen, USA) using a Qiagen Tissuelyser. Total RNA was extracted in accordance with the manufacturer's protocol and then quantified using a NanoDrop ND-1000 spectrophotometer (Thermo Fisher Scientific, Waltham, MA). RNA integrity of each sample was assessed by denaturing agarose gel electrophoresis.

RNA labeling and array hybridization

The expression of lncRNAs and mRNA was determined using Arraystar Human LncRNA Microarray v2.0 (CapitalBio, China). Sample labeling and array hybridization were performed according to the Agilent One-Color Microarray-Based Gene Expression Analysis protocol (Agilent Technology, USA) with minor modifications for all 12 samples. First, rRNA was removed from total RNA using mRNA-ONLY™ Eukaryotic mRNA Isolation Kit (Epicentre Biotechnologies, USA). Then, each sample was amplified and transcribed into fluorescent cRNA along the entire length of the transcripts without 3′ bias using the random priming method. The labeled cRNAs were purified using an RNeasy Mini Kit (Qiagen, Germany) and then hybridized with the specific probes on the Human LncRNA Array v2.0. Positive probes for housekeeping genes and negative probes are printed onto the array for quality control. The hybridized arrays were washed, fixed, and scanned with an Agilent DNA Microarray Scanner G2505C.

Table 1 Clinical characteristics of HCM patients (n = 7) and controls (n = 5)

Indices	HCM patients (N =7)							Controls (N = 5)					P-value
	1	2	3	4	5	6	7	1	2	3	4	5	
Gender	F	M	M	F	F	M	M	F	F	M	M	M	0.92
Age (years)	51	39	49	60	42	54	43	48	54	31	41	40	0.29
Family history of hypertrophic cardiomyopathy (Y or N)	Y	N	N	N	Y	Y	Y	N	N	N	N	N	0.04
Heart rate (bpm)	80	98	74	73	70	62	67	74	84	59	61	60	0.29
Previous angina pectoris	N	N	Y	Y	Y	N	N	N	N	N	Y	N	0.41
SBP (mmHg)	114	122	112	117	121	123	115	127	110	126	129	131	0.11
DBP (mmHg)	82	62	65	70	75	74	71	75	80	71	82	91	0.09
NYHA Classes	3	4	3	4	3	3	3	N.A.	N.A.	N.A.	N.A.	N.A.	

F female, M male, Y yes, N no, SBP systolic blood pressure, DBP diastolic blood pressure, NYHA New York Heart Association, N. A. not available

Microarray data analysis

Agilent Feature Extraction software (version 11.0.1.1) was used to analyze acquired array images. Quantile normalization and subsequent data processing were performed using the GeneSpring GX software package (version 11.5.1, Agilent Technologies). Differentially expressed lncRNAs and protein-coding mRNAs between patient group and control group were identified through Volcano Plot filtering (fold change > 2 and P < 0.05).

Real-time PCR

Single-strand cDNA was synthesized by AMV Reverse Transcriptase Kit (Promega, USA) in accordance with the manufacturer's instructions. Real-time PCR was performed using SsoFast EvaGreen Supermix (Bio-Rad, USA) on a CFX96 Real-Time PCR Detection System (Bio-Rad, USA). The PCR conditions included an initial step at 95 °C for 30 s, followed by 40 cycles of amplification and quantification (95 °C for 5 s, 60 °C for 5 s). Each DNA sample was performed in triplicates in a final volume of 25 µl containing 1 µl of cDNA and 400 nM of forward and reverse gene-specific primers. Relative gene expression levels were quantified based on the cycle threshold (Ct) values and ACTIN was used as an internal control. For quantitative results, expression of each gene was represented as a fold change using the following mathematical model: Fold change = $(E_{target})^{\Delta Cttarget\ (Control\ -\ Sample)}$/$(E_{ref})^{\Delta Ctref\ (Control\ -\ Sample)}$. E_{target} and E_{ref} are the PCR efficiency of target gene transcript and reference gene transcript, respectively; ΔCt_{target} is the Ct deviation of control – sample of the target gene transcript; ΔCt_{ref} is the Ct deviation of control – sample of the reference gene transcript. All primer pairs are available upon request.

Functional group analysis

Gene Ontology (GO) analysis was performed to explore the functions of differentially expressed coding genes identified in this study by using the Database for Annotation, Visualization and Integrated Discovery (DAVID; http://david.abcc.ncifcrf.gov/) [17, 18]. Pathway analysis was used to place differentially expressed coding genes according to Kyoto Encyclopedia of Genes and Genomes (KEGG), Biocarta and Reactome (http://www.genome.jp/kegg/). Generally, Fisher's exact test and v2 test were used to classify the GO category and select the significant pathway. Besides, the threshold of significance was defined by the P-value and false discovery rate (FDR).

Statistical analysis

The statistical significance of microarray data was analyzed in terms of fold change using the Student's t-test and FDR was calculated to correct the P-value. FC ≥ 2 and P < 0.05 were used to screen the differentially expressed lncRNAs and coding mRNAs. For other statistical analysis, GraphPad Prism 5 software and Microsoft Office software were applied. Stusent's t-test was applied for comparison of two groups and differences with P < 0.05 were considered statistically significant.

Results

Analysis of differentially expressed lncRNAs

In total, 8435 lncRNAs were detected by Arraystar Human LncRNA Microarray v2.0 (Additional file 1). From the lncRNA expression profiles, differentially expressed lncRNAs were discriminated between patients with HCM and controls. Hierarchical Clustering was performed to group lncRNAs based on their expression levels among samples (Fig. 1a). We set a threshold as fold-change >2.0, P-value < 0.05 and FDR < 0.05, and found that a total of 1426 lncRNAs were differentially expressed, consisting of 965 up-regulated lncRNAs and 461 down-regulated lncRNAs. The top 10 up-regulated and 10 down-regulated lncRNAs between two groups were listed in Table 2.

We summarized the classification and length distribution of dysregulated lncRNAs. Among the dysregulated lncRNAs, there were 705 intergenic, 315 antisense, 286 intronic and 120 divergent (Fig. 1b). These differentially expressed lncRNAs showed different length on chromosome (DNA) ranging from 86 bp to 506 kb and 753 lncRNAs (52.8 %) were between 200 bp and 5000 bp in length (Fig. 1c). Moreover, these differentially expressed lncRNAs were distributed across nearly all of the human chromosomes (Fig. 1d).

Analysis of differentially expressed mRNAs

From the analysis, we totally detected 8404 mRNAs, of which 1715 showed significantly different expression between HCM group and control group (FC > 2.0, P-value < 0.05 and FDR < 0.05) (Additional file 2). Among them, 819 mRNAs were down-regulated and 896 mRNAs were up-regulated. Their distinct expression patterns were presented by hierarchical clustering analysis (Fig. 2).

Real-time PCR validation of some differentially expressed lncRNAs and mRNAs

We randomly selected 10 dysregulated lncRNAs, including 5 up-regulated (ENST00000453100.1, ENST00000442794.1, ENST00000563521.1, uc.279+ and TCONS_00013406) and 5 down-regulated (HIT000075931, ENST00000508961.1, ENST00000504833.1, ENST00000420356.1 and ENST00000568819.1), for verification in these myocardial tissues samples. A general consistency between the real-time PCR and microarray analysis results was confirmed in 9 selected lncRNAs in terms of regulation direction (up-regulation or down-regulation) and significance except ENST00000420356.1 (Fig. 3a).

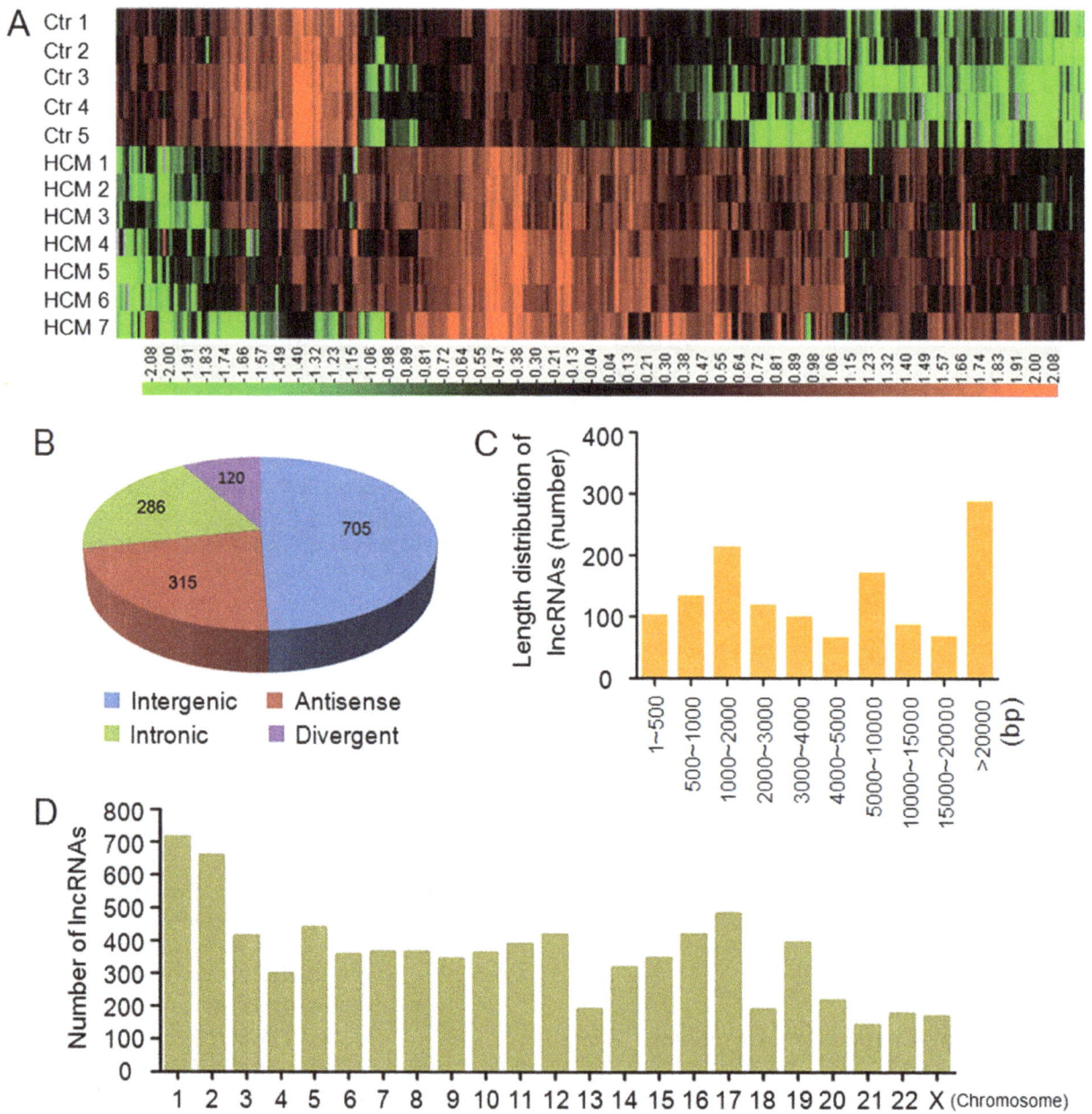

Fig. 1 Overview of lncRNAs microarray analysis. **a** The hierarchical clustering of partial differentially expressed lncRNAs between 7 HCM patients and 5 controls. 'Red' indicates high relative expression, and 'green' indicates low relative expression. Ctr: control. **b** Class distribution of dysregulated lncRNAs, including 705 intergenic, 315 antisense, 286 intronic and 120 divergent. **c** The length distribution of lncRNAs on Chromosome (DNA). The lncRNAs genes were mainly between 200 and 5000 bp in length. **d** Chromosomal distribution of dysregulated lncRNAs

Moreover, we randomly selected 10 dysregulated mRNAs, consisting of 5 up-regulated (TAS2R46, RFX3, HEMGN, SSH1 and SLC1A5) and 5 down-regulated (KLRB1, NDUFA6, ATP6V1G1, SMARCD1 and SDAD1). All the 10 mRNAs showed the same change patterns as shown in microarray analysis (Fig. 3b).

GO and pathway analysis for differentially expressed mRNAs
The GO categories for each gene were derived from the GO website (www.geneontology.org) and comprised of 3

structured networks: biological processes, cellular components and molecular function. Through GO analysis, we found that the differentially expressed mRNAs were principally enriched for translational elongation, translation, ribonuclearprotein complex biogenesis linked with biological processes (Fig. 4a), and ribonucleoprotein complex, ribosome, cytosolic ribosome involved in cellular components (Fig. 4b), as well as structural constituent of ribosome, structural molecule activity, RNA binding in molecular functions (Fig. 4c). Pathway analysis was carried out

Table 2 Top 10 up-regulated and 10 down-regulated lncRNAs between HCM patients and controls

lncRNA ID	FC (abs)	Regulation	FDR	Chrosome	Strand	Start[1]	End[1]	Class	Database
ENST00000472913.1	8.29	up	5.11E–19	3	+	155203591	155204910	Intronic	ENSEMBL
ENST00000588634.1	10.05	up	1.01E–15	19	+	11314303	11326844	Antisense	ENSEMBL
TCONS_00006679	12.76	up	1.99E–10	3	-	148164072	148173245	Intergenic	Human LincRNA Catalog
ENST00000440196.2	12.93	up	3.48E–21	1	-	529832	530597	Intergenic	ENSEMBL
TCONS_00024565	14.61	up	1.60E–18	16	-	3995946	4002465	Intergenic	Human LincRNA Catalog
ENST00000445814.1	14.90	up	1.28E–01	X	-	73047635	73051045	Intergenic	ENSEMBL
TCONS_00017343	15.20	up	8.42E–02	X	-	73040858	73061243	Intergenic	Human LincRNA Catalog
TCONS_00017432	27.97	up	6.45E–02	X	+	73045949	73047819	Intergenic	Human LincRNA Catalog
XR_110349.1	0.13	down	9.57E–15	12	-	49626572	49658539	Divergent	RefSeq
ENST00000450016.1	0.14	down	1.92E–07	7	+	44888657	44889164	Divergent	ENSEMBL
ENST00000443565.1	0.15	down	2.14E–04	1	+	81106968	81112473	Intergenic	ENSEMBL
HIT000075931	0.15	down	6.17E–22	5	-	172083325	172083570	Intronic	H-InvDB
TCONS_00022136	0.16	down	8.21E–09	13	+	20530916	20532202	Divergent	Human LincRNA Catalog
ENST00003376482.3	0.17	down	4.56E–16	7	+	99728586	99738062	Intergenic	ENSEMBL
uc.324-	0.19	down	5.29E–01	11	-	30557520	30557745	Antisense	UCR
TCONS_00014990	0.19	down	2.04E–16	8	-	41998257	41998755	Intergenic	Human LincRNA Catalog
TCONS_00014155	0.20	down	6.11E–14	7	+	65959182	65960476	Intergenic	Human LincRNA Catalog
ENST00000563833.1	0.20	down	3.97E–09	4	-	103421997	103422476	Divergent	ENSEMBL

FC fold change, *FDR* false discover rate
[1]Chromosomal positions based on GRCh38

based on the KEGG database. The dysregulated mRNAs were associated with 12 biological pathways, including ribosome, oxidative phosphorylation, parkinson's disease, huntington's disease, alzheimer's disease, as well as others (Fig. 4d).

Several lines of evidence revealed that most of lncRNAs may act in cis and regulate gene expressions within their chromosomal neighboring regions [19]. We first identified the nearest protein-coding neighbor within 100 kb of dysregulated lncRNA and then applied GO and pathway analysis to determine the roles of these closest coding genes. The neighbor coding gene function of dysregulated lncRNAs mainly involved: (1) biological process (protein metabolic process, gene expression, mRNA metabolic process, biosynthetic process, etc.); (2) cellular component (cytosolic ribosome, nucleus, cytosolic small ribosomal subunit, large ribosomal subunit, etc.); (3) molecular function (transcription factor binding, mRNA binding, oxidoreductase activity, structural constituent of ribosome, etc.) (Fig. 5a–c). The neighbor gene function of dysregulated lncRNAs mainly involved the following pathways: (1) oxidative phosphorylation;

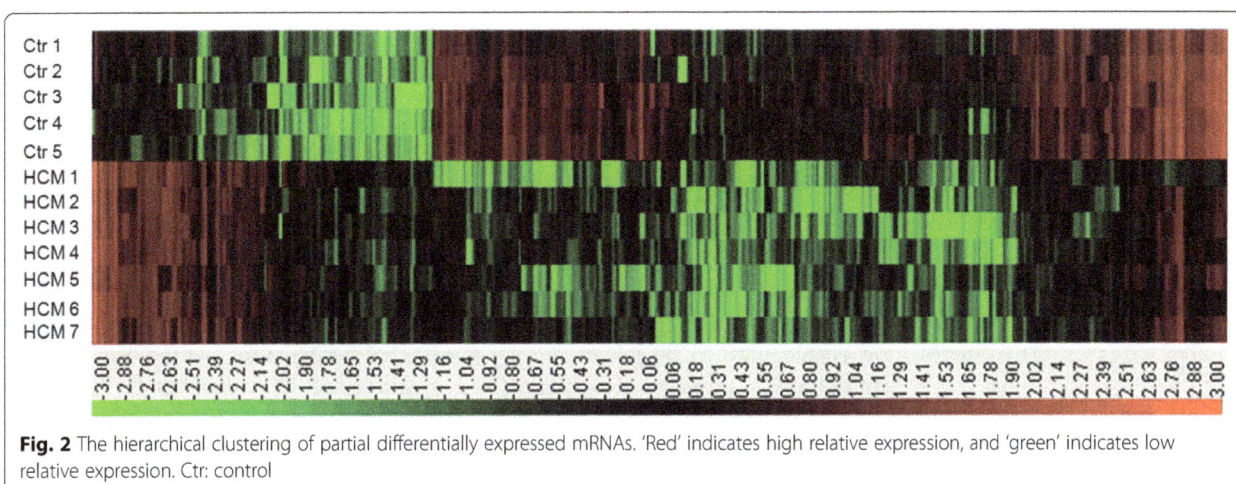

Fig. 2 The hierarchical clustering of partial differentially expressed mRNAs. 'Red' indicates high relative expression, and 'green' indicates low relative expression. Ctr: control

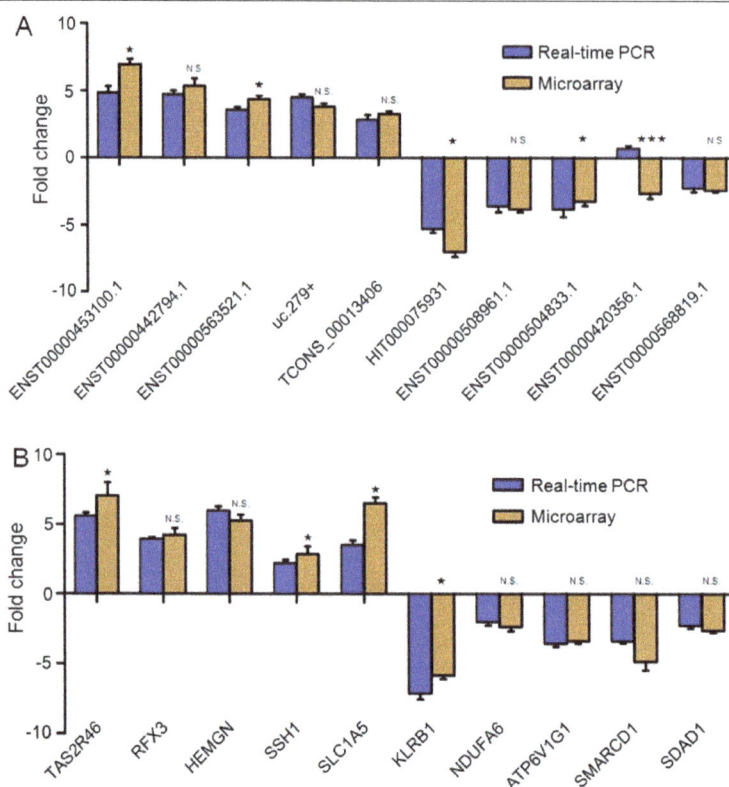

Fig. 3 Real-time PCR validation of some differentially expressed lncRNAs and mRNA from microarray data. **a** 10 lncRNAs were randomly chosen for real-time PCR validation. **b** 10 mRNAs were randomly chosen for real-time PCR validation. Fold changes were calculated by the $2^{-\triangle\triangle Ct}$ method. Data shown are representative of 7 patients and 5 controls; error bars represent means ± SEM, ★$P < 0.05$, ★★$P < 0.01$, ★★★$P < 0.001$, N.S. not significant (student t test). Apart from ENST00000420356.1, the real-time PCR validation results of all lncRNAs and mRNAs were generally consistent with microarray data

(2) renin-angiotensin system; (3) spliceosome; (4) cardiac muscle contraction; (5) apoptosis; (6) p53 signaling pathway (Fig. 5d).

Discussion

In the present study, we performed a comprehensive analysis of dysregulated lncRNAs by comparing the transcriptome profiles of hypertrophied myocardial tissues from HCM patients and normal myocardial tissues. A total of 8435 lncRNAs and 8404 mRNAs were detected. We identified 965 up-regulated and 461 down-regulated lncRNAs, and summarized their general characteristics and functional annotations. Thus, our study could provide a comprehensive understanding of lncRNAs in HCM patients and help to elucidate the molecular mechanisms of HCM.

To our knowledge, several proteomic and transcriptome profiling of HCM have been performed and a number of dysregulated genes have been identified before [20–23] (Additional file 3). For example, Lim et al. identified 36 dysregulated genes involved in cytoskeletal proteins, protein synthesis, redox system, ion channels and those with unknown function in HCM [20]. We

compared the list of HCM-related genes between our study and previous studies and found that some genes appeared both in our study and previous studies, including *AFG3L2, AGPAT9, CDC14B, CMKLR1, COX4I1, GFM1, GLUD1, LDHB, LYRM4, MRPL22, NCAM1, SLC25A46, SS18L2, TACO1, TMEM135, TMEM41B and ZFAND1.*

However, there were also many genes which occurred only in previous studies but not in our study. We believed that discrepancy of expression profiling of mRNA and lncRNA between our study and previous studies was mainly derived from the following several reasons. First, as we know, the RNA and protein profiling fluctuated dramatically during different stages of diseases' progress [24, 25]. In different progess stage of HCM, the RNA profiling might be variable and this would be the major reason. Second, time-dependent degradation of nucleic acids confers great difficulty to expression analysis when postmortem tissues were used. In our study, the normal myocardial tissues were excised from healthy formalin-fixed postmortem individuals 3–7 days after death, which might lead to significant RNA degradation [26, 27]. Inhomogenous RNA degradation would result in the change of relative expression of RNAs, Third,

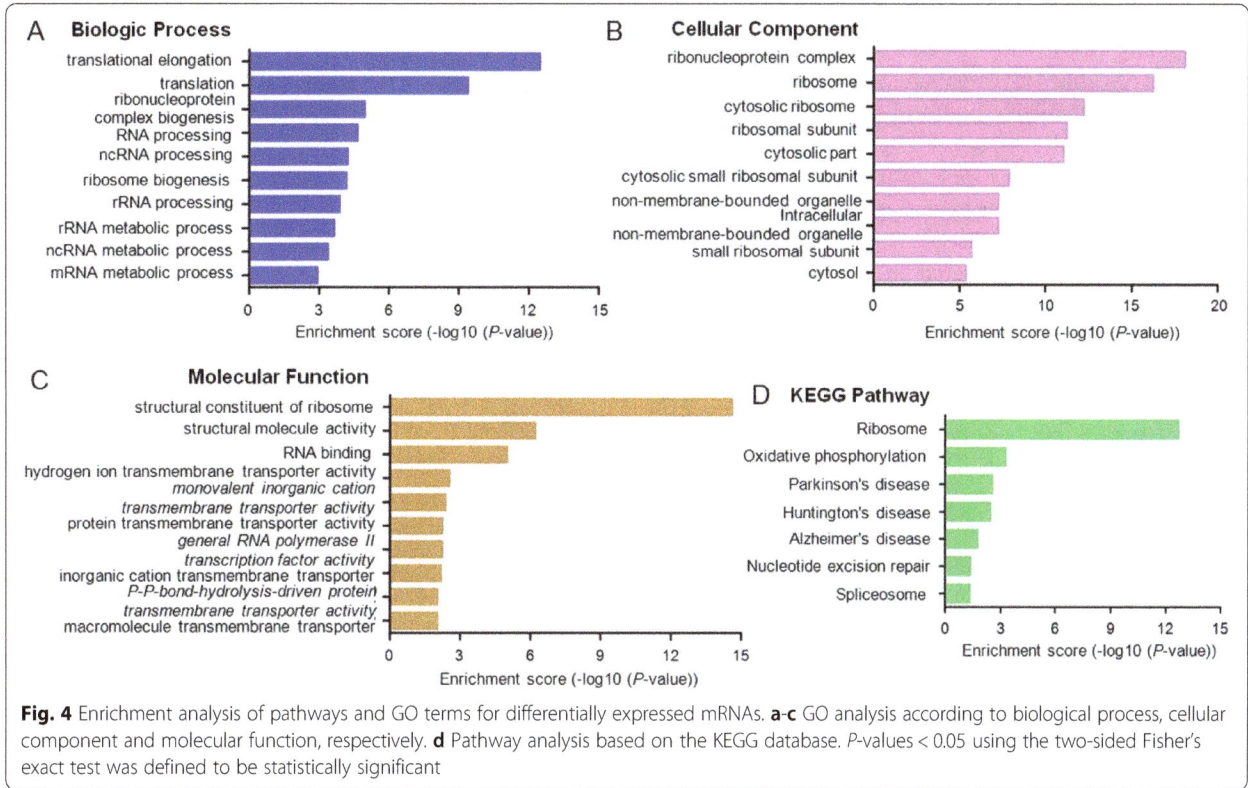

Fig. 4 Enrichment analysis of pathways and GO terms for differentially expressed mRNAs. **a-c** GO analysis according to biological process, cellular component and molecular function, respectively. **d** Pathway analysis based on the KEGG database. *P*-values < 0.05 using the two-sided Fisher's exact test was defined to be statistically significant

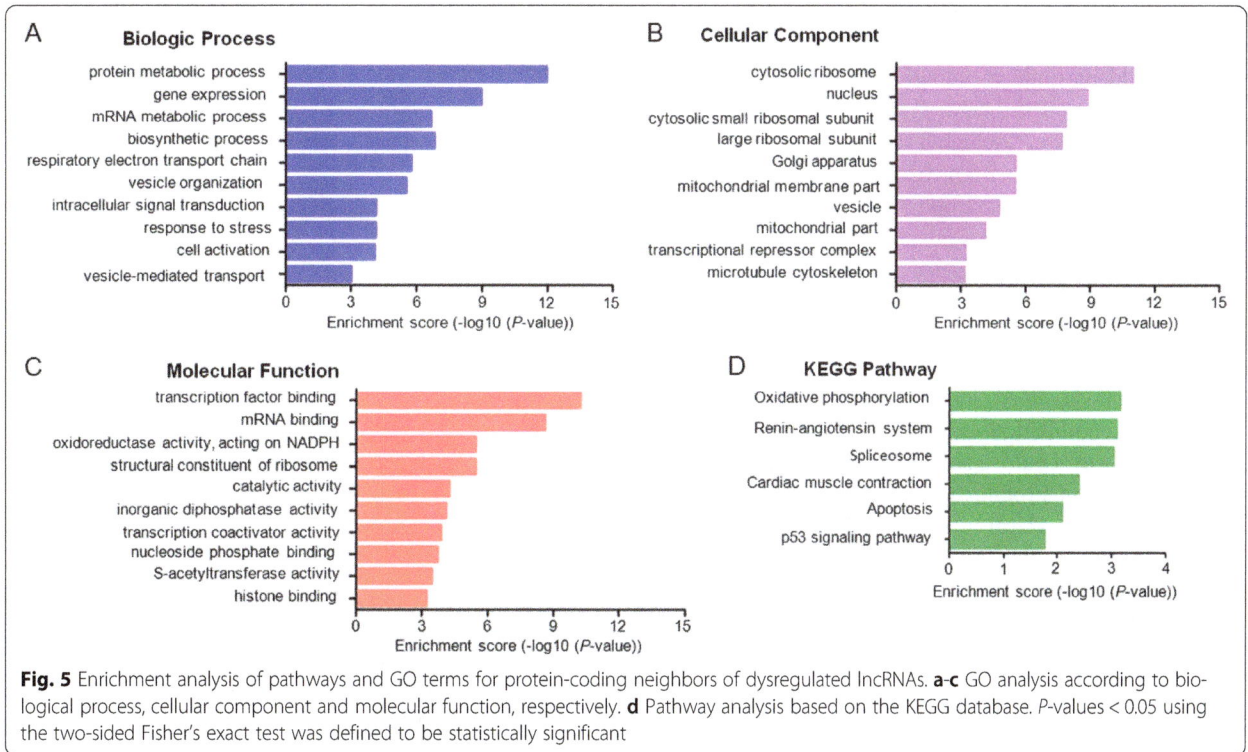

Fig. 5 Enrichment analysis of pathways and GO terms for protein-coding neighbors of dysregulated lncRNAs. **a-c** GO analysis according to biological process, cellular component and molecular function, respectively. **d** Pathway analysis based on the KEGG database. *P*-values < 0.05 using the two-sided Fisher's exact test was defined to be statistically significant

different detection platforms may have huge impact on the profiling result and this is why subsequent experimental verification is essential. Most of the previous studies used Affymetrix platform for profiling analysis, while, in our study, Arraystar Human LncRNA Microarray v2.0 was used. The molecular mechanisms responsible for HCM have been extensively explored. However the pathogenesis of this disease is still largely unknown. Most of the genes discovered in HCM were protein-coding while non-coding genes were scarcely reported. Technological improvements have contributed to reveal the importance of lncRNA underling various diseases [28]. Up till now, both transcriptome sequencing [29] and microarrays [30] have been applied to identify differential lncRNA expression. To the best of our knowledge, only one lncRNA, *Myheart*, was reported to be involved in cardiac hypertrophy in previous studies. *Myheart* could protect heart from pathological hypertrophy by its interaction with chromatin [31, 32]. Our study could greatly enrich the lncRNAs spectrums involved in the pathogenesis of HCM.

The Gene Ontology project provides a controlled vocabulary to describe gene attributes unbiasedly [18]. Interestingly, in our study, these dysregulated genes were mainly involved in translational regulation, including translational elongation, ribonucleoprotein complex, ribosome and structural constituent of ribosome. As we know, once the translational process was disrupted, the levels of numerous proteins would be influenced, which might have profound effects on normal physiological processes [33, 34]. However, no previous study of HCM was concentrated on translational regulation and we hold the opinion that it would be quite meaningful to investigate translational dysregulation in HCM. Pathway analysis identified 7 distinct pathways, including ribosome and oxidative phosphorylation. `It has been reported that CREB contributes to physiological hypertrophy by enhancing expression of genes in complex I of oxidative phosphorylation [35]. Many more studies are needed to fully understand the molecular mechanisms of HCM in the future.

Conclusion

LncRNAs are involved in the pathogenesis of HCM through the modulation of multiple pathogenetic pathways. Our study could also provide clinic evidence for the diagnosis and prognostic management of HCM patients, as well as medical intervening for HCM.

Competing interests
The authors declare that they have no competing interests.

Authors' contributions
WY and HXW conceived of this study and participated in the design of the study. HXW oversaw all aspects of the research. WY, YL and FWH performed

RNA extraction and real-time PCR analysis. WY analyzed the microarray data and drew figures and tables. WY performed statistic analysis and wrote the manuscript; HXW revised it. All authors contributed to and have approved the final manuscript.

Acknowledgments
We would like to thank all of the subjects for their active participation in this work. We thank S. Rao for helpful discussions, and Y. Zhai for technical assistance. This work was supported by Health and Family Planning Commission of Sichuan Province (130227).

References
1. Ho CY. Hypertrophic cardiomyopathy in 2012. Circulation. 2012;125(11):1432–8.
2. Maron BJ. Hypertrophic cardiomyopathy: an important global disease. Am J Med. 2004;116(1):63–5.
3. Maron BJ, Maron MS. Hypertrophic cardiomyopathy. Lancet. 2013;381(9862):242–55.
4. Maron BJ. Hypertrophic cardiomyopathy: a systematic review. JAMA. 2002;287(10):1308–20.
5. Maron BJ, Thompson PD, Puffer JC, McGrew CA, Strong WB, Douglas PS, et al. Cardiovascular preparticipation screening of competitive athletes: addendum: an addendum to a statement for health professionals from the Sudden Death Committee (Council on Clinical Cardiology) and the Congenital Cardiac Defects Committee (Council on Cardiovascular Disease in the Young), American Heart Association. Circulation. 1998;97(22):2294.
6. Maron MS, Olivotto I, Betocchi S, Casey SA, Lesser JR, Losi MA, et al. Effect of left ventricular outflow tract obstruction on clinical outcome in hypertrophic cardiomyopathy. N Engl J Med. 2003;348(4):295–303.
7. Maron BJ, Maron MS, Semsarian C. Genetics of hypertrophic cardiomyopathy after 20 years: clinical perspectives. J Am Coll Cardiol. 2012;60(8):705–15.
8. Efthimiadis GK, Pagourelias ED, Gossios T, Zegkos T. Hypertrophic cardiomyopathy in 2013: Current speculations and future perspectives. World J Cardiol. 2014;6(2):26–37.
9. Nishimura RA, Ommen SR. Hypertrophic cardiomyopathy: the search for obstruction. Circulation. 2006;114(21):2200–2.
10. Roma-Rodrigues C, Fernandes AR. Genetics of hypertrophic cardiomyopathy: advances and pitfalls in molecular diagnosis and therapy. Appl Clin Genet. 2014;7:195–208.
11. Guttman M, Amit I, Garber M, French C, Lin MF, Feldser D, et al. Chromatin signature reveals over a thousand highly conserved large non-coding RNAs in mammals. Nature. 2009;458(7235):223–7.
12. Derrien T, Johnson R, Bussotti G, Tanzer A, Djebali S, Tilgner H, et al. The GENCODE v7 catalog of human long noncoding RNAs: analysis of their gene structure, evolution, and expression. Genome Res. 2012;22(9):1775–89.
13. Mattick JS. The genetic signatures of noncoding RNAs. PLoS Genet. 2009;5(4), e1000459.
14. Rinn JL, Chang HY. Genome regulation by long noncoding RNAs. Annu Rev Biochem. 2012;81:145–66.
15. Ge X, Chen Y, Liao X, Liu D, Li F, Ruan H, et al. Overexpression of long noncoding RNA PCAT-1 is a novel biomarker of poor prognosis in patients with colorectal cancer. Med Oncol. 2013;30(2):588.
16. Barry G, Briggs JA, Vanichkina DP, Poth EM, Beveridge NJ, Ratnu VS, et al. The long non-coding RNA Gomafu is acutely regulated in response to neuronal activation and involved in schizophrenia-associated alternative splicing. Mol Psychiatry. 2014;19(4):486–94.
17. Dennis Jr G, Sherman BT, Hosack DA, Yang J, Gao W, Lane HC, et al. DAVID: Database for Annotation, Visualization, and Integrated Discovery. Genome Biol. 2003;4(5):3.
18. Ashburner M, Ball CA, Blake JA, Botstein D, Butler H, Cherry JM, et al. Gene ontology: tool for the unification of biology. The Gene Ontology Consortium. Nat Genet. 2000;25(1):25–9.
19. Guttman M, Donaghey J, Carey BW, Garber M, Grenier JK, Munson G, et al. lincRNAs act in the circuitry controlling pluripotency and differentiation. Nature. 2011;477(7364):295–300.
20. Lim DS, Roberts R, Marian AJ. Expression profiling of cardiac genes in human hypertrophic cardiomyopathy: insight into the pathogenesis of phenotypes. J Am Coll Cardiol. 2001;38(4):1175–80.
21. Wei BR, Simpson RM, Johann DJ, Dwyer JE, Prieto DA, Kumar M, et al.

Proteomic profiling of H-Ras-G12V induced hypertrophic cardiomyopathy in transgenic mice using comparative LC-MS analysis of thin fresh-frozen tissue sections. J Proteome Res. 2012;11(3):1561–70.

22. Lam L, Tsoutsman T, Arthur J, Semsarian C. Differential protein expression profiling of myocardial tissue in a mouse model of hypertrophic cardiomyopathy. J Mol Cell Cardiol. 2010;48(5):1014–22.

23. Rajan S, Pena JR, Jegga AG, Aronow BJ, Wolska BM, Wieczorek DF. Microarray analysis of active cardiac remodeling genes in a familial hypertrophic cardiomyopathy mouse model rescued by a phospholamban knockout. Physiol Genomics. 2013;45(17):764–73.

24. Gonzalez-Dominguez R, Garcia A, Garcia-Barrera T, Barbas C, Gomez-Ariza JL. Metabolomic profiling of serum in the progression of Alzheimer's disease by capillary electrophoresis-mass spectrometry. Electrophoresis. 2014;35(23):3321–30.

25. Fan Y, Wei C, Xiao W, Zhang W, Wang N, Chuang PY, et al. Temporal profile of the renal transcriptome of HIV-1 transgenic mice during disease progression. PLoS One. 2014;9(3), e93019.

26. Bauer M, Gramlich I, Polzin S, Patzelt D. Quantification of mRNA degradation as possible indicator of postmortem interval–a pilot study. Leg Med. 2003;5(4):220–7.

27. Young ST, Wells JD, Hobbs GR, Bishop CP. Estimating postmortem interval using RNA degradation and morphological changes in tooth pulp. Forensic Sci Int. 2013;229(1–3):163.e1-6.

28. Spizzo R, Almeida MI, Colombatti A, Calin GA. Long non-coding RNAs and cancer: a new frontier of translational research? Oncogene. 2012;31(43):4577–87.

29. Gibb EA, Vucic EA, Enfield KS, Stewart GL, Lonergan KM, Kennett JY, et al. Human cancer long non-coding RNA transcriptomes. PLoS One. 2011;6(10), e25915.

30. Liu Z, Li X, Sun N, Xu Y, Meng Y, Yang C, et al. Microarray profiling and co-expression network analysis of circulating lncRNAs and mRNAs associated with major depressive disorder. PLoS One. 2014;9(3), e93388.

31. Han P, Li W, Lin CH, Yang J, Shang C, Nurnberg ST, et al. A long noncoding RNA protects the heart from pathological hypertrophy. Nature. 2014;514(7520):102–6.

32. Liu J, Wang DZ. An epigenetic "LINK(RNA)" to pathological cardiac hypertrophy. Cell Metab. 2014;20(4):555–7.

33. Gonzalez C, Sims JS, Hornstein N, Mela A, Garcia F, Lei L, et al. Ribosome profiling reveals a cell-type-specific translational landscape in brain tumors. J Neurosci. 2014;34(33):10924–36.

34. Boczonadi V, Horvath R. Mitochondria: impaired mitochondrial translation in human disease. Int J Biochem Cell Biol. 2014;48:77–84.

35. Watson PA, Reusch JE, McCune SA, Leinwand LA, Luckey SW, Konhilas JP, et al. Restoration of CREB function is linked to completion and stabilization of adaptive cardiac hypertrophy in response to exercise. Am J Physiol Heart Circ Physiol. 2007;293(1):H246–59.

5

Elevated expression of periostin in diabetic cardiomyopathy and the effect of valsartan

Jun Guan[1], Wen-Qi Liu[1,2,4], Ming-Qing Xing[3], Yue Shi[2], Xue-Ying Tan[2,4], Chang-Qing Jiang[5] and Hong-Yan Dai[1*]

Abstract

Background: Periostin, an extracellular matrix protein, plays a significant role in adverse cardiac remodeling. However, no report has documented the function of periostin in left ventricular remodeling of streptozototin (STZ)-induced diabetic rats. The aim of the present study was to observe the expression of periostin in Wistar rat's myocardium of diabetic cardiomyopathy (DCM) and the effect of valsartan on it.

Methods: Immunohistochemistry, real-time polymerase chain reaction, and Western blot analysis were used to determine the degree of expression and location of periostin, transforming growth factor (TGF)-β1, TGF-β1 type II receptor (TGF-β1 R II), and Type I and III collagens in the myocardium of STZ-induced diabetic rats.

Results: Periostin, TGF-β1, TGF-β1 R II, and Type I and III collagens were significantly increased in the myocardium of diabetic rats compared with control group on both messenger ribonucleic acid and protein levels. In addition, diabetic rats treated with valsartan could have reduced expression of periostin and improved cardiac remodeling of DCM.

Conclusions: Periostin may play a crucial role in cardiac remodeling and myocardial interstitial fibrosis process of DCM and it could be one of the important mechanisms for valsartan to improve the ventricular remodeling of DCM.

Background

Diabetes mellitus remains a highly prevalent and a vigorous independent risk factor for cardiovascular disease. Recently, an accumulating number of evidence has demonstrated that the presence of abnormal myocardial structure and myocardial dysfunction in patients with diabetes in the absence of epicardial coronary artery disease (CAD), hypertension, and congestive heart failure after adjusting left ventricular hypertrophy [1–3]. This hypothesis was originally recognized in 1972 by Rubler S, who described data from patients with diabetes and heart failure without any evidence of CAD, valvular heart disease, hypertension, or congenital heart disease. This phenomenon has led to the increased recognition of a distinct disease process defined as "diabetic cardiomyopathy" (DCM). Multifactorial mechanisms were thought to be involved in the pathogenesis of DCM. Predominantly, myocardial fibrosis and myocyte hypertrophy are the significant mechanisms to explain the cardiac changes of DCM [4].

Periostin, a 90-KDa secretory protein within the extracellular matrix (ECM), has been derived from studies of bone development wherein it is expressed in both the periodontal ligament and the cortical bone periosteum of adult mice [5]. The association between periostin and myocardium was first reported in the context of mature valves and endocardial cushion development [6]. Recently, numerous studies have described a strong relationship between periostin overexpression and cardiac remodeling in human [7] and rat failing heart or myocardial heart [8–11]. Significantly, periostin is sensitive to transforming growth factor (TGF)-β activation and has emerged to play an important role in collagen fibrillogenesis [12–14]. All of these findings suggest that periostin is an important novel factor in the pathogenesis of cardiovascular disease and in the evolution of cardiac remodeling. Meanwhile in vitro study showed that high glucose increased periostin expression in adult rat cardiac fibroblasts [15]. So it is valuable to elucidate the expression level and possible function of periostin in DCM.

Valsartan, an Angiotensin II (Ang II) receptor blocker, has been reported to protect against diabetic cardiomyopathy [16]. Blockage of Ang II AT1 receptor is thought

* Correspondence: daihy9@163.com
[1]Department of Cardiology, Qingdao Municipal Hospital, Qingdao, Shandong, China
Full list of author information is available at the end of the article

to be the main mechanism of valsartan's protection on cardiac remodeling. But is there any other mechanism involved? In previous studies, it has been demonstrated the existence and activation of a cardiac renin-angiostensin system (RAS) in the hearts in diabetes [17]. Ang II could stimulate the periostin expression in both fibroblasts and cardiac myocytes in vitro, and this increase was inhibited partially, but significantly, by valsartan [11, 18]. Periostin can induce fibroblast proliferation and myofibroblast persistence in vitro [19]. In vivo, valsartan can also significantly attenuate the increased periostin expression, accompanied by improvement of cardiac dysfunction in acute myocardial infarction rat models [11]. But whether periostin takes part in the valsartan-induced protection of DCM is still unknown.

So it is worth clarifying the role of periostin in cardiac remodeling of DCM as no studies yet documented the relation between the periostin and DCM. In the present study, the changes of periostin expressions in cardiac remodeling of DCM and the effects of valsartan on the regulation of periostin expression were examined.

Methods

Induction of diabetes

Male healthy Wister-Albino rats (6-week-old; 180-220 g; n = 60) were purchased from the animal center of Lu-kang corporation. All experimental procedures were performed in accordance with the institutional animal care guidelines. Rats were housed in an air-conditioned room at a constant temperature of 20 ± 2 °C and were fed with a standard diet and water at liberty. Following one week of acclimatization, the rats were assigned randomly to a control group (n = 10) and a diabetic group (n = 50). All rats were weighed, then blood glucose levels were measured initially before the experiment and then weekly once throughout the experiment. Diabetes was induced by a single intraperitoneal injection of streptozotocin (STZ) (60 mg/kg body weight; Sigma, USA) dissolved in 0.1 mmol/L sodium citrate buffer (pH adjusted to 4.2), whereas rats in control group were injected with 0.1 mmol/L citrate buffer alone. All rats were given the same weight of normal (non-high fat and sugar) diet and the same volume of water. Three weeks after the injection of STZ, blood was collected from tail vein and samples were analyzed for blood glucose using a glucometer. Rats with random fasting blood glucose levels greater than 16.7 mmol/L were considered as the distribution criteria of type 1 diabetic rat. In addition, the eligible diabetic rats were randomly assigned to two groups: diabetes group (n = 21) and diabetes plus valsartan group (n = 20). Rats in diabetes plus valsartan group were given valsartan by gavage using a suitable intubation cannula at 30 mg/kg/day dose levels to soluble in 5 mL distilled water, whereas rats in the

diabetes group were administered with the same amount of distilled water each day. No additional treatments were given to control rats.

After 16 weeks, all animals from each group were euthanized using pentobarbital and fresh hearts were harvested immediately. Then, weight of the left ventricle was noted in order to observe the degree of left ventricular hypertrophy. Furthermore, a transversal cross-section block was cut from the left ventricle, soaked in 4 % paraformaldehyde, and remained frozen in liquid nitrogen until mechanical testing.

Hematoxylin eosin (HE) and Masson's trichrome stain of myocardial tissue

After 48 h of treatment with 4 % paraformaldehyde, the tissues were dehydrated and the transparent tissues were embedded in paraffin. The tissues were cut into 6-μm slices, heated at 60 °C for 3 h, dewaxed, and stained with HE and Masson's trichrome dyeing kits. Each slice was analyzed under a microscope at 400× magnification. The collagen volume fraction was determined as the ratio of interstitial collagen area to myocardial area.

Immunohistochemistry

For immunohistochemical analysis, the transversal sections of the left ventricle were cut into 5-μm sections and the endogenous peroxidase activity was quenched by incubation with 3 % hydrogen peroxide for 15 min. The sections were then blocked using 5 % bovine serum albumin to prevent the nonspecific staining with the secondary antibodies. After overnight incubation at 4 °C with primary antibodies (anti-periostin, anti-TGF-β1, anti-TGF-β1 RII, and anti-collagen I and III antibodies were used at 1:100 dilutions), the sections were exposed to the secondary antibody conjugated with horseradish peroxidase. The reaction was visualized using a light microscopy with 3, 3'-diamno-benzidine tetrahydrochloride.

Western blot analysis

Protein fractions were isolated in ice-cold radioimmunoprecipitation assay lysis buffer (Beyotime, China) and protein concentrations were determined using the enhanced bicinchoninic acid protein assay kit (Beyotime, China). Protein fractions were denatured in a loading buffer, and 100 μg of each sample was loaded into alternating lane of 10 % sodium dodecyl sulfate -polyacrylamide gel. Protein blots were transferred to polyvinylidene fluoride membranes (Milipore, USA). After blocking with 5 % non-fat milk, the blots were washed with a mixture of Tris-buffered saline and Tween 20 (TBST) and incubated overnight at 4 °C with an appropriate primary antibody (anti-β-actin, anti-periostin, anti-TGF-β1, anti-TGF-β1 II R, and anti-collagen I and III antibodies were used at 1:1000, 1:500, 1:400, 1:2000, 1:2000, and 1:5000 dilutions, respectively). Membranes were washed with TBST and then incubated at room temperature for 1 h with an appropriate secondary antibody conjugated to horseradish peroxidase and washed again. Finally, the protein blots were visualized using an enhanced chemiluminescence kit (Millipore, USA). Relative intensities of protein bands were measured using Gel-Pro analyzer. β-actin was used as a control.

Real-time polymerase chain reaction (RT-PCR) analysis

The total RNA was extracted from the frozen myocardial tissues using Trizol reagent (Invitrogen, USA), according to the manufacturer's instructions. The concentration of extracted total RNA was quantified using spectrophotometry. The reverse transcription of RNA to complementary deoxyribonucleic acid (cDNA) was performed using Sensiscript RT kit (TaKaRa Biotechnology, China). Total cDNA was amplified with LightCycler-FastStart DNA Master SYBR Green I (TaKaRa Biotechnology, China). Primers for rats periostin, TGF-β1, TGF-β1 R II, Type I collagen, Type III collagen, and β-actin were designed by TaKaRa Biotechnology Corporation: Periostin S: 5'-GGCTGAAGA CTGCCTTGAATGAC-3, A: 5'-CGTGGCAGCACCTTC AAAGA-3'; TGF-β1 S: 5'-AGGTAACGCCAGGAATTGT TGCTA-3, A: 5'-CATTGCTGTCCCGTGCAGA-3'; TGF-β1 R II S: 5'-CTACAAGGCCAAGCTGAAGC-3, A: 5'-A GCCAATGGAAGTAGACATCCG-3'; collagen I S: 5'-AG GGACCCTTAGGCCATTGTGTA-3, A: 5'-GACATGTT CAGCTTTGTGGACCTC-3'; collagen III S: 5'-GACAG ATCCCGAGTCGCAGA-3, A: 5'-TTTGGCACAGCAGT CCAATGTA-3'; and β-actin S: 5'-AGACCTTCAACACC CCAG-3, A: 5'-CACGATTTCCCTCTCAGC-3'. Amplification process included an initial denaturation step of 30s at 95 °C followed by 40 cycles of three-step procedure (denaturation at 95 °C for 5 s, annealing at 60 °C for 30s, and extension at 60 °C for 30s) and then a melting-curve procedure at 60 °C for 1 min. At the end of each cycle, fluorescence emitted by the SYBR Green I dye was measured. For each PCR product, a single narrow peak was obtained through melting curve analysis at a specific melting-curve temperature, indicating specific amplifications. The amount of periostin, TGF-β1, TGF-β1 R II, Type I and Type III collagens, and β-actin transcripts was calculated from their respective standard curves using the Light Cycler software. Samples were tested for three times, and the average values were used for quantification. Ultimately, the relative expression levels of each target gene were normalized to the messenger RNA (mRNA) of the internal standard gene β-actin.

Statistical analysis

All data were expressed as mean ± standard error of the mean. Comparisons between two groups were performed using paired student's t test. One-way analysis of variance was used to compare more than two groups. A value of P less than 0.05 was considered statistically significant.

Results and discussion
General characteristics of the experimental rats

At the end of the experiment, 21 STZ-induced diabetic rats, 20 diabetic rats with valsartan, and 10 control rats were survived, and the rest of 9 diabetic rats were died due to infection. Blood glucose levels were significantly increased in diabetic rats compared with control rats at the end of one week after STZ injection, the difference has statistically significant ($p = 0.0002$). Meanwhile, the glucose levels of diabetic rats were decreased by valsartan treatment at the end of nine weeks, the difference between diabetic group and diabetic plus valsartan have statistically significant ($p = 0.0197$) (see Fig. 1). The STZ-induced diabetic rats were at a diabetic state of polydipsia, polyphagia, and polyuria with lowered body weights.

Degree of left ventricular hypertrophy

Left ventricular coefficient, used to assess the extent of cardiac hypertrophy, which can calculated by comparing the left ventricular weight and body weight [20]. The left ventricular coefficient of diabetic rats was higher than control rats ($p = 0.003$), whereas it was lower in the valsartan-treated diabetic rats than the diabetic rats without valsartan ($p = 0.006$), those differences have statistically significant (see Fig. 2).

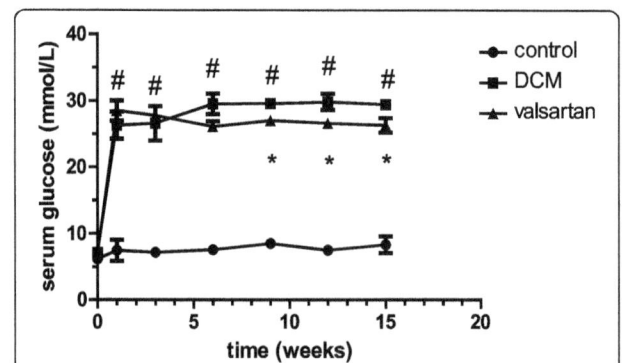

Fig. 1 Serum glucose levels of experimental animals. The first week: control (7.513 ± 1.589) vs DCM (26.534 ± 0.684) #p = 0.0002. The third week: control (7.085 ± 0.527) vs DCM (25.940 ± 0.661) #p = 0.0001. The sixth week: control (7.703 ± 0.454) vs DCM (28.811 ± 0.448) #p = 0.0001. The ninth week: control (9.282 ± 0.167) vs DCM (29.441 ± 0.406) vs valsartan (27.303 ± 0.398) #p = 0.0001,*p = 0.0197. The twelfth week: control (7.948 ± 0.242) vs DCM (29.129 ± 0.591) vs valsartan (26.887 ± 0.832) #p = 0.0001, *p = 0.0332. The fifteenth week: control (8.949 ± 0.579) vs DCM (29.101 ± 0.599) vs valsartan (26.554 ± 0.542) #p = 0.0001, *p = 0.0347

HE and Masson's stains of myocardium

Through light microscope, it was observed that the diabetic rats had increased sizes as well as disordered arrangement of cardiocytes compared with control rats, while the myocardial distribution of valsartan-treated group obviously improved than DCM group. The cardiac collagen deposition was dramatically increased in the diabetic rats than control rats. However, the amount of collagen in valsartan-treated rats was markedly alleviated than diabetic rats (see Fig. 3).

Immunohistochemical analysis

Immunohistochemical analysis revealed that the enhanced staining of periostin occurred in fibroblast, endothelial cells, inflammatory cells, and myocytes in hearts of diabetic rats, whereas little periostin protein expression was found in the control rats. Similarly, weak collagen I and III protein expressions were found in the control rats, whereas the diabetic rats showed strong collagen deposition in hearts. Furthermore, strong TGF-β1 and TGF-β1 R II expressions were also obviously found in diabetic rats; however, there was little or no expression in the control rats. Moreover, in valsartan-treated diabetic group, the expression of periostin, TGF-β1, TGF-β1 R II, and Type I and III collagens were alleviated compared to DCM group (see Fig. 4).

Western blot analysis

The present study results revealed that the expression of periostin was extremely upregulated in DCM rats compared to control rats. And the overexpression of periostin was inhibited by the valsartan treatment. In addition, TGF-β1, TGF-β1 R II, and Type I and III collagens were regarded as a marker reflecting the activation of cardiac fibrosis [21, 22]. All these markers were expressed abundantly in the hearts of diabetic rats compared with control rats, and all these marker expressions were reduced after the valsartan treatment (see Fig. 5).

Myocardial mRNA expression

The RT-PCR analysis revealed that a remarkable increase in periostin mRNA expression in the diabetic rats compared with control rats. In addition, the mRNA expressions in valsartan-treated rats were significantly decreased compared to diabetic rats after 8 weeks. Furthermore, TGF-β1, TGF-β1 R II, and Type I and III collagen mRNA expressions in DCM group were significantly increased compared with control rats. While in valsartan-treated group, the mRNA expressions were decreased compared to the DCM group (see Fig. 6).

Conclusions

The DCM is associated with a significant myocardial remodeling which consists of cardiac hypertrophy, interstitial fibrosis, and changes in the cardiac metabolism [23]. Abundant evidences from experimental models of DCM indicated that the cardiac interstitial fibrosis and cardiac hypertrophy were the pathological substrate features of DCM [24, 25]. In the present study, Wister rats were made severely and chronically diabetic for 16 weeks with a single intraperitoneal injection of STZ (60 mg/kg body weight), and at the end of three weeks after STZ injection, the diabetic group rats were at a state of hyperglycemic, unfortunately, eight rats in diabetic group were died due to diabetic ketoacidosis, infection, fighting each other or digestive complications. In addition, there was one rat, which blood glucose does not meet the model standard, removed. Therefore, preventing acidosis caused by high blood sugar, keeping the environment clean and treating infections as well as other complications to ensure the quality and quantity of rats is very significant in this kind of trials. Moreover, changes in the cellular morphology and structural abnormalities of myocardium were found in the experiment. From HE and Masson's staining of myocardium, it was found that the cardiomyocytes were disorganized with abundant myocardial collagen deposition, accompanied by a markedly increased left ventricular mass index. These salient endings of the present study demonstrated that 16 weeks of hyperglycemia contributes to a successful experimental Type 1 DCM with the development of cardiac hypertrophy and fibrosis.

Previous studies had demonstrated the pathophysiological role of periostin in myocardial fibrosis and cardiac remodeling *in vivo* and *in vitro*. Oka T, et al [26] found mice lacking the gene encoding periostin showed less fibrosis and better ventricular performance after a myocardial infarction, while inducible overexpression of

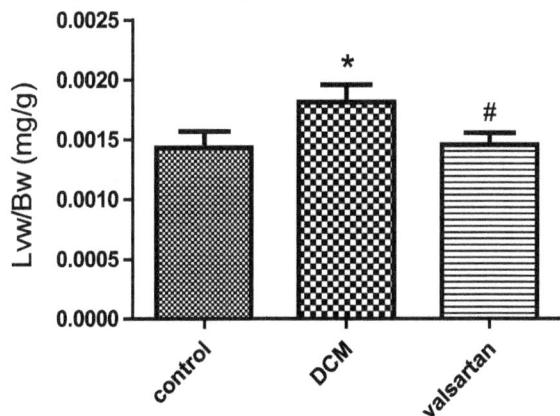

Fig. 2 The degree of left ventricular hypertrophy of experimental animals. Control (1.43 ± 0.08) vs DCM (1.81 ± 0.8) vs valsartan (1.52 ± 0.55) #$p = 0.0295$, *$p = 0.0427$

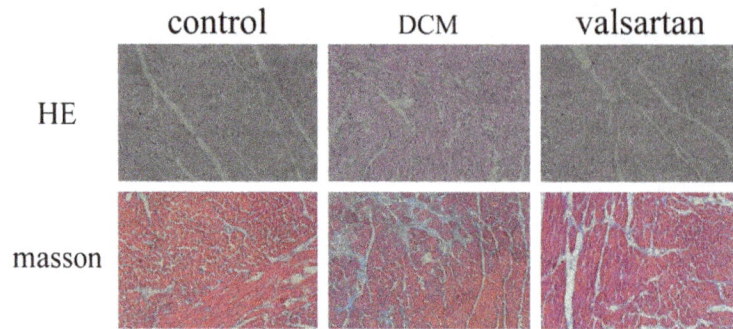

Fig. 3 Hematoxylin and eosin stained (*purple* and *red*) rat's myocardium. The cardiomyocytes size and quantity were increased in DCM rats compared with control rats, whereas it was obviously alleviated in the valsartan-treated diabetic rats than DCM rats (×400). Masson's trichrome staining of rat's myocardium revealed that the collagen deposition was obviously enhanced in the myocardium of diabetic rats than control rats; however, the myocardial fibrosis was markedly decreased in the valsartan-treated rats than DCM rats (×400)

periostin in the heart induced spontaneous hypertrophy with aging. In both animal and human models, periostin is closely associated with pressure overload-induced left ventricular hypertrophy (LVH) and LVH regression [9]. In vitro study found periostin is a profibrogenic matricellular protein that promotes collagen fibrogenesis, inhibits differentiation of progenitor cells into cardiomyocytes [27]. Periostin can also induce fibroblast proliferation and myofibroblast persistence in vitro [28]. In the present study, a high level of mRNA and protein expressions of periostin was found in the hearts of diabetic rats, consistent with the study of Zou P [15]. Periostin expression

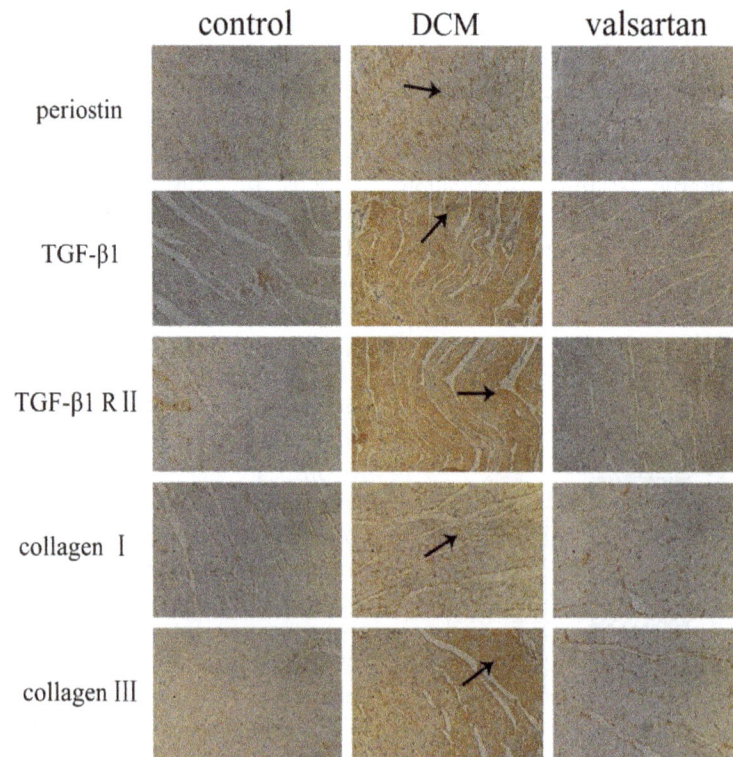

Fig. 4 Immunohistochemical staining of periostin, TGF-β1, TGF-β1 R II, and Type I and III collagens in the control, DCM, and valsartan-treated group. The representative images of *brown* grain deposition showed the localization of the proteins. In contrast to the little or no protein staining in the control rat's myocardium, the DCM rats displayed increased expression of above mentioned proteins in the heart, while the protein expressions were decreased in the valsartan-treated diabetic rats comparted to DCM group (×200)

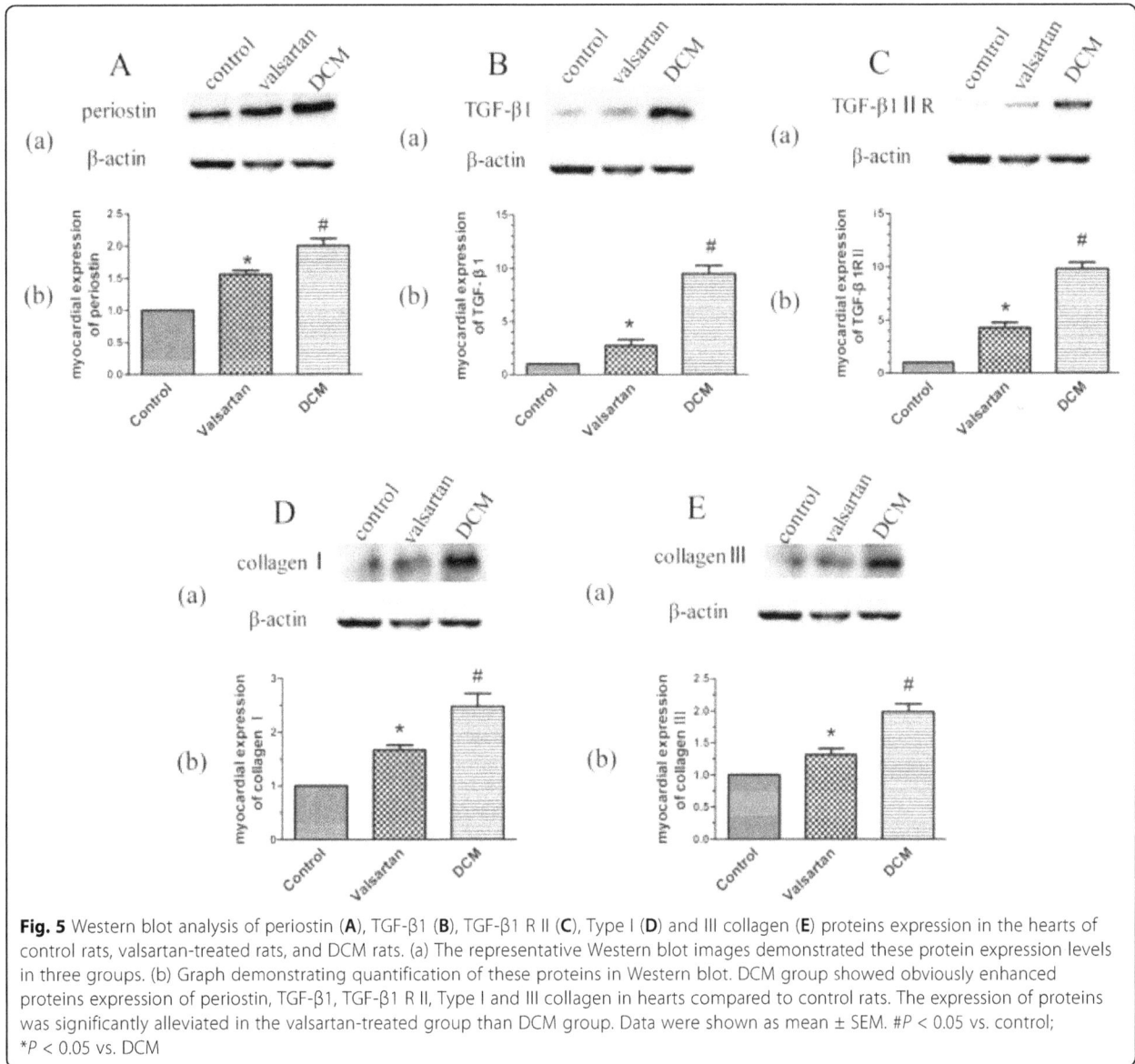

Fig. 5 Western blot analysis of periostin (**A**), TGF-β1 (**B**), TGF-β1 R II (**C**), Type I (**D**) and III collagen (**E**) proteins expression in the hearts of control rats, valsartan-treated rats, and DCM rats. (a) The representative Western blot images demonstrated these protein expression levels in three groups. (b) Graph demonstrating quantification of these proteins in Western blot. DCM group showed obviously enhanced proteins expression of periostin, TGF-β1, TGF-β1 R II, Type I and III collagen in hearts compared to control rats. The expression of proteins was significantly alleviated in the valsartan-treated group than DCM group. Data were shown as mean ± SEM. #$P < 0.05$ vs. control; *$P < 0.05$ vs. DCM

is localized to fibroblast, endothelial cells, inflammatory cells, and myocytes of the damaged heart. These results suggest that periostin might play an important role in the pathogenesis of DCM. Furthermore, in the DCM process, its myocardial cells metabolic disorders include glucose metabolism and lipid metabolism. The carbohydrate oxidation for energy is reduced and the use of lipid oxidation is increased as well as the material for the energy transferred from glucose to fatty acids, so the free fatty acid is elevated caused by lipid metabolism disorders has been widely accepted [29]. In addition, Carley et al [30] have shown that fatty acid, the endogenous ligand of Peroxisome Proliferator Activated Receptors α (PPARα), which uptake and utilization in the regulation of PPARα. Morever, the energy metabolism

signaling pathway of PPARα-FFA in cardiomyocytes may joint with ventricular remodeling, which are important reasons for the pathogenesis of diabetic cardiomyopathy [31]. More study is needed to demonstrate if there is any relationship between FFA-metabolism and periostin on diabetic cardiomyopathy.

Experiment has demonstrated the existence and activation of a cardiac rennin-angiostensin system (RAS) in the hearts in diabetes [17]. In diabetic hearts, both the density and mRNA levels of Ang II receptors are increased [32, 33]. Blockage of RAS by Ang II receptor (AT1R) blockers prevents diabetes-induced heart dysfunction [34]. In our study, varstan, an AT1R antagonist, not only alleviated cardiac remodeling in DCM, but also reduced periostin expression. Together with

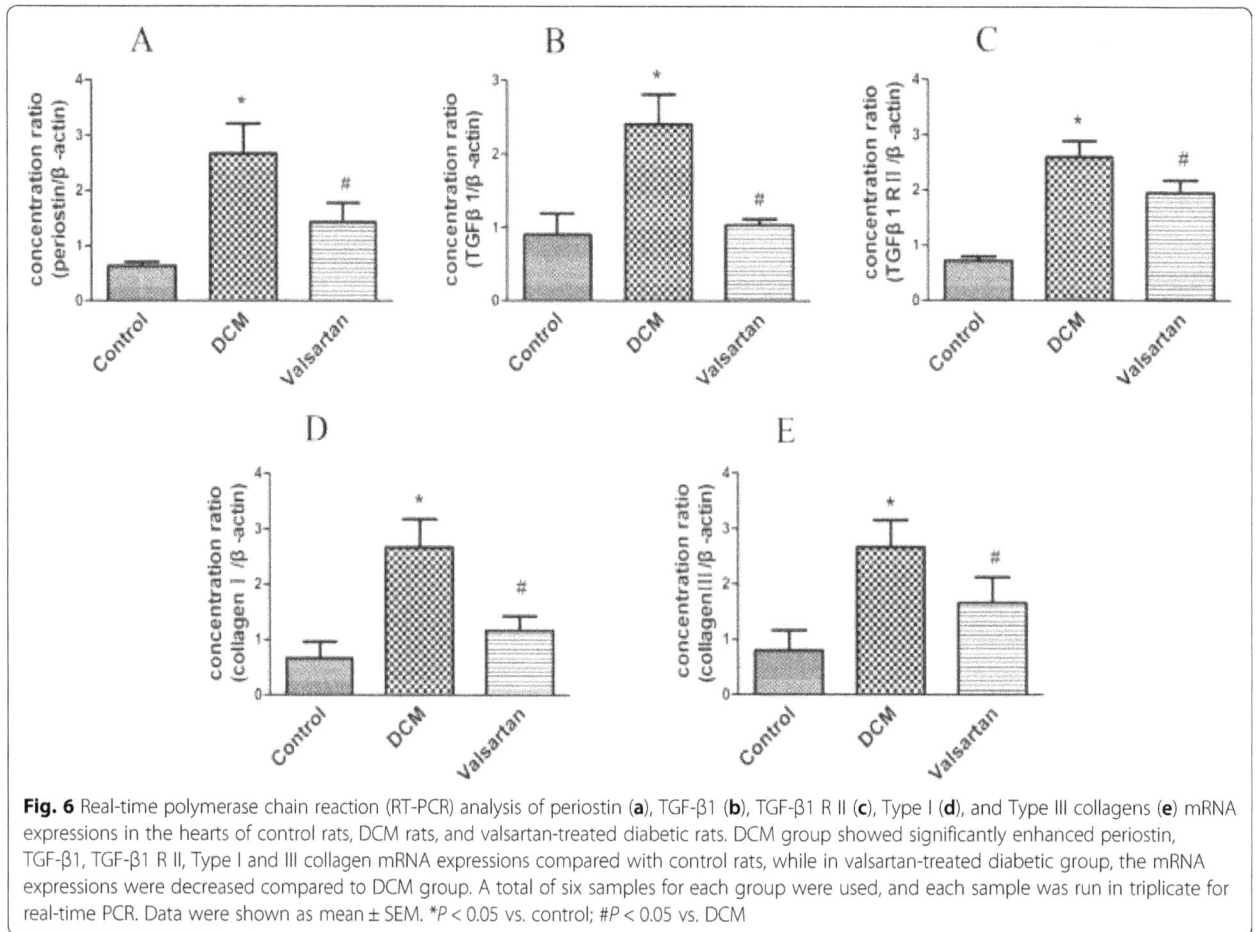

Fig. 6 Real-time polymerase chain reaction (RT-PCR) analysis of periostin (**a**), TGF-β1 (**b**), TGF-β1 R II (**c**), Type I (**d**), and Type III collagens (**e**) mRNA expressions in the hearts of control rats, DCM rats, and valsartan-treated diabetic rats. DCM group showed significantly enhanced periostin, TGF-β1, TGF-β1 R II, Type I and III collagen mRNA expressions compared with control rats, while in valsartan-treated diabetic group, the mRNA expressions were decreased compared to DCM group. A total of six samples for each group were used, and each sample was run in triplicate for real-time PCR. Data were shown as mean ± SEM. *$P < 0.05$ vs. control; #$P < 0.05$ vs. DCM

the knowledge that Ang II could promote the mRNA and protein expression of periostin in vivo and in vitro [11], and periostin has been proved to take part in cardiac remodeling, we can conclude that valsartan could attenuate the cardiac remodeling in the DCM rats partly via down-regulating the expression of periostin. Periostin may become a new therapeutic target for DCM.

In addition, the present study data also revealed that the blood glucose levels of valsartan-treated diabetic rats were improved compared with diabetic rats. This result was accordant with the study of Chan P et al [35], which indicated that valsartan, not only decreased the systolic blood pressure but also improved the glucose utilization.

In conclusion, the present study findings confirmed up-regulated expression of periostin in DCM and provided strong evidence that valsartan protects against the cardiac remodeling in DCM rats which may partly related to the down-regulation of periostin protein, and provides a new insight into the potential therapeutic strategy of cardiac remodeling in DCM.

Abbreviations

STZ: streptozototin; DCM: Diabetic cardiomyopathy; TGF-β1: Transforming growth factor; TGF-β1 R II: TGF-β1 type II receptor; CAD: Coronary artery disease; ECM: extracellular matrix; Ang II: Angiotensin II; RAS: Renin-angiostensin system; HE: Hematoxylin eosin; RT-PCR: Real-time polymerase chain reaction; LVH: Left ventricular hypertrophy.

Competing interests

The authors declare that they have no competing interests.

Authors' contributions

JG, WQL made substantial contributions to conception and design, MQX, YS made acquisition of data, XYT analysis of data, CQJ interpretation of data, WQL be involved in drafting the manuscript, HYD revise the manuscript and give final approval of the version to be published. All authors read and approved the final manuscript.

Acknowledgements

We want to thank Mrs. Mingqing Xing, Mrs Xueying Tan, Mrs. Changqing Jiang, Mrs Xiaoping Wu, Miss Jie Zhang, Mr Hui He for their technical assistance in this research work.

This study was supported by a Project of Qingdao Municipal Science and Technology Commission (Grant No. 13-1-4-140-jch) and National Natural Science Foundation of China (Grant No. 81200175). In addition to, our study is approved by the ethical committee of Qingdao Municipal Hospital.

Author details

[1]Department of Cardiology, Qingdao Municipal Hospital, Qingdao, Shandong, China. [2]Qingdao University Medical College, Qingdao, Shandong,

China. ³Department of Clinical laboratory, Qingdao Municipal Hospital, Qingdao, Shandong, China. ⁴Key Laboratory of cellular transplantation , Chinese Ministry of Public Health, Qingdao Municipal Hospital, Qingdao, Shandong, China. ⁵Department of pathology department, Qingdao Municipal Hospital, Qingdao, Shandong, China.

References

1. Rubler S, Dlugash J, Yuceoglu YZ, Kumral T, Branwood AW, Grishman A. New type of cardiomyopathy associated with diabetic glomerulosclerosis [J]. Am J Cardiol. 1972;30(6):595–602.
2. Aneja A, Tang WH, Bansilal S, Garcia MJ, Farkouh ME. Diabetic cardiomyopathy: insights into pathogenesis, diagnostic challenges, and therapeutic options [J]. Am J Med. 2008;121(9):748–57.
3. Fang ZY, Prins JB, Marwick TH. Diabetic cardiomyopathy: evidence, mechanisms, and therapeutic implications [J]. Endocr Rev. 2004;25(4):543–67.
4. Fischer VW, Barner HB, Larose LS. Pathomorphologic aspects of muscular tissue in diabetes mellitus [J]. Hum Pathol. 1984;15(12):1127–36.
5. Horiuchi K, Amizuka N, Takeshita S, Takamatsu H, Katsuura M, Ozawa H, et al. Identification and characterization of a novel protein, periostin, with restricted expression to periosteum and periodontal ligament and increased expression by transforming growth factor β [J]. J Bone Miner Res. 1999;14(7):1239–49.
6. Kruzynska-Frejtag A, Machnicki M, Rogers R, Markwald RR, Conway SJ. Periostin (an osteoblast-specific factor) is expressed within the embryonic mouse heart during valve formation [J]. Mech Dev. 2001;103(1):183–8.
7. Zhao S, Wu H, Xia W, Chen X, Zhu S, Zhang S, et al. Periostin expression is upregulated and associated with myocardial fibrosis in human failing hearts [J]. J Cardiol. 2014;63(5):373–8.
8. Katsuragi N, Morishita R, Nakamura N, Ochiai T, Taniyama Y, Hasegawa Y, et al. Periostin as a novel factor responsible for ventricular dilation [J]. Circulation. 2004;110(13):1806–13.
9. Stansfield WE, Andersen NM, Tang RH, Selzman CH. Periostin is a novel factor in cardiac remodeling after experimental and clinical unloading of the failing heart [J]. Ann Thorac Surg. 2009;88(6):1916–21.
10. Ladage D, Yaniz-Galende E, Rapti K, Ishikawa K, Tilemann L, Shapiro S, et al. Stimulating myocardial regeneration with periostin Peptide in large mammals improves function post-myocardial infarction but increases myocardial fibrosis [J]. PLoS One. 2013;8(5):e59656.
11. Iekushi K, Taniyama Y, Azuma J, Katsuragi N, Dosaka N, Sanada F, et al. Novel mechanisms of valsartan on the treatment of acute myocardial infarction through inhibition of the antiadhesion molecule periostin [J]. Hypertension. 2007;49(6):1409–14.
12. Conway SJ, Molkentin JD. Periostin as a heterofunctional regulator of cardiac development and disease [J]. Curr Genomics. 2008;9(8):548.
13. Norris RA, Moreno-Rodriguez R, Hoffman S, Markwald RR. The many facets of the matricelluar protein periostin during cardiac development, remodeling, and pathophysiology [J]. Journal of cell communication and signaling. 2009;3(3-4):275–86.
14. Snider P, Standley KN, Wang J, Azhar M, Doetschman T, Conway SJ. Origin of cardiac fibroblasts and the role of periostin [J]. Circ Res. 2009;105(10):934–47.
15. Zou P, Wu LL, Wu D, Fan D, Cui XB, Zhou Y, et al. High glucose increases periostin expression and the related signal pathway in adult rat cardiac fibroblasts [J]. Sheng Li Xue Bao. 2010;62(3):247–54.
16. Yang ZH, Peng XD. Effects of valsartan on diabetic cardiomyopathy in rats with type 2 diabetes mellitus [J]. Chin Med J (Engl). 2010;123(24):3640–3.
17. Fiordaliso F, Li B, Latini R, Sonnenblick EH, Anversa P, Leri A, et al. Myocyte death in streptozotocin-induced diabetes in rats in angiotensin II-dependent [J]. Lab Invest. 2000;80:513–27.
18. Li L, Fan D, Wang C, Wang JY, Cui XB, Wu D, et al. Angiotensin II increases periostin expression via Ras/p38 MAPK/CREB and ERK1/2/TGF-β1 pathways in cardiac fibroblasts [J]. Cardiovasc Res. 2011;91(1):80–9.
19. Crawford J1, Nygard K, Gan BS, O'Gorman DB. Periostin induces fibroblast proliferation and myofibroblast persistence in hypertrophic scarring [J]. Exp Dermatol. 2014 Nov 24. doi:10.1111/exd.12601.
20. Hai-feng ZHANG, Feng WANG, Hong Sun, Mingming Xue. Effects of Pioglitazone on AngII、SOD、NO in Cardiac Hypertrophic Rats [J]. Inner Mongolia Med J. 2013;45(9):1031–3.
21. Westermann D, Walther T, Savvatis K, Escher F, Sobirey M, Riad A, et al. Gene deletion of the kinin receptor B1 attenuates cardiac inflammation and fibrosis during the development of experimental diabetic cardiomyopathy [J]. Diabetes. 2009;58(6):1373–81.
22. Porter KE, Turner NA. Cardiac fibroblasts: at the heart of myocardial remodeling [J]. Pharmacol Ther. 2009;123(2):255–78.
23. Murarka S, Movahed MR. Diabetic cardiomyopathy [J]. J Card Fail. 2010;16(12):971–9.
24. TSCHÖPE C, Walther T, KÖNIGER J, Spillmann F, Westermann D, Escher F, et al. Prevention of cardiac fibrosis and left ventricular dysfunction in diabetic cardiomyopathy in rats by transgenic expression of the human tissue kallikrein gene [J]. FASEB J. 2004;18(7):828–35.
25. Dai HY, Guo XG, Ge ZM, Li ZH, Yu XJ, Tang MX, et al. Elevated expression of urotensin II and its receptor in diabetic cardiomyopathy [J]. J Diabetes Complications. 2008;22(2):137–43.
26. Oka T, Xu J, Kaiser RA, Melendez J, Hambleton M, Sargent MA, et al. Genetic manipulation of periostin expression reveals a role in cardiac hypertrophy and ventricular remodeling [J]. Circ Res. 2007;101(3):313–21.
27. Norris RA, Borg TK, Butcher JT, Baudino TA, Banerjee I, Markwald RR. Neonatal and adult cardiovascular pathophysiological remodeling and repair: developmental role of periostin [J]. Ann N Y Acad Sci. 2008;1123:30–40.
28. Crawford J, Nygard K, Gan BS, O'Gorman DB. Periostin induces fibroblast proliferation and myofibroblast persistence in hypertrophic scarring [J]. Exp Dermatol. 2014 Nov 24. doi:10.1111/exd.12601.
29. Ren J, Davidoff AJ. Diabetes rapidly induces contractile dysfunctionsin isolated ventricular myocytes [J]. Am J Physiol Heart Circ Physiol. 1997;272:148–58.
30. Carley AN, DL S s. Fatty acid metabolism is enhanced in type 2 diabetic hearts [J]. Biochim Biophys Acta JT-Biochimicaet Biophysica Acta. 2005;1734(2):112.
31. Feng Z, Qiutang Z, Bingong L, Shuguo L. The alterations of peroxisome proliferator-activated receptor alpha (PPARα) and free fatty acids in STZ-induced diabetic cardiomyopathy rats [J]. Central China Medical Journal. 2007;31(5):364–6.
32. Khatter JC, Sadri P, Zhang M, Hoeschen RJ. Myocardial angiotensin II (Ang II) receptors in diabetic rats [J]. Ann N Y Acad Sci. 1996;793:466–72.
33. Sechi LA, Griffin CA, Schambelan M. The cardiac renin–angiotensin system in STZ-induced diabetes. Diabetes [J]. 1994;43:1180–4.
34. Kim S, Wanibuchi H, Hamaguchi A, Miura K, Yamanaka S, Iwao H. Angiotensin blockade improves cardiac and renal complications of type II diabetic rats [J]. Hypertension. 1997;30:1054–61.
35. Chan P, Wong KL, Liu IM, Tzeng TF, Yang TL, Cheng JT. Anti-hyperglycemic action of angiotensin II receptor antagonist, valsartan, in streptozotocin-induced diabetic rats [J]. J Hypertens. 2003;21(4):761–9.

6

Recurrent Tako-Tsubo cardiomyopathy (TTC) in a pre-menopausal woman: late sequelae of a traumatic event?

Jochen Hefner[1*], Herbert Csef[1], Stefan Frantz[2,3], Nina Glatter[4] and Bodo Warrings[4]

Abstract

Background: "Tako-Tsubo cardiomyopathy" (TTC) is a syndrome characterized by left ventricular (LV) wall motion abnormalities, usually without coronary artery disease, mimicking the diagnosis of acute coronary syndrome. It most often affects post-menopausal women and TTC tends to run a benign course with very low rates of recurrence, complications or mortality. The condition is also called "stress-induced cardiomyopathy" because acute physical or emotional stress appears to be frequently related to its onset. The pathogenic role of premorbid or comorbid psychiatric illnesses has been discussed controversially. For the first time, we present a case of fourfold recurrent TTC with severe complications in a pre-menopausal woman. Furthermore, a long history of flaring posttraumatic stress symptoms anteceded the first event.

Case presentation: A 43-year old, pre-menopausal Caucasian woman was hospitalized with symptoms of acute coronary syndrome. Clinical examination revealed hypokinetic wall motion in the apical ventricular region with no signs of coronary artery disease and diagnosis of TTC was established. She experienced recurrence three times within the following ten months, which led to thrombembolism and myocardial scarring among others. The circumstances of chronic distress were striking. 16 years ago she miscarried after having removed a myoma according to her doctor's suggestion. Since then, she has suffered from symptoms of posttraumatic distress which peaked annually at the day of abortion. Chronic distress became even more pronounced after the premature birth of a daughter some years later. The first event of TTC occurred after a family dispute about parenting.

Conclusion: This is the first case report of fourfold TTC in a pre-menopausal woman. From somatic perspectives, the course of the disease with recurrences and complications underlines the fact that TTC is not entirely benign. Furthermore, it is the first case report of long lasting symptoms of traumatic stress anteceding TTC. Close connections between adrenergic signaling and late onset of clinical stress symptoms are well known in the psychopathology of traumatization. Although larger clinical trials are needed to elucidate possible interactions of premorbid psychiatric illnesses and TTC, cardiologists should be vigilant especially in cases of recurrent TTC.

Keywords: Recurrent Tako-Tsubo cardiomyopathy, Chronic distress, Gene-environment interaction, Comprehensive psychosomatic assessment

Background

Tako-Tsubo cardiomyopathy is a syndrome first described by Sato et al. in 1991 [1] consisting of transient wall motion abnormalities most often involving the apical ventricle. Abnormalities of the electrocardiogram (ECG) and myocardial enzyme release may mimic acute coronary

syndrome (ACS) in the angiographic absence of coronary artery disease [2]. The estimated prevalence is 2.5% in patients with ACS and post-menopausal women are most often affected [2,3]. Usually, TTC subsides rapidly without somatic complications [4]. But a growing number of recent reports demonstrate that TTC is not entirely benign [5,6]. For example, prolongation of the QT-interval is a well known finding in patients with acute TTC [7]. In a subgroup of patients, the severe prolongation of the QT-interval (QTc > 500 ms) may be a marker for the risk of sudden death [7]. Furthermore, in patients with pre-

* Correspondence: hefner_j@ukw.de
[1]Section of Psychosomatic Medicine and Psychotherapy, Department of Internal Medicine II, Julius-Maximilian-University of Wuerzburg, Oberduerrbacher Str. 6, D- 97080 Wuerzburg, Germany
Full list of author information is available at the end of the article

existing long QT syndrome or concomitant psychiatric diseases and respective medication, TTC may lead to lethal arrhythmias [8]. The in-hospital mortality rate is 1.1% and incidence of recurrence is recently reported to be 2.9 – 10% [4,9,10]. Left ventricular thrombus occurs in about 5% of patients, 1.6% suffer from nonfatal cardioembolic outcomes [11]. In a subgroup of patients, cardiac MRI late enhancement may be present and last over time [12]. Late enhancement consistent with myocardial scarring has been reported sporadically and scars were not associated with adverse long term outcomes [5,13]. The exact pathomechanisms of TTC have not been elucidated [14,15]. Five different etiological mechanisms of TTC are discussed [16]. There is evidence for (1) multi-vessel epicardial spasms [17], (2) microcirculatory dysfunction [18], (3) obstruction of the left ventricular outflow [19] and (4) endocrine effects like increased vulnerability of postmenopausal women to hormonal and sympathetic stimuli [20]. Most pathophysiological models point to (5) elevated catecholamine levels in TTC patients which are higher compared to patients with myocardial infarction of corresponding Killip classes [21]. In latest reports, a hypothetical association of concurrent sympathetic over activity and vagal withdrawal has been proposed [22]. As acute episodes of physical or mental stress antecede an event in 7 out of 10 cases, stress induced peaks of catecholamine levels acting on differently localized and sensitized adrenergic receptors are thought of setting off an event [2,23-27]. In several recent reports, a high prevalence of anxiety and depression (21 – 66%) has been found in TTC patients [28-32]. Furthermore, anxiety and depression show effects on catecholamine metabolism. For example, levels of systemic and cardiac catecholamines are elevated and noradrenaline reuptake is reduced in depressed patients [33]. Additionally, noradrenaline responses to emotional stress are correlated with the extent of depressive symptoms [34]. In patients with panic disorders, epinephrine is released from the heart at rest and during spontaneous attacks [35]. Due to a norepinephrine transporter impairment, patients with panic disorder show a reduced uptake of nor-/epinephrine during transit to the heart [36,37]. In sum, the high prevalence of psychological illnesses in TTC patients led to the assumption that psychosocial stress concomitant with abnormalities in catecholamine signaling may be a risk factor whereas acute physical or emotional stress may ultimately trigger the event [28,30-32,38-40]. But the key question of cause and effect of psychiatric disorders in the context of TTC remains. Most of the studies could not determine the timeline of psychiatric disorders, and it may well be that the circumstances after the onset of TTC led to psychiatric comorbidity. In an unprecedented study, a high prevalence (56%) of chronic anxiety disorder anteceding TTC has been reported [32]. The authors

hypothesized that premorbid chronic psychiatric conditions may not only be risk factors for TTC but also for recurrences [32].

There is very little documentation of posttraumatic stress disorder (PTSD) in the context of TTC are very rare. At the same time, stressful events antecede the first onset of PTSD and symptoms are often chronic (>90%) and unremitting (>30%) [41]. Hyperarousal is one major clinical sign and the condition is closely linked to neuroendocrine alterations [42,43]. To our knowledge, there is only one case report of TTC in a postmenopausal patient with a 5 year history of PTSD [44]. The patient recovered fully and there was no report of recurrences or complications [44]. We present a unique case of recurrent TTC with complications in a pre-menopausal woman. Furthermore, it is the first description of chronic symptoms of posttraumatic stress peaking right before the first onset of TTC.

Case presentation

A 43 year-old Caucasian woman with a history of hypertension and nicotine abuse was hospitalized with acute onset of chest pain, nausea, and dizziness. Shortly before, she had a vigorous argument with her partner about child education. In the course of the altercation, she was accused to be "a bad mother". The patient was overwhelmed by the allegations that instantly lead to perceptions of tension, fear and derealisation. At the hospital she appeared anxious with a blood pressure of 168/78 mmHg, a pulse of 78 bpm, shallow breathing and oxygen saturation of 96%. The physical exam and a chest x-ray showed normal findings. Tentative diagnosis was non-STEMI myocardial infarction as ECG was normal and Troponin T levels rose to 0.22 ng/ml. A coronary angiogram revealed no obstructive coronary artery disease or plaque rupture. A left ventriculography demonstrated hypokinetic apical, diaphragmal, and posterobasal segments (Figure 1). The diagnosis of Tako-Tsubo cardiomyopathy (TTC) was established and medication with beta blocker, ACE inhibitor, and aspirin was initiated. An echocardiography five days later showed normal wall movement and an ejection fraction of 72% on echocardiography. The patient was discharged after declining psycho-somatic support.

Six months later, weekly recurrent chest pain increased dramatically while reading a newspaper. Following hospitalization, all results of an examination were very similar to the first event and the diagnosis of recurrent TTC was established.

Nine months after the first cardiac event the patient was admitted to the emergency ward again after dyspnoea, chest pain, nausea, and vertigo had increased for several days. This time, the physical exam revealed rales in the right lung field. ECG showed T-wave inversions in leads V2-V3 (Figure 2), and Troponin T levels were at 0.14 ng/ml. Echocardiography demonstrated normal left

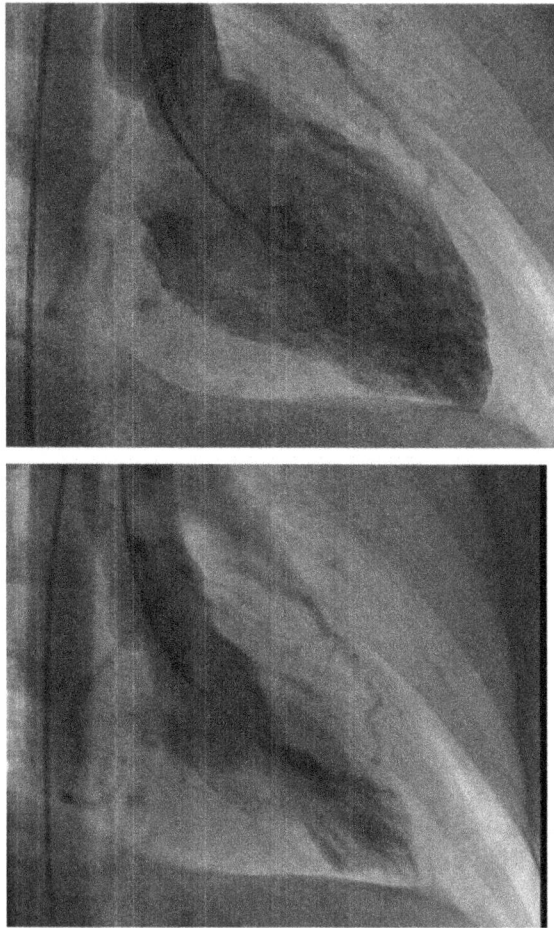

Figure 1 Left ventriculogram with hypokinetic segments (apical, diaphragmal, and posterobasal) indicative of Tako-Tsubo Cardiomyopathy at first admission to the hospital (upper: diastole; lower: systole).

ventricle function (LVEF > 55%), akinesia of apical segments (septal, lateral, anterior, inferior), and a thrombus of 19 × 11 mm in the left ventricle. Despite administering an anticoagulant, thrombembolism to the right lower leg occurred and had to be surgically removed. After normalized echocardiographic and angiographic results, the patient was discharged a few days later. The last event of TTC emerged another four weeks later. The patient suffered from dyspnoea and pain of the chest and both arms. Physical examination was normal, ECG showed ST depression in leads V2-V4, Troponin T level was 0.06 ng/ml. Cardio-MRI revealed normal left ventricular function (LVEF = 70%) and hypokinetic wall movement of apical and lateral segments. Nonischemic patchy late enhancement was present in the apical, apical inferior septal and lateral regions. A month later late enhancement demonstrated inhomogeneous, inferior-apical transmural scar tissue

(Figure 3) which did not change significantly at another follow-up after 9 months. During the fourth event and due to a depressive syndrome, psychosomatic support was once again recommended. This time the patient agreed and for the first time, an antidepressant was administered. Because of latest reports of TTC associated with the use of serotonine and noradrenaline reuptake inhibitors, we selected Mirtazapine in order to avoid increased plasma catecholamine concentrations [45-47]. The psychosomatic history revealed several chronic stress factors. At the age of 27, the patient was pregnant (gestational age 14 weeks) and was advised to undergo surgery of the uterus due to a fast growing myoma. 4 months later fetal death was diagnosed and the pregnancy had to be interrupted shortly before calculated date of birth. This was experienced as a traumatic event by the patient. Since then, she suffered from recurrent solitary symptoms indicative of post traumatic stress disorder (occasional flashbacks, hyperarousal) which did not qualify for a diagnosis of PTSD according to diagnostic manuals. Additionally she described a prolonged grief reaction with rumination about the loss of her child, peaking annually in the month of the fetal death. Three years later, the patient gave birth to a healthy premature child. The patient experienced the incident as a distressing life-event as well and felt chronically concerned about her daughter. Therefore, final diagnoses were recurrent TTC, a chronic posttraumatic stress syndrome with solitary symptoms of PTSD, and a prolonged grief disorder with depressive anniversary reactions.

Conclusion

Recurrent TTC in pre-menopausal women is very unusual. On the somatic level, a total of four episodes with distinct complications like thromboembolism and scarring of the left ventricle are among the unique peculiarities of this case. Especially the last finding may challenge the diagnosis of TTC. But from our perspective, all symptoms point to unidentified pathomechanisms and to a broader clinical spectrum of TTC [5,13,14,48]. The chronic mental distress of our patient is another remarkable feature of our case. Retrospectively, she suffered from solitary posttraumatic symptoms accompanied by depressive anniversary reactions since the stillbirth 16 years ago. The first event of TTC occurred right after an intense argument about parenting. The psycho-somatic connections underlying TTC are far from clear [14,15,39]. In a case study published recently in this journal, Waldenborg et al. even proposed to avoid terms as "stress-induced cardiomyopathy" or "broken heart syndrome" for TTC [49]. They detected symptoms of acute posttraumatic stress in 9 out of 13 (69%) TTC patients (2 patients qualified for

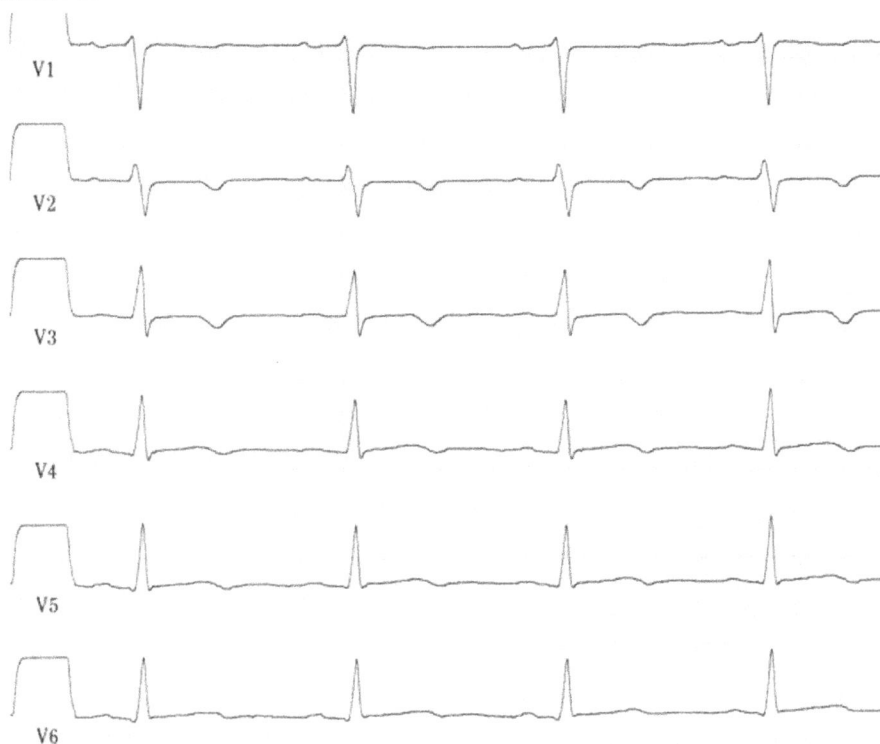

Figure 2 Electrocardiogram showing T-wave inversions in leads V2-V3 during the second event of Tako-Tsubo cardiomyopathy.

having PTSD) and similar numbers of acute distress can be found in patients with acute myocardial infarction [49]. From our point of view, it needs to be taken into account that only one patient had a history of mental illness (manic-depressive disorder), symptoms of borderline or definite PTSD were absent before TTC and recurrences were not reported in a 3 month follow-up [49]. We are aware that the literature on TTC mainly consists of case reports and hypotheses about new pathomechanisms are therefore prone to valid objection. But in line with other researchers we believe that chronic distress may act as a risk factor of TTC and recurrences [32]. Specifically in PTSD, close interactions between trauma and adrenergic signaling do exist [41]. Even on the genetic level, traumatic events may lead to subthreshold endocrine modifications [50,51]. They in turn may facilitate repeating adrenergic surges many years later [50,51], even with recurrent cardiac consequences in pre-menopausal women. Despite the practical difficulties, prospective and much larger clinical trials are needed in order to test for these hypotheses. But we believe that already clinicians should be aware of possible connections to long preceding distress or traumatic events especially in cases of recurrent TTC.

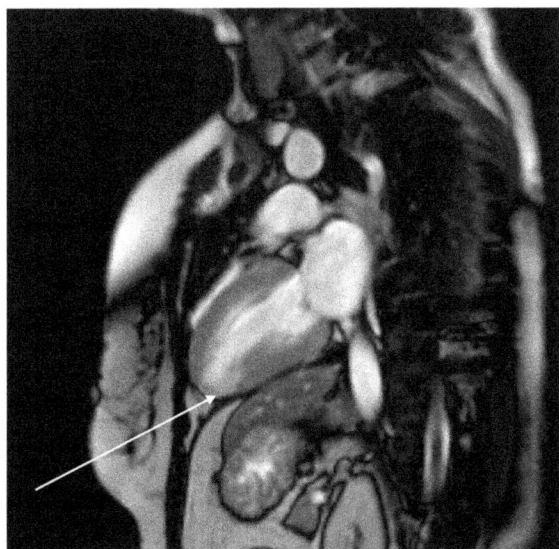

Figure 3 Cardiac magnetic resonance imaging after fourth event of TTC: transmural scar tissue (inferior apical; white arrow).

Consent

Written informed consent was obtained from the patient for publication of this case report and any accompanying images. A copy of the written consent is available for review by the Editor of this journal.

Competing interests
The authors declare that they have no competing interests.

Authors' contributions
JH, SF, NG and BW gathered patient data. HC, SF, NG and BW treated the patient. All authors contributed to the conception of the report. JH wrote the report and HC, SF, NG and BW assisted with critical revision. All authors gave their final acceptance to the submission of this report. All authors read and approved the final manuscript.

Author details
¹Section of Psychosomatic Medicine and Psychotherapy, Department of Internal Medicine II, Julius-Maximilian-University of Wuerzburg, Oberduerrbacher Str. 6, D- 97080 Wuerzburg, Germany. ²Unit of Cardiology, Department of Internal Medicine I, Julius-Maximilian-University of Wuerzburg, Wuerzburg, Germany. ³Comprehensive Heart Failure Center, Julius-Maximilian-University of Wuerzburg, Wuerzburg, Germany. ⁴Department of Psychiatry, Psychosomatics and Psychotherapy, Julius-Maximilian-University of Wuerzburg, Wuerzburg, Germany.

References

1. Sato H, Tateishi H, Uchida T, Dote K, Ishihara M. Stunned Myocardium with specific (tsubo-type) Left Ventriculographic Configuration due to Multivessel Spasm. In: Kodama K, Haze K, Hori M, editors. Clinical Aspects of Myocardial Injury: From Ischemia to Heart Failure. Tokyo: Kagakuhyouronsya Co; 1990. p. 56–64.
2. Bossone E, Savarese G, Ferrara F, Citro R, Mosca S, Musella F, et al. Takotsubo cardiomyopathy: overview. Heart Fail Clin. 2013;9:249–66.
3. Mansencal N, Auvert B, N'Guetta R, Esteve JB, Zarca K, Perrot S, et al. Prospective assessment of incidence of Tako-Tsubo cardiomyopathy in a very large urban agglomeration. Int J Cardiol. 2013;168:2791–5.
4. Gianni M, Dentali F, Grandi AM, Sumner G, Hiralal R, Lonn E. Apical ballooning syndrome or takotsubo cardiomyopathy: a systematic review. Eur Heart J. 2006;27:1523–9.
5. Sharkey SW, Windenburg DC, Lesser JR, Maron MS, Hauser RG, Lesser JN, et al. Natural history and expansive clinical profile of stress (tako-tsubo) cardiomyopathy. J Am Coll Cardiol. 2010;55:333–41.
6. Singh K, Carson K, Usmani Z, Sawhney G, Shah R, Horowitz J. Systematic review and meta-analysis of incidence and correlates of recurrence of takotsubo cardiomyopathy. Int J Cardiol. 2014;174:696–701.
7. Behr ER, Mahida S. Takotsubo cardiomyopathy and the long-QT syndrome: an insult to repolarization reserve. Europace. 2009;11:697–700.
8. Rotondi F, Manganelli F, Lanzillo T, Candelmo F, Lorenzo ED, Marino L, et al. Tako-tsubo cardiomyopathy complicated by recurrent torsade de pointes in a patient with anorexia nervosa. Intern Med. 2010;49:1133–7.
9. Elesber AA, Prasad A, Lennon RJ, Wright RS, Lerman A, Rihal CS. Four-year recurrence rate and prognosis of the apical ballooning syndrome. J Am Coll Cardiol. 2007;50:448–52.
10. Summers MR, Prasad A. Takotsubo cardiomyopathy: definition and clinical profile. Heart Fail Clin. 2013;9:111–22.
11. de Gregorio C. Cardioembolic outcomes in stress-related cardiomyopathy complicated by ventricular thrombus: a systematic review of 26 clinical studies. Int J Cardiol. 2010;141:11–7.
12. Naruse Y, Sato A, Kasahara K, Makino K, Sano M, Takeuchi Y, et al. The clinical impact of late gadolinium enhancement in Takotsubo cardiomyopathy: serial analysis of cardiovascular magnetic resonance images. J Cardiovasc Magn Reson. 2011;13:67.
13. Bellera MN, Ortiz JT, Caralt MT, Perez-Rodon J, Mercader J, Fernandez-Gomez C, et al. Magnetic resonance reveals long-term sequelae of apical ballooning syndrome. Int J Cardiol. 2010;139:25–31.
14. Ghadri JR, Ruschitzka F, Luscher TF, Templin C. Takotsubo cardiomyopathy: still much more to learn. Heart. 2014;100:1804–12.
15. Tranter MH, Wright PT, Sikkel MB, Lyon AR. Takotsubo cardiomyopathy: the pathophysiology. Heart Fail Clin. 2013;9:187–96.
16. Maldonado JR, Pajouhi P, Witteles R. Broken heart syndrome (Takotsubo cardiomyopathy) triggered by acute mania: a review and case report. Psychosomatics. 2013;54:74–9.
17. Pilgrim TM, Wyss TR. Takotsubo cardiomyopathy or transient left ventricular apical ballooning syndrome: A systematic review. Int J Cardiol. 2008;124:283–92.
18. Bybee KA, Prasad A, Barsness GW, Lerman A, Jaffe AS, Murphy JG, et al. Clinical characteristics and thrombolysis in myocardial infarction frame counts in women with transient left ventricular apical ballooning syndrome. Am J Cardiol. 2004;94:343–6.
19. El Mahmoud R, Mansencal N, Pilliere R, Leyer F, Abbou N, Michaud P, et al. Prevalence and characteristics of left ventricular outflow tract obstruction in Tako-Tsubo syndrome. Am Heart J. 2008;156:543–8.
20. Ueyama T, Kasamatsu K, Hano T, Tsuruo Y, Ishikura F. Catecholamines and estrogen are involved in the pathogenesis of emotional stress-induced acute heart attack. Ann N Y Acad Sci. 2008;1148:479–85.
21. Wittstein IS, Thiemann DR, Lima JA, Baughman KL, Schulman SP, Gerstenblith G, et al. Neurohumoral features of myocardial stunning due to sudden emotional stress. N Engl J Med. 2005;352:539–48.
22. Mohammad M, Patel AK, Koirala A, Asirvatham SJ. Tako-tsubo cardiomyopathy following colonoscopy: insights on pathogenesis. Int J Cardiol. 2011;147:e46–49.
23. Nef HM, Mollmann H, Hilpert P, Masseli F, Kostin S, Troidl C, et al. Sympathoadrenergic overstimulation in Tako-Tsubo cardiomyopathy triggered by physical and emotional stress. Int J Cardiol. 2008;130:266–8.
24. Bybee KA, Kara T, Prasad A, Lerman A, Barsness GW, Wright RS, et al. Systematic review: transient left ventricular apical ballooning: a syndrome that mimics ST-segment elevation myocardial infarction. Ann Intern Med. 2004;141:858–65.
25. Akashi YJ, Musha H, Kida K, Itoh K, Inoue K, Kawasaki K, et al. Reversible ventricular dysfunction takotsubo cardiomyopathy. Eur J Heart Fail. 2005;7:1171–6.
26. Eitel I, von Knobelsdorff-Brenkenhoff F, Bernhardt P, Carbone I, Muellerleile K, Aldrovandi A, et al. Clinical characteristics and cardiovascular magnetic resonance findings in stress (takotsubo) cardiomyopathy. JAMA. 2011;306:277–86.
27. Tsuchihashi K, Ueshima K, Uchida T, Oh-mura N, Kimura K, Owa M, et al. Transient left ventricular apical ballooning without coronary artery stenosis: a novel heart syndrome mimicking acute myocardial infarction. Angina Pectoris-Myocardial Infarction Investigations in Japan. J Am Coll Cardiol. 2001;38:11–8.
28. Mudd JO, Kass DA. Reversing chronic remodeling in heart failure. Expert Rev Cardiovasc Ther. 2007;5:585–98.
29. Regnante RA, Zuzek RW, Weinsier SB, Latif SR, Linsky RA, Ahmed HN, et al. Clinical characteristics and four-year outcomes of patients in the Rhode Island Takotsubo Cardiomyopathy Registry. Am J Cardiol. 2009;103:1015–9.
30. Vidi V, Rajesh V, Singh PP, Mukherjee JT, Lago RM, Venesy DM, et al. Clinical characteristics of tako-tsubo cardiomyopathy. Am J Cardiol. 2009;104:578–82.
31. Nguyen SB, Nugent K, Otahbachi M, Roonsritong C, Kumar A, Meyerrose G, et al. Transient left ventricular apical ballooning syndrome. J Invest Med. 2007;55:S256.
32. Summers MR, Lennon RJ, Prasad A. Pre-morbid psychiatric and cardiovascular diseases in apical ballooning syndrome (tako-tsubo/stress-induced cardiomyopathy): potential pre-disposing factors? J Am Coll Cardiol. 2010;55:700–1.
33. Barton DA, Dawood T, Lambert EA, Esler MD, Haikerwal D, Brenchley C, et al. Sympathetic activity in major depressive disorder: identifying those at increased cardiac risk? J Hypertens. 2007;25:2117–24.
34. Mausbach BT, Dimsdale JE, Ziegler MG, Mills PJ, Ancoli-Israel S, Patterson TL, et al. Depressive symptoms predict norepinephrine response to a psychological stressor task in Alzheimer's caregivers. Psychosom Med. 2005;67:638–42.
35. Wilkinson DJ, Thompson JM, Lambert GW, Jennings GL, Schwarz RG, Jefferys D, et al. Sympathetic activity in patients with panic disorder at rest, under laboratory mental stress, and during panic attacks. Arch Gen Psychiatry. 1998;55:511–20.
36. Alvarenga ME, Richards JC, Lambert G, Esler MD. Psychophysiological mechanisms in panic disorder: a correlative analysis of noradrenaline spillover, neuronal noradrenaline reuptake, power spectral analysis of heart rate variability, and psychological variables. Psychosom Med. 2006;68:8–16.
37. Shioiri T, Kojima-Maruyama M, Hosoki T, Kitamura H, Tanaka A, Yoshizawa M, et al. Dysfunctional baroreflex regulation of sympathetic nerve activity in remitted patients with panic disorder. A new methodological approach. Eur Arch Psychiatry Clin Neurosci. 2005;255:293–8.
38. Nguyen SB, Cevik C, Otahbachi M, Kumar A, Jenkins LA, Nugent K. Do comorbid psychiatric disorders contribute to the pathogenesis of tako-tsubo syndrome? A review of pathogenesis. Congest Heart Fail. 2009;15:31–4.
39. Goldfinger JZ, Nair A, Sealove BA. Brain-heart interaction in takotsubo cardiomyopathy. Heart Fail Clin. 2013;9:217–23.

Recurrent Tako-Tsubo cardiomyopathy (TTC) in a pre-menopausal woman: late sequelae of a traumatic...

51

40. Ziegelstein RC. Depression and tako-tsubo cardiomyopathy. Am J Cardiol. 2010;105:281–2.

41. Schnurr PP, Friedman MJ, Bernardy NC. Research on posttraumatic stress disorder: epidemiology, pathophysiology, and assessment. J Clin Psychol. 2002;58:877–89.

42. Gamo NJ, Arnsten AF. Molecular modulation of prefrontal cortex: rational development of treatments for psychiatric disorders. Behav Neurosci. 2011;125:282–96.

43. Yehuda R. Advances in understanding neuroendocrine alterations in PTSD and their therapeutic implications. Ann N Y Acad Sci. 2006;1071:137–66.

44. Primus C, Auer J. Atypical "mid-ventricular" Tako-tsubo cardiomyopathy in a patient suffering from posttraumatic stress disorder: A case report. Wien Klin Wochenschr. 2011;123:562–5.

45. Christoph M, Ebner B, Stolte D, Ibrahim K, Kolschmann S, Strasser RH, et al. Broken heart syndrome: Tako Tsubo cardiomyopathy associated with an overdose of the serotonin-norepinephrine reuptake inhibitor Venlafaxine. Eur Neuropsychopharmacol. 2010;20:594–7.

46. Rotondi F, Manganelli F, Carbone G, Stanco G. "Tako-tsubo" cardiomyopathy and duloxetine use. South Med J. 2011;104:345–7.

47. Neil CJ, Chong CR, Nguyen TH, Horowitz JD. Occurrence of Tako-Tsubo cardiomyopathy in association with ingestion of serotonin/noradrenaline reuptake inhibitors. Heart Lung Circ. 2012;21:203–5.

48. Pelliccia F, Greco C, Vitale C, Rosano G, Gaudio C, Kaski JC. Takotsubo Syndrome (Stress Cardiomyopathy): An Intriguing Clinical Condition in Search of Its Identity. Am J Med. 2014;127:699–704.

49. Waldenborg M, Soholat M, Kahari A, Emilsson K, Frobert O. Multidisciplinary assessment of tako tsubo cardiomyopathy: a prospective case study. BMC Cardiovasc Disord. 2011;11:14.

50. McGowan PO. Epigenomic mechanisms of early adversity and HPA dysfunction: considerations for PTSD Research. Front Psychiatry. 2013;4:110.

51. Mehta D, Binder EB. Gene x environment vulnerability factors for PTSD: the HPA-axis. Neuropharmacology. 2012;62:654–62.

7

Neuroticism, depression and anxiety in takotsubo cardiomyopathy

Thomas Emil Christensen[1,2*], Lia E. Bang[1], Lene Holmvang[1], Philip Hasbak[2], Andreas Kjær[2], Per Bech[3] and Søren Dinesen Østergaard[4,5]

Abstract

Background: Takotsubo cardiomypathy (TTC) causes acute reversible heart failure. Prior studies have indicated that the syndrome is associated with traits such as social inhibition, chronic psychological stress, and anxio-depressive disorders. The objective of this study was to further characterize key psychological/psychopathological traits of patients with TTC.

Methods: A survey of three groups was conducted: I) Female post-recovery TTC patients admitted between October 1st 2009 and December 10th 2014, II) Age, gender and geographically matched ST-elevation myocardial infarction (STEMI) patients, and III) Age, gender and geographically matched individuals from the background population. The following questionnaires were used in the survey: the WHO-5 Well-Being Index, Eysenck's Neuroticism Scale, the Major Depression Inventory, and the anxiety subscale of Symptoms Checklist (SCL-90).

Results: In total, 173 of 230 invitees (75 %) participated in the study. In comparison to the background controls, TTC patients reported significantly less well-being, more neuroticism, more depression, and more anxiety. The levels of well-being, depression and neuroticism were comparable between TTC and STEMI patients, but the level of anxiety was higher in the TTC patients. There was a negative correlation between the time since TTC admission and the total scores on the psychopathology rating scales.

Conclusions: Patients with TTC reported significantly higher anxiety levels compared to both STEMI patients and background controls. However, unlike the STEMI patients, the TTC patients appeared to improve psychologically during the post-recovery phase. This may be a consolation for TTC patients in acute psychological distress.

Keywords: Takotsubo cardiomyopathy, Well-being, Neuroticism, Depression, Anxiety

Background

Takotsubo cardiomypathy (TTC) is an increasingly recognized cause of acute heart failure mainly affecting elderly females [1]. The onset of TTC is often preceded by an emotional stressor [2], and catecholamine induced cardiomyopathy has been suggested as the underlying cause [3, 4]. TTC patients typically have elevated cardiac biomarkers, electrocardiographic abnormalities including ST-elevations, but absence of a coronary culprit lesion on angiography. Left ventricle contractility is abnormal with characteristic akinesia of the apical-midventricular segments, and basal normo- or hyperkinesia ('apical ballooning') [5]. Complete remission usually occurs within 1 month [6] and it was previously thought that TTC patients had an excellent prognosis. However, recent reports indicate a poor outcome similar to myocardial infarction [7].

It is well established that affective disorders constitute an independent risk factor for cardiovascular disease [8]. In the case of TTC, studies indicate that the syndrome is linked to psychopathological traits such as social inhibition, chronic psychological stress, and anxio-depressive disorders [9–12]. However, most studies have been conducted within a few months of initial admission, and thus recent life events related to the onset of TTC may have confounded the results. Therefore, the

* Correspondence: thomas.emil.christensen@regionh.dk
[1]Department of Cardiology, Copenhagen University Hospital, Rigshospitalet, Copenhagen, Denmark
[2]Department of Clinical Physiology, Nuclear Medicine & PET and Cluster for Molecular Imaging, Copenhagen University Hospital, Rigshospitalet and University of Copenhagen, Copenhagen, Denmark
Full list of author information is available at the end of the article

aim of this study was to characterize key psychological/ psychopathological traits in a large, carefully diagnosed cohort of post-recovery TTC patients using well-validated psychometric tools. For comparison, we included one group of patients with previous ST elevation myocardial infarction (STEMI), and one group of background population controls. We hypothesized that specific psychopathological traits were more pronounced in the patients with TTC compared to the STEMI patients and the individuals in the background control group.

Method
Participants
A total of 45 TTC patients were prospectively recruited among female patients admitted at the Department of Cardiology, Copenhagen University Hospital from October 1st 2009 to December 10th 2014. Inclusion criteria were (1) acute onset of symptoms, (2) no culprit lesion on coronary angiography, (3) typical 'apical ballooning', (4) elevated cardiac biomarkers, and (5) normalized left ventricle systolic function on follow-up echocardiography. The STEMI patients were 95 age- and geographically matched females with previous one-vessel disease and STEMI that had received primary coronary intervention at Copenhagen University Hospital within the TTC inclusion period. The background controls were 90 age- and geographically matched females randomly selected from the Danish Civil Registration Registry [13].

Survey
The survey was conducted between February and April 2015. A questionnaire for self-reporting was mailed to the invitees' home addresses, and a maximum of two reminders were sent by letter if invitees did not respond to the first questionnaire. The questionnaire consisted of the following self-rating scales: The 5-item WHO-5 Well-Being Index (WHO-5) [14], the 23-item Eysenck's Neuroticism Scale (ENS) [15, 16], the 10-item Major Depression Inventory (MDI) [17], and the 8-item anxiety subscale of Hopkin's Symptoms Checklist (ASS) [18]. These self-rating scales are well-validated measures of well-being, neuroticism, depression, and anxiety, respectively. Not all questionnaires were fully filled out by the participants. If >20 % of the item scores on one of the four self-rating scales were missing, this entire scale was excluded from further analysis. If ≤20 % of the item scores were missing on a self-rating scale, the missing scores were replaced by the mean value of the completed item scores of this scale.

Statistics
Unless stated otherwise, results are presented as median (interquartile range). The total score for each of the four rating scales was compared pair-wise between groups by

means of the Wilcoxon-Mann-Whitney test. Correlations between rating scale total scores and age, and time since admission respectively, were tested by Spearman rank (r) correlation analysis. Both the Wilcoxon-Mann-Whitney test and the r correlation analyses were performed using SAS Statistical software® (version 9.0) with the level of significance set at two-tailed $p < 0.05$. As we intended to use the total scores of each of the four self-rating scales as measures for overall well-being (WHO-5) or syndrome severity (END, MDI, and ASS), we tested the scalability of these scales. Scalability is present when each of the individual item scores of a scale contributes unique information regarding the dimension of interest. Only when this is the case can the individual item scores be summed to a meaningful total score [19]. The analysis of scalability was performed using the Mokken non-parametric item response theory model, where the degree of scalability is expressed by the coefficient of homogeneity. A coefficient of 0.40 or higher indicates acceptable scalability [20]. The Mokken analysis was performed with the dedicated MSP 3.0 software [21].

Ethics
The study was approved by the regional ethics committee, and all participants provided written consent.

Results
The flow of participants in the survey is depicted in Fig. 1. In total, 173 of 230 (75 %) invitees, 40 TTC patients (89 % of invitees), 71 STEMI patients (75 % of invitees) and 62 background controls (69 % of invitees), participated in the study. Age in years was 70 (64; 76) for the TTC patients, 72 (64; 77) for the STEMI patients, and 67 (64; 70) for the background controls. The age of the TTC and the STEMI patients was comparable ($p = 0.79$), whereas the background controls were significantly younger than both the TTC patients (p = 0.02), and the STEMI patients ($p = 0.003$). The time from initial admission to the survey was 24 (8; 36) months and 26 (22; 32) months for TTC and STEMI patients, respectively, with no statistically significant difference between the two groups ($p = 0.70$). The Mokken analysis showed that all of the self-rating scales included in the survey had acceptable coefficients of homogeneity (≥0.40): WHO-5 0.65, ENS 0.40, ASS 0.66, and MDI 0.53. This entails that the total scores of the scales are valid (scalable) measures of the psychological/psychopathological dimensions being investigated [19].

The results of the survey are presented in Fig. 2. Well-being and depression scores were comparable between the TTC and STEMI groups (WHO-5: 64 (40; 80) vs. 68 (52; 80), $p = 0.57$. MDI: 8 (3; 16) vs. 7 (3; 14), $p = 0.72$). ENS score tended to be higher in the TTC group (ENS: 9 (3; 13) vs. 5 (2; 11), $p = 0.08$), but the difference was

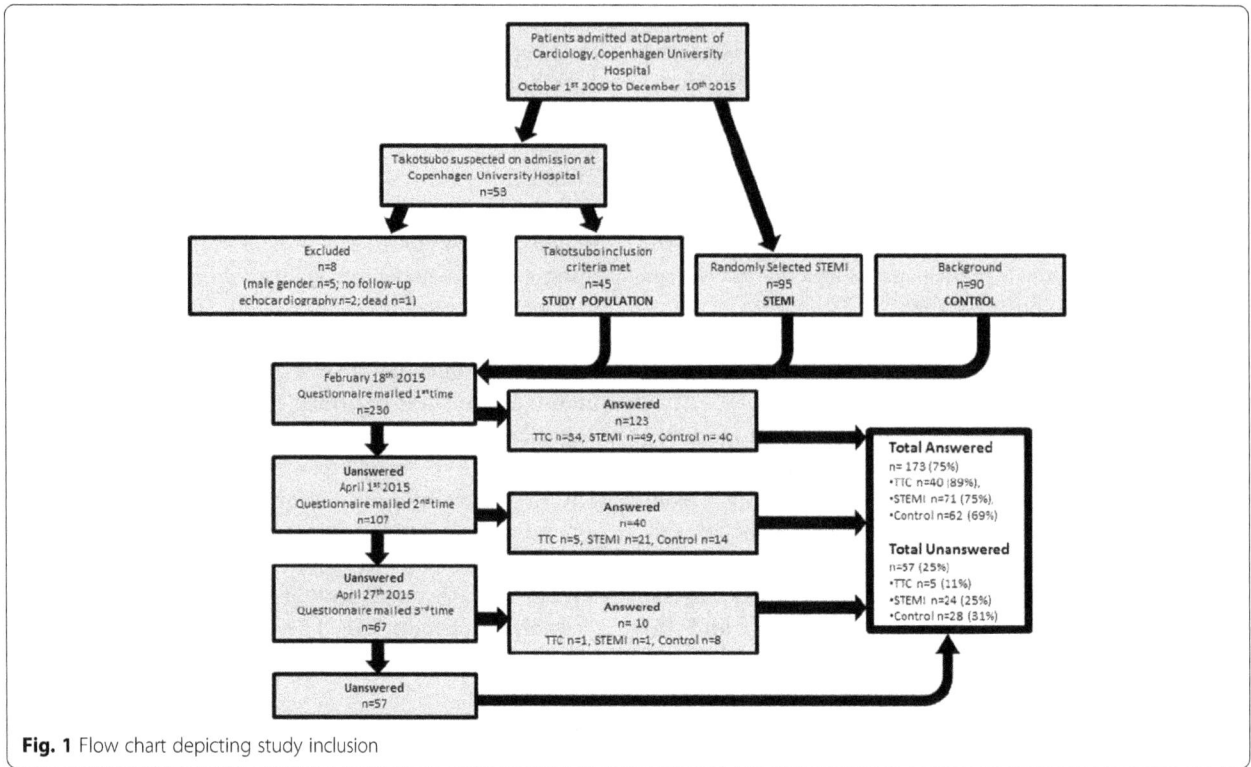

Fig. 1 Flow chart depicting study inclusion

not statistically significant. The anxiety score was significantly higher in the TTC than the STEMI group (ASS: 2 (1; 7) vs. 1 (0; 3), $p = 0.007$). When compared to the control group, TTC patients reported significantly less well-being (WHO-5: 76 (68; 84) vs. 64 (40; 80), $p = 0.02$),

higher neuroticism (ENS: 3 (0; 9) vs. 9 (3; 13), $p = 0.0002$), more depression (MDI: 4 (1; 9) vs. 8.0 (3; 16), $p = 0.007$), and more anxiety (ASS: 1 (0; 2) vs. 2 (1; 7), $p = 0.0001$). Compared to the background controls, the STEMI patients reported less well-being (WHO-5: 76 [68; 84] vs.

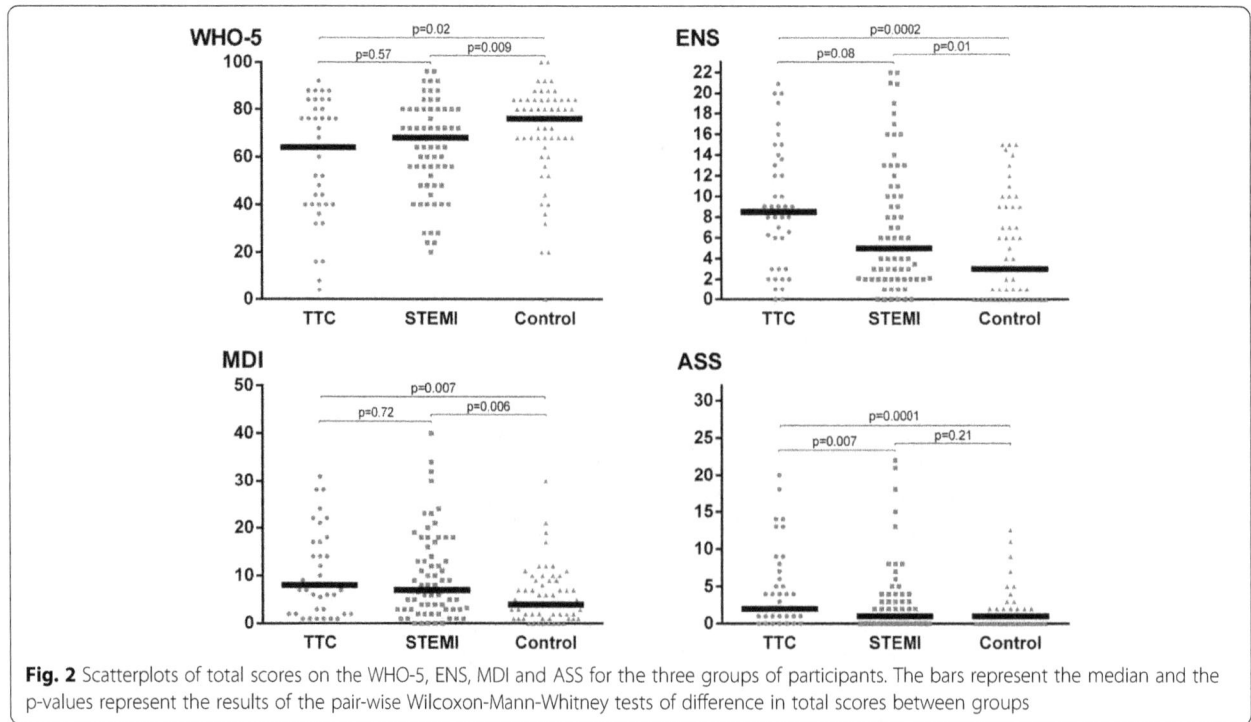

Fig. 2 Scatterplots of total scores on the WHO-5, ENS, MDI and ASS for the three groups of participants. The bars represent the median and the p-values represent the results of the pair-wise Wilcoxon-Mann-Whitney tests of difference in total scores between groups

68 [52; 80], $p = 0.009$), more neuroticism (ENS: 3 [0; 9] vs. 5[2; 11], $p = 0.01$), more depression (MDI: 4 [1; 9] vs. 7 [3; 14], $p = 0.006$), whereas the level of anxiety was similar (ASS: 1[0; 2] vs. 1 [0; 3], $p = 0.21$). There was no significant correlation between age and any of the total scores on the four self-rating scales (Age and WHO-5: $r = 0.06$, $p = 0.46$, $n = 173$; Age and ENS: $r = 0.01$, $p = 0.94$, $n = 169$;

Age and MDI: $r = 0.01$, $p = 0.94$, $n = 173$; Age and ASS: $r = -0.01$, $p = 0.93$, $n = 171$).

In Fig. 3, the time between admission and survey participation is plotted against the total scores of the WHO-5, ENS, MDI and ASS for the TTC and STEMI patients, respectively. For the STEMI patients, there was no significant correlation between time and total scores

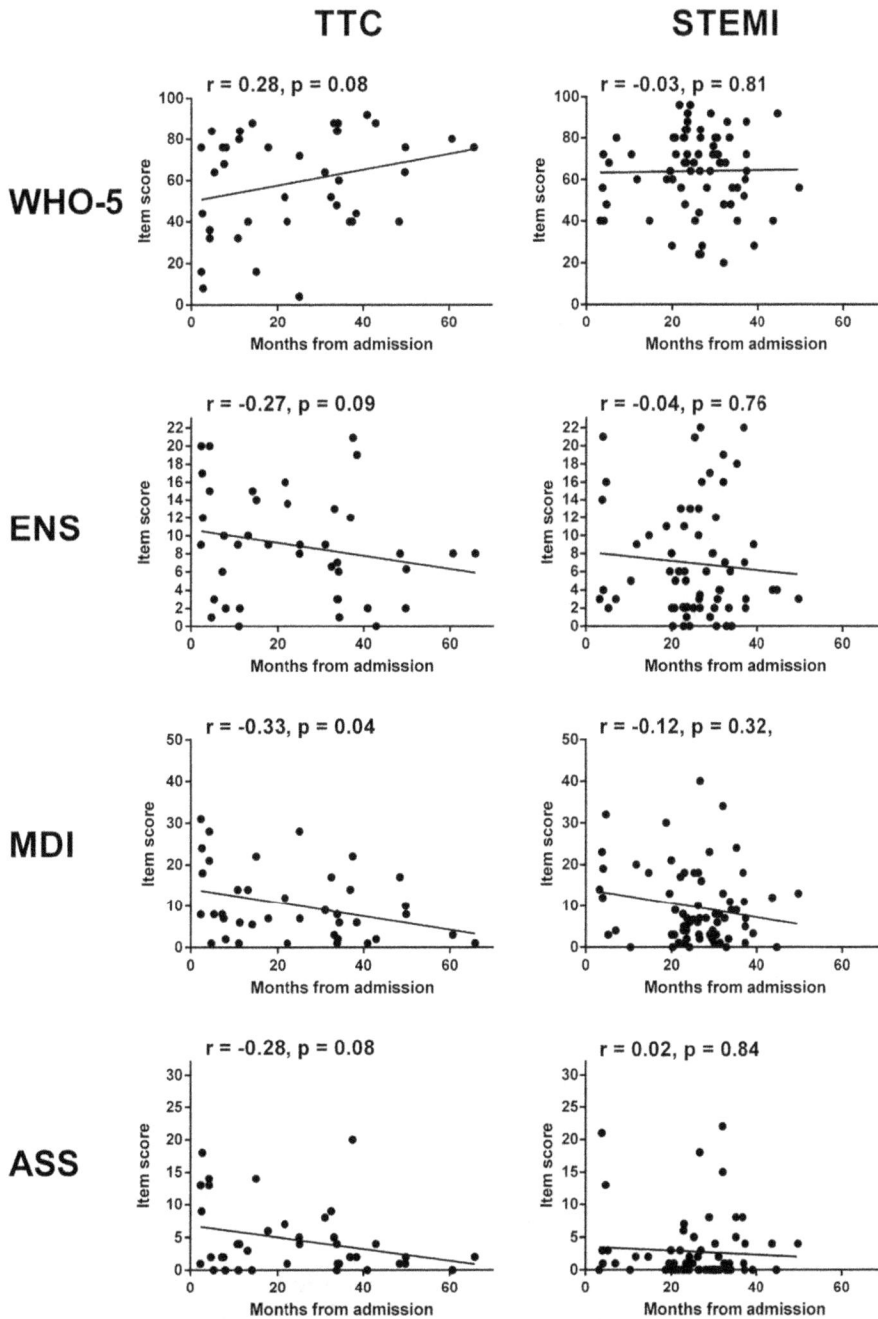

Fig. 3 The time (in months) between admission and survey participation (*x-axis*) plotted against the total score (*y-axis*) on each of the four rating scales for the TTC (left) and STEMI (*right*) patients respectively. The fitted line of least squares is depicted. The Spearman rank coefficient (r) and the associated p-value are shown for each correlation

(Time and WHO-5: $r = -0.03$, $p = 0.81$, $n = 70$; Time and ENS: $r = -0.04$, $p = 0.76$, $n = 69$; Time and MDI: $r = -0.12$, $p = 0.32$, $n = 70$; Time and ASS: $r = 0.02$, $p = 0.84$, $n = 68$). Conversely, the same correlations were either significant or near-significant ($p < 0.1$) for the TTC patients (Time and WHO-5: $r = 0.28$, $p = 0.08$, $n = 40$; Time and ENS: $r = -0.27$, $p = 0.09$, $n = 40$; Time and MDI: $r = -0.33$, $p = 0.04$, $n = 40$; Time and ASS: $r = -0.28$, $p = 0.08$, $n = 40$), which is indicative of psychological improvement in the post-recovery phase of TTC.

Discussion

We examined four psychological/psychopathological dimensions in post-recovery female TTC patients, age- and geographically matched female STEMI patients and age- and geographically matched females from the background population. As expected, the results showed that TTC patients reported significantly less well-being, more neuroticism, more depression, and more anxiety than the background controls. The level of well-being, depression and neuroticism in TTC patients was comparable to that of the STEMI patients, but the TTC patients were significantly more anxious than the STEMI patients. These findings are consistent with previous studies of the psychological/psychopathological profile of patients with TTC. Specifically, Compare et al. compared the prevalence of Type D personality in TTC patients with an emotional trigger to TTC patients without an emotional trigger and to STEMI patients. Type D personality is characterized by negative affect and social inhibition, and the frequency of Type D personality was higher in the TTC patients with an emotional trigger than in the two other groups [9]. Similarly, Delmas et al. showed that anxio-depressive disorders and chronic psychological stress was common in TTC patients and occurred more often than in patients with coronary disease [10]. Finally, Kastaun et al. found that TTC patients showed impaired cortisol release in response to stress, and were more anxious, worried and socially inhibited when compared to STEMI and healthy controls [11].

In contrast to STEMI, TTC leaves no permanent myocardial damage [22]. Thus, TTC patients are generally not considered to be chronically ill. Despite this fact, both the present study and the literature in general indicate that TTC is associated with more pronounced psychopathology compared to chronic ischemic heart disease. However, the results of our study also indicated that TTC patients, as opposed to STEMI patients, tend to improve psychologically during the post-recovery phase. To our knowledge, this is a novel finding, which may be a consolation for TTC patients in psychological distress in the acute phase.

Limitations to this study warrant a mention. First and foremost, since our survey was conducted post-TTC, we were not able to investigate the direction of causality of the psychopathology-TTC association, i.e., whether individuals develop TTC because they are psychologically vulnerable, or whether they develop psychopathology because of TTC? Since TTC is believed to be caused by sympathetic hyperactivity [3, 4] and patients with anxiety disorders show increased sympathetic reactivity in response to stress [23, 24], it seems plausible that the direction of causality goes from psychopathology to TTC. This hypothesis is supported by a small retro-perspective study by Summers et al. [12] in which past medical records of TTC patients were reviewed and compared to those of STEMI patients and background controls. Compared to the two other groups, the TTC patients had a much higher prevalence of anxiety disorders in their pre-cardiac-illness medical history. However, definitive prospective studies of this association are lacking from the literature. This is probably due to the fact that with the relatively low incidence of TTC (approximately 2 % of patients admitted on suspicion of acute coronary syndrome [1]), it will require extremely large surveys with very long follow-up to obtain pre-morbid psychological/psychopathological data on a sufficient number of TTC patients. Consistently, the small sample size is also a limitation of the present retrospective study.

Another limitation of our study is the risk of self-selection-bias as not all invitees completed the survey. Indeed, the age of the controls was slightly lower than that of the TTC and STEMI patients, but the Spearman rank correlation analysis revealed no significant correlation between age and rating scale total scores. It therefore seems unlikely that the lower age of the background controls has biased the results. Since many baseline data were not collected, we cannot exclude that confounders such as differences in educational or income level between groups have contributed to our results.

Conclusion

In conclusion, we found that post-recovery TTC patients reported levels of well-being, neuroticism, and depression that are comparable to those of STEMI patients. However, TTC patients reported higher levels of anxiety than STEMI patients. In contrast to STEMI patients, the TTC patients appear to improve psychologically during the post-recovery phase. This may be a consolation for patients in psychological distress in the acute phase of TTC.

Abbreviations

ASS, 8-item anxiety subscale of Hopkin's Symptoms Checklist; ENS, 23-item Eysenck's Neuroticism Scale; MDI, 10-item Major Depression Inventory; STEMI, ST-elevation myocardial infarction; TTC, Takotsubo cardiomyopathy; WHO-5, World Health Organization-5 Well-Being Index.

Acknowledgements
The authors are grateful to the study participants.

Funding
Søren Dinesen Østergaard was funded by a grant from the Lundbeck Foundation. The remaining authors were funded by their respective departments.

Authors' contributions
All authors contributed to the design and conduct of this study. The manuscript was drafted by Thomas Emil Christensen and Søren Dinesen Østergaard, and was critically revised by the remaining authors. The final version of the manuscript was approved by all authors prior to submission.

Competing interests
The authors declare that they have no competing interests.

Author details
[1]Department of Cardiology, Copenhagen University Hospital, Rigshospitalet, Copenhagen, Denmark. [2]Department of Clinical Physiology, Nuclear Medicine & PET and Cluster for Molecular Imaging, Copenhagen University Hospital, Rigshospitalet and University of Copenhagen, Copenhagen, Denmark. [3]Psychiatric Research Unit, Psychiatric Center North Zealand, Copenhagen University Hospital, Hillerød, Denmark. [4]Department of Clinical Medicine, Aarhus University Hospital, Aarhus, Denmark. [5]Department P - Research, Aarhus University Hospital, Risskov, Denmark.

References
1. Akashi YJ, Nef HM, Lyon AR. Epidemiology and pathophysiology of Takotsubo syndrome. Nat Rev Cardiol. 2015;12:387–97.
2. Akashi YJ, Goldstein DS, Barbaro G, Ueyama T. Takotsubo cardiomyopathy: a new form of acute, reversible heart failure. Circulation. 2008;118:2754–62.
3. Wittstein IS. Stress cardiomyopathy: a syndrome of catecholamine-mediated myocardial stunning? Cell Mol Neurobiol. 2012;32:847–57.
4. Lyon AR, Rees PS, Prasad S, Poole-Wilson PA, Harding SE. Stress (Takotsubo) cardiomyopathy–a novel pathophysiological hypothesis to explain catecholamine-induced acute myocardial stunning. Nat Clin Pract Cardiovasc Med. 2008;5:22–9.
5. Madhavan M, Prasad A. Proposed Mayo Clinic criteria for the diagnosis of Tako-Tsubo cardiomyopathy and long-term prognosis. Herz. 2010;35:240–3.
6. Ako J, Sudhir K, Farouque HM, Honda Y, Fitzgerald PJ. Transient left ventricular dysfunction under severe stress: brain-heart relationship revisited. Am J Med. 2006;119:10–7.
7. Redfors B, Vedad R, Angeras O, et al. Mortality in takotsubo syndrome is similar to mortality in myocardial infarction - A report from the SWEDEHEART registry. Int J Cardiol. 2015;185:282–9.
8. Fiedorowicz JG. Depression and cardiovascular disease: an update on how course of illness may influence risk. Curr Psychiatry Rep. 2014;16:492.
9. Compare A, Bigi R, Orrego PS, Proietti R, Grossi E, Steptoe A. Type D personality is associated with the development of stress cardiomyopathy following emotional triggers. Ann Behav Med. 2013;45:299–307.
10. Delmas C, Lairez O, Mulin E, et al. Anxiodepressive disorders and chronic psychological stress are associated with Tako-Tsubo cardiomyopathy- New Physiopathological Hypothesis. Circ J. 2013;77:175–80.
11. Kastaun S, Schwarz NP, Juenemann M, et al. Cortisol awakening and stress response, personality and psychiatric profiles in patients with takotsubo cardiomyopathy. Heart. 2014;100:1786–92.
12. Summers MR, Lennon RJ, Prasad A. Pre-morbid psychiatric and cardiovascular diseases in apical ballooning syndrome (tako-tsubo/stress-induced cardiomyopathy): potential pre-disposing factors? J Am Coll Cardiol. 2010;55:700–1.
13. Pedersen CB. The Danish civil registration system. Scand J Public Health. 2011;39(7 Suppl):22–5.
14. Topp CW, Ostergaard SD, Sondergaard S, Bech P. The WHO-5 Well-Being Index: a systematic review of the literature. Psychother Psychosom. 2015; 84:167–76.
15. Eysenck HJ, Eysenck SBG. Manual of the eysenck personality questionnaire. London: Hodder Stoughton; 1975.
16. Bech P, Jorgensen B, Jeppesen K, Loldrup PD, Vanggaard T. Personality in depression: concordance between clinical assessment and questionnaires. Acta Psychiatr Scand. 1986;74:263–8.
17. Bech P, Rasmussen NA, Olsen LR, Noerholm V, Abildgaard W. The sensitivity and specificity of the Major Depression Inventory, using the Present State Examination as the index of diagnostic validity. J Affect Disord. 2001;66:159–64.
18. Bech P, Bille J, Moller SB, Hellstrom LC, Ostergaard SD. Psychometric validation of the Hopkins Symptom Checklist (SCL-90) subscales for depression, anxiety, and interpersonal sensitivity. J Affect Disord. 2014;160:98–103.
19. Bech P. Clinical psychometrics. 1st ed. Oxford: Wiley Blackwell; 2012.
20. Mokken RJ. Theory and practice of scale analysis. Berlin: Mouton; 1971.
21. Molenaar IWDPSK. User's manual MSP, a program for mokken scale analyses for polytomous items (Version 3.0). Groeningen: ProGAMMA; 1994.
22. Ahtarovski KA, Iversen KK, Christensen TE, et al. Takotsubo cardiomyopathy, a two-stage recovery of left ventricular systolic and diastolic function as determined by cardiac magnetic resonance imaging. Eur Heart J Cardiovasc Imaging. 2014;15:855–62.
23. Nutt DJ. Neurobiological mechanisms in generalized anxiety disorder. J Clin Psychiatry. 2001;62 Suppl 11:22–7.
24. Kalk NJ, Nutt DJ, Lingford-Hughes AR. The role of central noradrenergic dysregulation in anxiety disorders: evidence from clinical studies. J Psychopharmacol. 2011;25:3–16.

8

N-Acetyl Cysteine improves the diabetic cardiac function: possible role of fibrosis inhibition

Cong Liu[1†], Xiao-Zhao Lu[2†], Ming-Zhi Shen[2], Chang-Yang Xing[1], Jing Ma[1], Yun-You Duan[1*] and Li-Jun Yuan[1*]

Abstract

Background: Diabetic cardiomyopathy is one of the leading causes of death in diabetes mellitus (DM) patients. This study aimed to explore the therapeutic implication of N-acetyl-L-cysteine (NAC, an antioxidant and glutathione precursor) and the possible underlying mechanism.

Methods: Thirty five 12-week-old male C57BL/6 mice were included. Twenty-five diabetic mice were induced by intraperitoneal injection of streptozocin (STZ, 150 mg/kg, Sigma-Aldrich) dissolved in a mix of citrate buffer after overnight fast. Mice with a blood glucose level above 13.5 mmol/L were considered diabetic. As a non-DM (diabetic) control, mice were injected with equal volume of citrate buffer. The 25 diabetic mice were divided into 5 groups with 5 animals in each group: including DM (diabetes without NAC treatment), and 4 different NAC treatment groups, namely NAC1, NAC3, NAC5 and NAC7, with the number defining the start time point of NAC treatment. In the 10 non-DM mice, mice were either untreated (Ctrl) or treated with NAC for 5 weeks (NAC only). Echocardiography was performed 12 weeks after STZ injection. Heart tissue were collected after echocardiography for Hematoxylin Eosin (HE) and Trichrome staining and ROS staining. Cardiac fibroblast cells were isolated, cultured and treated with high glucose plus NAC or the vehicle. qPCR analysis and CCK-8 assay were performed to observe fibrotic gene expression and cell proliferation.

Results: We found that both cardiac systolic function and diastolic function were impaired, coupled with excessive reactive oxygen stress and cardiac fibrosis 12 weeks after STZ induction. NAC significantly reduced ROS generation and fibrosis, together with improved cardiac systolic function and diastolic function. Strikingly, NAC1 treatment, which had the earlier and longer treatment, produced significant improvement of cardiac function and less fibrosis. In the cardiac fibroblasts, NAC blocked cardiac fibroblast proliferation and collagen synthesis induced by hyperglycemia.

Conclusions: Our study indicates that NAC treatment in diabetes effectively protects from diabetic cardiomyopathy, possibly through inhibiting the ROS production and fibrosis, which warrants further clarification.

Keywords: Diabetic cardiomyopathy, Fibrosis, Reactive oxygen species, N-acetyl-L-cysteine, Cardiac function

Background

Diabetes mellitus (DM) is one of the most common chronic diseases in nearly all countries, and by 2030 people with diabetes is expected to rise to 552 million [1]. It has become a fast-growing global problem with huge social, health, and economic consequences. Among the diabetic complications, diabetic cardiomyopathy (mainly manifested as two interconnected pathological processes: cardiac hypertrophy and fibrosis) is considered as one of the leading causes of death [2–5]. It is well established that diabetes increases oxygen stress, which have a causative role in cardiac dysfunction [6]. N-Acetylcysteine (NAC) is a thiol-containing radical scavenger and glutathione precursor. Several studies have demonstrated that antioxidant treatment using NAC may attenuate the myocardial damage by protecting cardiomyocyte and endothelium from cell death [7, 8]. Taken together, role of ROS in diabetic cardiomyopathy is still evasive, especially how ROS involved in the cardiac fibrosis.

This study aimed to explore the therapeutic implication of NAC and the possible underlying mechanism. We evaluated the efficacy of anti-oxidative NAC in preventing cardiac fibrosis and ventricular functional remodeling in the

---

* Correspondence: duanyy@fmmu.edu.cn; yuanlj@fmmu.edu.cn

†Equal contributors

[1]Department of Ultrasound Diagnostics, Tangdu Hospital, Fourth Military Medical University, #569 Xinsi RoadBaqiao District, Xi'an 710038, China

Full list of author information is available at the end of the article

mouse model of STZ-induced diabetes at different time points. We found that early treatment of NAC in STZ induced diabetic mice resulted in better outcome, while later treatment produced less beneficial results, suggesting that diabetic cardiomyopathy is an irreversible process or alternatively NAC is incapable to reverse the pathological process. Mechanisitically, we found that NAC blocked hyperglycemia promoted induced cardiac fibroblast proliferation and myofibroblast differentiation via inhibition of ROS. Our study revealed an irreversible role of ROS in cardiac fibrosis and related cardiac dysfunction, shedding light on anti-oxidative therapy in protecting from diabetic cardiomyopathy.

Methods

All experiments involving animals were performed in adherence with the Guide for the Care and Use of Laboratory Animals, and approved by the Fourth Military Medical University Committee on Animal Care.

Diabetes model and treatments

Twelve-week-old male C57BL/6 mice from the Experimental Animal Center of the Fourth Military Medical University were housed five/cage under a temperature of 25 ± 1 °C, 50 ± 5 % humidity, with an alternating 12 hrs light–dark cycle and free access to food and water ad libitum. The type of housing facility was specific pathogen free (SPF), and the cage is 30 cm (width) × 40 cm (depth) × 20 cm (height). For STZ induced diabetes model, mice were injected intraperitoneally with streptozocin (150 mg/kg, Sigma-Aldrich) dissolved in a mix of citrate buffer (citric acid and sodium citrate, pH 4.8) or vehicle (citrate buffer) after overnight fast similar as described before [9]. Blood glucose was checked 5 days later via tail vein; mice with a blood glucose level above 13.5 mmol/L were considered diabetic. As a control, mice were injected with equal volume of citrate buffer. In total, 35 mice were include in this study, which were divided into 7 groups with 5

animals in each group: including control, NAC only, DM (diabetes without NAC treatment), and 4 different NAC treatment groups. The 4 NAC treatment groups, namely NAC1, NAC3, NAC5 and NAC7, define the start time point when NAC treatments start. For example, in the NAC1 groups, diabetic mice were treated with NAC (A9165, Sigma-Aldrich) from 1 week after STZ induction at the dose of 1.0 g/kg body weight per day in drinking water. In the NAC only group, control mice were further treated with NAC for five weeks. No obvious adverse events were seen in each experimental group. The detailed procedure described in Fig. 1.

Echocardiography

Echocardiography was performed from week 12 after STZ injection. Transthoracic 2-dimensional (2D), M-mode and Doppler echocardiographic studies were performed with Mylab 50 (Esaote, Italy) using a high-resolution transducer (SL3116) with frequency of 22 MHz. Briefly, each mouse was anesthetized by injecting intraperitoneally with 10 % chloral hydrate at the dose of 350 mg/kg body weight before echocardiographic study [10], which had an onset of sedation within 5–10 minutes and was maintained for about 30–40 minutes. Heart rates were monitored and generally maintained around 450 beats per minute. The chest hairs were removed using Depilatory creams. The mouse was then placed on a warm pad to keep the body temperature around 36 ± 0.5°C. Warmed echo gel was placed on the shaved chest as a coupling medium while the mouse lay on the warm pad at a supine position. Images were acquired and analyzed by an operator blinded to mouse treatment.

Interventricular septal thickness and LV posterior wall thickness during diastole (IVSd, LVPWd), LV internal dimensions during diastole (LVIDd) and systole (LVIDs) were measured from M-mode images at the level of the papillary muscles at LV short-axis view (Additional file 1: Figure S1a). Representative images were digitally acquired and stored on the internal

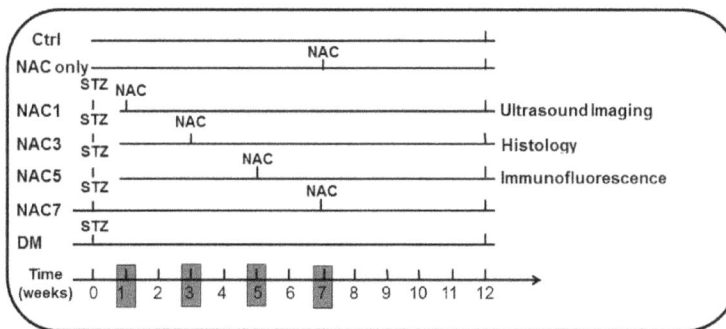

Fig. 1 Schematic representation of the experimental procedure. Diabetic mouse model was induced by streptozotocin (STZ) injection. NAC treatment was done via drinking water starting from week 1, week 3, week 5 and week 7 STZ injection till the end of the week 12, respectively. Cardiac function and structure were analyzed by both echocardiography and histology

hard disk and USB Mass Storage Device for off-line analysis. LV ejection fraction (EF), LV fractional shortening (FS) were calculated according to the recommendation of the American Society of Echocardiography Committee [11].

Transmitral inflow Doppler was obtained from the apical 4-chamber view. The sample volume was placed just below the level of the mitral annulus and adjusted to the position at which the velocity was maximal. The angle correction was kept less than 20 degree. LV diastolic function was evaluated using the methods described previously [12]. In brief, the left ventricular isovolumic relaxation time (IVRT) and the acceleration and deceleration times of the early peak (E) wave (E_{AT} and E_{DT}, respectively) were derived respectively from the Doppler waveform (Additional file 1: Figure S1b).

Tissue collection and histology

After echocardiography, the heart was excised from the chest, trimmed of atria and large vessels and weighed. Half of the hearts (in the long axis view) were formalin-fixed for Hematoxylin Eosin (HE) and Trichrome staining, while the other half were mounted with OCT directly for ROS staining. For histological analysis, excised hearts were washed with saline solution, placed in 10 % formalin, and embedded in paraffin. Then, 5-µm thick sections were prepared and stained with Masson Trichrome staining for detecting the myocardial fibrosis [13]. To determine myocardial ROS generation, dihydroethidium (DHE) staining was included by probing for the ROS on the 5-µm frozen myocardial sections [14].

Cardiac fibroblast cell isolation and culture

Fibroblasts were isolated from the hearts of normal P7 (postnatal day 7) male C57/Bl6 mice similar as previously described [15]. Briefly, 3 hearts were isolated and vessels and atria were removed before transferred to 1 mL of collagenase buffer. In the buffer, the ventricles were quickly minced into small pieces and digested for about 1 hour. Cell suspension were filtered with 100 µm filter and then centrifuged. The cell pellet was re-suspended and plated on a T75 tissue-culture flask (Corning Corp) in full medium supplemented with 10 % of fetal bovine serum (HyClone) and antibiotic-antimycotic solution. Non-adherent cells were removed after overnight culture, and adherent cells were cultivated as cardiac fibroblast. Only fibroblasts at passage 1 to 5 were used for the following experiments.

qPCR analysis

Cardiac fibroblast cells were cultured in the serum free medium containing either 5.5 mM (normal glucose, NG) or 25 mM glucose (HG) with 10 ng/ml TGFβ1 and without insulin for 24 hrs. In the HG group, cells were further added with control or NAC (5 mM). RNA was isolated with TriZOL (Invitrogen). Reverse transcription was performed with the Superscript III First Strand Synthesis kit (Invitrogen). SYBR Green Mix I (Takara) was used for amplification, and samples were run on an ABI7500 Instrument (AB, USA). Gapdh was used as internal control. 2– ΔΔCt method was used for analysis (n = 3). The primers are listed as follows: Gapdh forward, 5′-TGGCCTTCCGTGTTCCTACCC-3′, Gapdh reverse, 5′-AGCCCAAGATGCCCTTCAGTG-3′; Col1a1 forward, Col1a1 reverse, 5′-GGAATCCATCGGTCATGC TCT-3′; CTGF forward, 5′-CCACCCGAGTTACCAA TGACA-3′, CTGF reverse, 5′-CTTGGCGATTTTAG GTGTCCG-3′.

Cell proliferation assay

Cardiac fibroblast cells were seeded in 96-well plates at a density of 1.5×10^3 cells per well and treated as indicated. Cell numbers were analyzed by Cell Counting Kit-8 (Sigma-Aldrich) at 450-nm absorbance.

Statistical analysis

All data were expressed as mean ± SD. The mean data of six groups were compared with one-way ANOVA. The intra-and inter-observer variability were analyzed using 2-tailed Student's t-test and linear regression analysis. A P-value < 0.05 was considered statistically significant.

Results

Anatomical weights and physiological parameters of mice in different groups

We first analyzed anatomical weights and other physiological parameters in mice with different treatments. As shown in Table 1, the body weight in diabetic group was much lower than that in the control group at the time of sacrifice. However there were no significant differences among all the diabetic mice either with or without NAC treatment. Similar as the body weight, all the diabetic mice either with or without NAC treatments had significant higher blood glucose levels than the control mice, while there were no significant differences among the NAC treatment groups (Fig. 2). All of these data suggest that NAC did not alter the body weight and blood glucose levels.

The heart weight and heart weight index in untreated DM group were significantly lower than in the control group, which was at least partially rescued by NAC treatment (Table 1). Notably, there was no significant decrease of HWI in NAC1 group compared with the control group.

Table 1 Physiological parameters of mice in all groups

	Initial weight (g)	Terminal weight (g)	HW (mg)	HWI (mg/kg, %)	HR (bpm)
Control	24.32 ± 1.89	27.56 ± 2.33	168.12 ± 8.37	6.11 ± 0.22	446 ± 11
NAC only	23.44 ± 0.89	25.40 ± 0.54	160.40 ± 7.12	6.31 ± 0.21	448 ± 9
NAC1	23.22 ± 1.02	24.54 ± 0.65[*]	150.56 ± 7.07[*△]	6.10 ± 0.18[△]	445 ± 14
NAC3	23.67 ± 2.03	24.36 ± 1.91[*]	144.32 ± 13.42[*]	5.80 ± 0.25[*]	453 ± 21
NAC5	24.72 ± 1.31	24.45 ± 0.97[*]	144.00 ± 5.48[*]	5.78 ± 0.23[*]	440 ± 11
NAC7	24.86 ± 1.96	24.92 ± 1.83[*]	143.57 ± 8.94[*]	5.77 ± 0.14[*]	451 ± 19
DM	24.19 ± 1.60	24.84 ± 0.79[*]	138.00 ± 4.47[*]	5.56 ± 0.26[*]	441 ± 9
p value[a]	0.347	0.940	0.668	0.066	0.61

Notes: No significant differences were found between control and NAC only group; *Compared with control, $p < 0.05$; △NAC treatment groups compared with DM group, $p < 0.05$; No significant difference was seen in initial weight and heart rate among all groups. a, ANOVA test among the NAC1, NAC3, NAC5 and NAC7 four groups, no significant difference was seen among the four groups. HW, heart weight; HWI, heart weight index; HR, heart rate. (n = 5 in each group)

NAC treatments improve cardiac systolic and diastolic function in diabetic mice

The cardiac morphology and function differences among the 7 groups were measured by echocardiography and compared using ANOVA (Table 2).

Compared with the control group, NAC only group had similar cardiac function, indicating that NAC did not change the normal cardiac function (Table 2). As expected, DM group displayed much lower left ventricular ejection fraction (LVEF) and left ventricular fractional shortening (LVFS), indicating significant decrease of systolic function. Coupled with the decreased systolic function in diabetic group, LV diastolic function was also significantly reduced, as seen by the increased IVRT, E_{AT} and E_{DT} in DM group (Table 2). In addition, DM group displayed thinner IVSd and LVPWd, which was consistent with the lower HWI.

NAC supplement improved the LVFS and LVEF. Notably, there was even no significant difference between control and NAC1 and NAC3 groups, indicating that NAC1 and NAC3 treatments significantly improved cardiac systolic function in mice with diabetic cardiomyopathy.

Similar to the improved cardiac systolic function, NAC treatments also increased the diastolic function. The values of IVRT, E_{AT} and E_{DT} in NAC1 group were close to the control group, while those in NAC7 group were close to the DM group (Table 2).

NAC treatments inhibit ROS production and cardiac fibrosis

We next explored the mechanism how NAC improved the cardiac function, mainly focused on ROS generation and cardiac fibrosis. ROS generation was determined in the frozen section of the myocardial tissues by DHE fluorescence. Diabetic heart displayed robust increase of ROS all over the heart (Fig. 3a-b), which was efficiently cleared in all the NAC treatment groups (Fig. 3c-f). Quantification data were shown in Fig. 3g.

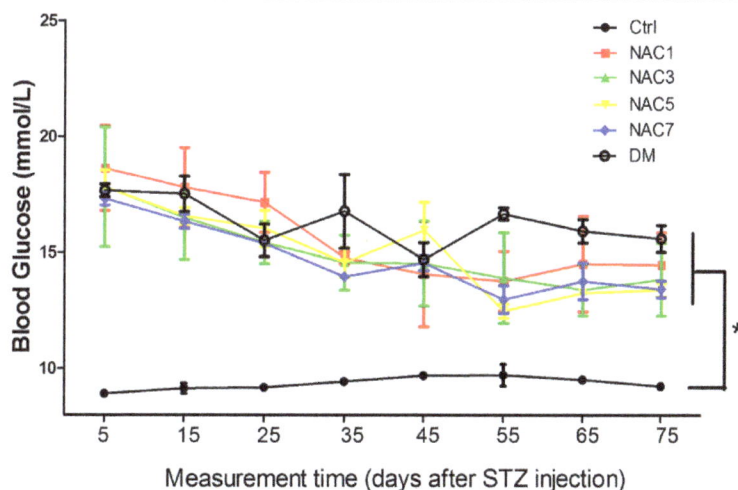

Fig. 2 Blood glucose levels among all groups. Blood glucose levels of all the groups were compared and *denoted significant differences. (n = 5 in each group)

Table 2 Comparison of echocardiographic morphological, systolic and diastolic functional indices

	IVSd (mm)	LVPWd (mm)	LVIDd (mm)	LVIDs (mm)	LVEF (%)	LVFS (%)	IVRT (ms)	E_{DT} (ms)	E_{AT} (ms)
Control	0.72 ± 0.04	0.70 ± 0.01	3.42 ± 0.31	1.98 ± 0.28	81.08 ± 4.6	42.31 ± 3.8	11.56 ± 1.74	11.00 ± 0.71	33.06 ± 3.27
NAC only	0.66 ± 0.05	0.67 ± 0.04	3.48 ± 0.08	2.06 ± 0.09	79.72 ± 2.58	40.80 ± 1.48	11.08 ± 0.66	11.80 ± 0.97	34.06 ± 2.48
NAC1	0.66 ± 0.05$^{△}$	0.65 ± 0.05$^{△}$	3.44 ± 0.05$^{△}$	2.00 ± 0.70$^{△}$	80.79 ± 2.3$^{△}$	41.86 ± 1.6$^{△}$	14.86 ± 0.78$^{*△}$	13.86 ± 1.49$^{*△}$	33.84 ± 2.67$^{△}$
NAC3	0.66 ± 0.05$^{△}$	0.65 ± 0.05$^{△}$	3.62 ± 0.04$^{△}$	2.12 ± 0.13$^{△}$	79.80 ± 3.1$^{△}$	41.45 ± 3.1$^{△}$	15.00 ± 0.71$^{*△}$	14.60 ± 0.89$^{*△}$	34.24 ± 3.74$^{△}$
NAC5	0.64 ± 0.05$^{*△}$	0.59 ± 0.02$^{*△}$	3.92 ± 0.17$^{*△}$	2.44 ± 0.15$^{*△}$	75.89 ± 1.4$^{*△}$	37.78 ± 1.2$^{*△}$	18.14 ± 1.33$^{*△}$	17.14 ± 2.02$^{*△}$	35.56 ± 3.56$^{△}$
NAC7	0.62 ± 0.04$^{*△}$	0.56 ± 0.04*	4.10 ± 0.25$^{*△}$	2.84 ± 0.21$^{*△}$	66.69 ± 3.1$^{*△}$	30.74 ± 2.2$^{*△}$	20.74 ± 1.02*	20.38 ± 1.07*	37.18 ± 2.84
DM	0.52 ± 0.07*	0.53 ± 0.07*	4.76 ± 0.28*	3.58 ± 0.24*	57.21 ± 5.3*	24.75 ± 3.2*	21.08 ± 0.99*	21.22 ± 3.14*	48.60 ± 2.30*
p value[a]	0.585	0.008	<0.0001	<0.0001	<0.0001	<0.0001	<0.0001	<0.0001	0.384

Notes: No significant differences were found between control and NAC only group; *Compared with control, p < 0.05; $^{△}$NAC treatment groups compared with DM group, p < 0.05; a, ANOVA test among the NAC1, NAC3, NAC5 and NAC7 four groups; IVSd and LVEPWd, interventricular septal thickness and left ventricular posterior wall thickness during diastole; LVIDd and LVIDs, left ventricular internal diameter during diastole and systole; LVEF, left ventricular ejection fraction; LVFS, left ventricular fractional shortening; IVRT, isovolumic relaxation time; E_{DT}, descending time of the transmitral Doppler E wave; E_{AT}, acceleration time of the transmitral Doppler E wave

Approximately 27 % of cells in the myocardium are fibroblasts [16], indicating that increased ROS in fibroblasts might be important in fibrosis and subsequent cardiac dysfunction. Consistent with the increase of NAC in DM group, Masson Trichrome staining revealed that the fibrotic area was significantly larger than that in the control group. NAC1 nearly attenuated the fibrosis induced by diabetes, while NAC3, NAC5 and NAC7 groups had weaker effects (Fig. 4a-g).

NAC inhibits high glucose induced fibroblast proliferation and collagen synthesis

Per the overt effects of NAC on cardiac fibrosis, we next tested the role of NAC on cardiac fibroblast proliferation and collagen synthesis. Isolated cardiac fibroblast cells were cultured in normal and high glucose medium. Compared with the normal glucose medium, high glucose slightly stimulated the fibroblast proliferation, which was totally blocked by NAC treatment (Fig. 5a). Besides the pro-proliferative role of high glucose on cardiac fibroblasts, high glucose also increased TGFβ1 induced expression of Col1a1 and CTGF (Fig. 5b-c). Again,

NAC attenuated the Col1a1 and CTGF expression induced by TGFβ1.

Discussion

By using the STZ induced diabetes mouse model, we systematically analyzed the function of NAC, a potent inhibitor of ROS, in preventing cardiac dysfunction. To our knowledge, we for the first time revealed that: earlier and longer NAC treatment improves both the systolic and diastolic function, which is coincided with the reduced ROS generation and fibrosis.

It has been suggested that oxidative stress plays a critical role in inducing cardiomyopathy and heart failure in chronic diabetes [17–19]. Oxidative stress results from an imbalance between the generation of oxygen derived radicals and the organism's antioxidant potential [20]. Various studies have shown that DM is associated with increased formation of free radicals and decrease in antioxidant potential. Increased oxidative stress has been suggested to be a common pathway linking diverse mechanisms for the pathogenesis of complications in diabetes [21, 22]. Previous studies have showed

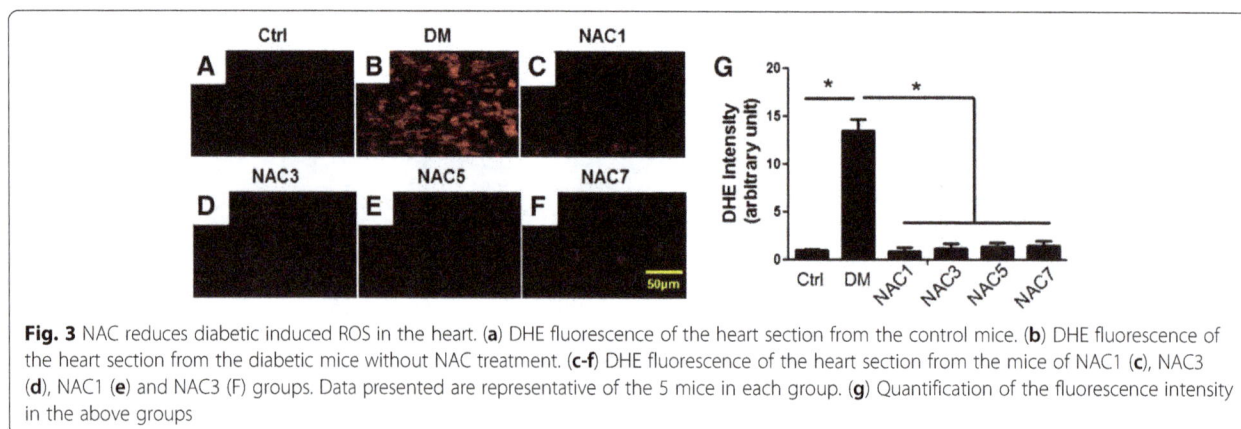

Fig. 3 NAC reduces diabetic induced ROS in the heart. (**a**) DHE fluorescence of the heart section from the control mice. (**b**) DHE fluorescence of the heart section from the diabetic mice without NAC treatment. (**c-f**) DHE fluorescence of the heart section from the mice of NAC1 (**c**), NAC3 (**d**), NAC1 (**e**) and NAC3 (F) groups. Data presented are representative of the 5 mice in each group. (**g**) Quantification of the fluorescence intensity in the above groups

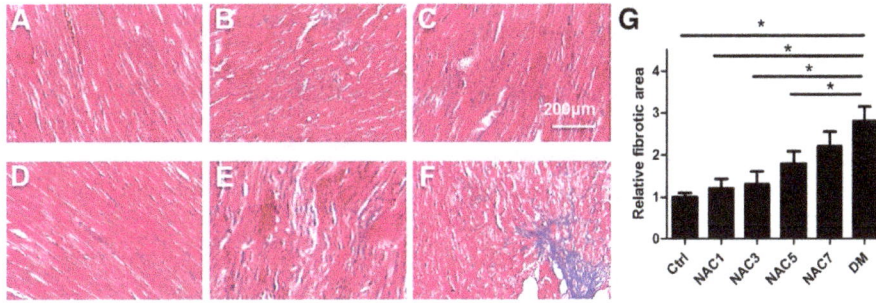

Fig. 4 Masson Trichrome staining of interstitial fibrosis in different groups. (a-f) Masson Trichrome staining of the heart section from control (a), NAC1 (b), NAC3 (c), NAC5 (d), NAC7 (e) and DM (f) groups. Data presented are representative of the 5 mice in each group. (g) Quantification data of Figure a-f

that increased ROS could lead to apoptosis in both endothelial cells and cardiomyocytes [8, 23], which are considered as the main causes of cardiac dysfunction. In fact, both endothelial and cardiomyocyte apoptosis would result in fibrosis, a kind of remodeling and repair. Our study here also found that ROS could directly promote fibrosis via promoting fibroblast proliferation and collagen synthesis in the setting of diabetes. In fact, the role of ROS in fibroblast activation has been found in the diseased prostatic stroma and other systems [24], further strengthening the role of ROS activated fibroblast in cardiac dysfunction. However, it is unknown how much fibrosis contributes to the diabetic cardiomyopathy, especially when endothelial cell and cardiomyocyte apoptosis is considered. It is highly possible that endothelium and cardiomyocyte apoptosis, and fibroblast activation form a viscous cycle that resulting in cardiomyopathy. And targeting the viscous is of therapeutic potential.

In this study, we found that NAC1 treatment group improved cardiac function much more than other NAC groups. Although previous studies have documented that NAC treatment suppressed ventricular structural and functional remodeling of the DM cardiomyopathy [5, 8]. Besides the evasive cardiac protection mechanism of NAC in the diabetic mice talked above, the time window of NAC action is unknown. The current study demonstrates that NAC 1 treatment, which NAC supplementation is earlier and longer results in the better cardiac outcomes than any other NAC treatment groups. One of the explanation is that toxic ROS generation begins and persists as early as onset of diabetes. In that case, longer and earlier NAC treatment would be beneficial.

Limitations

Notably, there are several limitations to this study. First, although we stress the importance of ROS in fibroblast and fibrosis, we still don't know how much the ROS-fibrosis contributes to the myocardiopathy in diabetes,

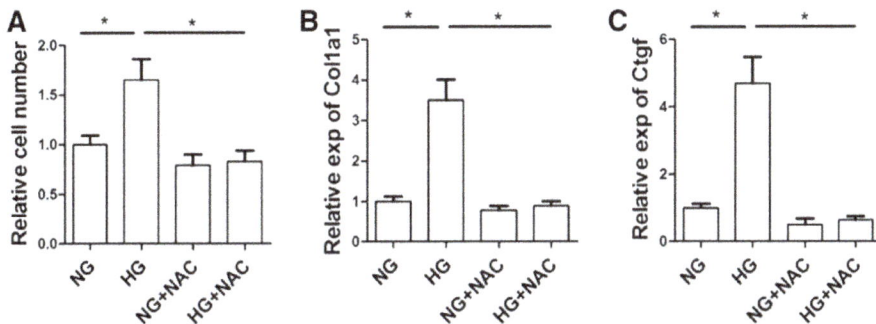

Fig. 5 Effects of NAC on high glucose induced fibroblast proliferation and collagen expression. (a) Cardiac fibroblast cells were cultured in 5.5 mM glucose (NG) and 25 mM glucose (HG) w/o 5 mM NAC. Viable cell numbers were calculated by CCK-8 kit. *p<0.05, n=3. (b) Col1a1 gene expression in cardiac fibroblasts cultured in serum free medium with 10 ng/ml TGFβ1 containing 5.5 mM glucose, 25 mM glucose with/o 5 mM NAC. *p<0.05, n=3. (c) CTGF gene expression in cardiac fibroblasts treated same as above. *p<0.05, n=3

especially their roles relative to the effects of ROS on cardiomyocytes and endothelial cells. Future studies by using fibrosis inhibitors would produce more informative data. Secondly, we haven't clarified the earlier or longer treatment of NAC in NAC1 group is better. Future studies comparing treatments with the same duration and different starting time point would possibly answer the question. Thirdly, we don't know whether NAC has a therapeutic function besides the preventive effects [17].

Conclusions

Increase of ROS plays an important role in the development of the ventricular remodeling and cardiomyopathy in the setting of diabetes. NAC treatment in diabetes effectively improves the cardiac function, either by preventing from diabetic cardiomyopathy or rescuing the cardiac function, which needs further clarification.

Abbreviations

DM: Diabetes Mellitus; ROS: Reactive Oxygen Species; NAC: N-Acetyl-L-Cysteine; STZ: Streptozocin; HE: Hematoxylin Eosin; IVSd: Interventricular Septal Thickness during Diastole; LVPWd: Left Ventricular Posterior Wall Thickness during Diastole; LVIDd: Left Ventricular Internal Dimensions during Diastole; LVIDs: Left Ventricular Internal Dimensions during Systole; LVEF: Left Ventricular Ejection Fraction; LVFS: Left Ventricular Fractional Shortening; IVRT: Isovolumic Relaxation Time; E: Peak Early Diastolic Transmitral Doppler Flow Velocity; E_{AT}: Acceleration Time of E wave; E_{DT}: Deceleration Time of E Wave; DHE: Dihydroethidium; HG: Glucose; HWI: Heart Weight Index.

Competing interests

The authors declare that they have no competing interests.

Authors' contributions

The contributions of individual authors to this paper were as follows. Dr. LC, LXZ, YLJ, DYY participated in 1. The conception and design, acquisition, analysis and interpretation of data, development of the hypothesis and research plan, establishment of methodology; 2. Drafting of the manuscript and critical revision of the manuscript for intellectual content and 3. Final approval of the version to be published. SMZ, XCY and MJ involved in 1. Acquisition of data, analysis and interpretation of data; 2. Assistance with revising the manuscript and 3. Final approval of the version to be published. All authors read and approved the final manuscript.

Acknowledgements

This study was supported by National Science Foundation of China (NSFC: 81101050, NSFC: 81170149 and NSFC: 81370275).

Author details

[1]Department of Ultrasound Diagnostics, Tangdu Hospital, Fourth Military Medical University, #569 Xinsi RoadBaqiao District, Xi'an 710038, China. [2]Department of Biochemistry and Molecular Biology, Fourth Military Medical University, Xi'an, China.

References

1. Whiting DR, Guariguata L, Weil C, Shaw J. IDF diabetes atlas: global estimates of the prevalence of diabetes for 2011 and 2030. Diabetes Res Clin Pract. 2011;94(3):311–21.
2. Rajesh M, Mukhopadhyay P, Batkai S, Mukhopadhyay B, Patel V, Hasko G, et al. Xanthine oxidase inhibitor allopurinol attenuates the development of diabetic cardiomyopathy. J Cell Mol Med. 2009;13(8B):2330–41.
3. Takeda N, Manabe I. Cellular Interplay between Cardiomyocytes and Nonmyocytes in Cardiac Remodeling. Int J Inflamm. 2011;2011:535241.
4. Brown RD, Ambler SK, Mitchell MD, Long CS. The cardiac fibroblast: therapeutic target in myocardial remodeling and failure. Annu Rev Pharmacol Toxicol. 2005;45:657–87.
5. Asbun J, Villarreal FJ. The pathogenesis of myocardial fibrosis in the setting of diabetic cardiomyopathy. J Am Coll Cardiol. 2006;47(4):693–700.
6. Tanaka K, Honda M, Takabatake T. Redox regulation of MAPK pathways and cardiac hypertrophy in adult rat cardiac myocyte. J Am Coll Cardiol. 2001;37(2):676–85.
7. Cailleret M, Amadou A, Andrieu-Abadie N, Nawrocki A, Adamy C, Ait-Mamar B, et al. N-acetylcysteine prevents the deleterious effect of tumor necrosis factor-(alpha) on calcium transients and contraction in adult rat cardiomyocytes. Circulation. 2004;109(3):406–11.
8. Fiordaliso F, Bianchi R, Staszewsky L, Cuccovillo I, Doni M, Laragione T, et al. Antioxidant treatment attenuates hyperglycemia-induced cardiomyocyte death in rats. Mol Cell Cardiol. 2004;37(5):959–68.
9. Luo M, Guan X, Luczak ED, Lang D, Kutschke W, Gao Z, et al. Diabetes increases mortality after myocardial infarction by oxidizing CaMKII. J Clin Invest. 2013;123(3):1262–74.
10. Tremoleda JL, Kerton A, Gsell W. Anaesthesia and physiological monitoring during in vivo imaging of laboratory rodents: considerations on experimental outcomes and animal welfare. EJNMMI Research. 2012;2(1):44.
11. Schiller NB, Shah PM, Crawford M, DeMaria A, Devereux R, Feigenbaum H, et al. Recommendations for quantitation of the left ventricle by two-dimensional echocardiography. American Society of Echocardiography Committee on Standards, Subcommittee on Quantitation of Two-Dimensional Echocardiograms. J Am Soc Echocardiogr. 1989;2(5):358–67.
12. Du J, Liu J, Feng HZ, Hossain MM, Gobara N, Zhang C, et al. Impaired relaxation is the main manifestation in transgenic mice expressing a restrictive cardiomyopathy mutation, R193H, in cardiac TnI. Am J Physiol Heart Circ Physiol. 2008;294(6):H2604–2613.
13. Connelly KA, Kelly DJ, Zhang Y, Prior DL, Martin J, Cox AJ, et al. Functional, structural and molecular aspects of diastolic heart failure in the diabetic (mRen-2)27 rat. Cardiovasc Res. 2007;76(2):280–91.
14. Yong QC, Thomas CM, Seqqat R, Chandel N, Baker KM, Kumar R. Angiotensin type 1a receptor-deficient mice develop diabetes-induced cardiac dysfunction, which is prevented by renin-angiotensin system inhibitors. Cardiovasc Diabetol. 2013;12:169.
15. Frangogiannis NG, Dewald O, Xia Y, Ren G, Haudek S, Leucker T, et al. Critical role of monocyte chemoattractant protein-1/CC chemokine ligand 2 in the pathogenesis of ischemic cardiomyopathy. Circulation. 2007;115(5):584–92.
16. Banerjee I, Fuseler JW, Price RL, Borg TK, Baudino TA. Determination of cell types and numbers during cardiac development in the neonatal and adult rat and mouse. Am J Physiol Heart Circ Physiol. 2007;293(3):H1883–1891.
17. Xu YJ, Tappia PS, Neki NS, Dhalla NS. Prevention of diabetes-induced cardiovascular complications upon treatment with antioxidants. Heart Fail Rev. 2014;19(1):113–21.
18. Dhalla NS, Rangi S, Zieroth S, Xu YJ. Alterations in sarcoplasmic reticulum and mitochondrial functions in diabetic cardiomyopathy. Exp Clin Cardiol. 2012;17(3):115–20.
19. Ceriello A, Motz E. Is oxidative stress the pathogenic mechanism underlying insulin resistance, diabetes, and cardiovascular disease? The common soil hypothesis revisited. Arterioscler Thromb Vasc Biol. 2004;24(5):816–23.
20. Abdollahi M, Ranjbar A, Shadnia S, Nikfar S, Rezaie A. Pesticides and oxidative stress: a review. Med Sci Monit. 2004;10(6):RA141–147.

21. Shih CC, Wu YW, Lin WC. Antihyperglycaemic and anti-oxidant properties of Anoectochilus formosanus in diabetic rats. Clin Exp Pharmacol Physiol. 2002;29(8):684–8.
22. Naziroglu M, Butterworth PJ. Protective effects of moderate exercise with dietary vitamin C and E on blood antioxidative defense mechanism in rats with streptozotocin-induced diabetes. Can J Appl Physiol. 2005;30(2):172–85.
23. Shaw A, Doherty MK, Mutch NJ, MacRury SM, Megson IL. Endothelial cell oxidative stress in diabetes: a key driver of cardiovascular complications? Biochem Soc Trans. 2014;42(4):928–33.
24. Sampson N, Koziel R, Zenzmaier C, Bubendorf L, Plas E, Jansen-Durr P, et al. ROS signaling by NOX4 drives fibroblast-to-myofibroblast differentiation in the diseased prostatic stroma. Mol Endocrinol. 2011;25(3):503–15.

9

Effects of ventricular conduction block patterns on mortality in hospitalized patients with dilated cardiomyopathy

Xiaoping Li[1,2*†], Rong Luo[3†], Wei Fang[1], Xiaolei Xu[4], Guodong Niu[2], Yixian Xu[5], Michael Fu[6], Wei Hua[2*] and Xiushan Wu[7]

Abstract

Background: Ventricular conduction blocks (VCBs) are associated with poor outcomes in patients with known cardiac diseases. However, the prognostic implications of VCB patterns in dilated cardiomyopathy (DCM) patients need to be evaluated. The purpose of this study was to determine all-cause mortality in patients with DCM and VCB.

Methods: This cohort study included 1119 DCM patients with a median follow-up of 34.3 (19.5–60.8) months, patients were then divided into left bundle branch block (LBBB), right bundle branch block (RBBB), intraventricular conduction delays (IVCD) and narrow QRS groups. The all-cause mortality was assessed using Kaplan-Meier survival curves and Cox regression.

Results: Of those 1119 patients, the all-cause mortality rates were highest in patients with IVCD (47.8, $n = 32$), intermediate in those with RBBB (32.9, $n = 27$) and LBBB (27.1 %, $n = 60$), and lowest in those with narrow QRS (19.9 %, $n = 149$). The all-cause mortality risk was significantly different between the VCB and narrow QRS group (log-rank $\chi2 = 51.564$, $P < 0.001$). The presence of RBBB, IVCD, PASP ≥ 40 mmHg, left atrium diameter and NYHA functional class were independent predictors of all-cause mortality in DCM patients.

Conclusions: Our findings indicate that RBBB and IVCD at admission,but not LBBB, were independent predictors of all-cause mortality in patients with DCM.

Keywords: Ventricular conduction block, Dilated cardiomyopathy, Pulmonary hypertension, Survival, Prognosis

Background

Dilated cardiomyopathy (DCM), a leading cause of heart failure and arrhythmia, is a disease of the heart muscle characterized by ventricular dilation and impaired systolic function. The prognosis in patients with DCM is poor. However, the clinical spectrum is wide, and it is difficult for physicians to predict which clinical course an individual patient may follow.

Patients with DCM present with an increase in the QRS duration in the presence of a ventricular conduction block (VCB) [1–3]. There is controversy regarding the type of bundle branch block (BBB) that is associated with poorer outcomes in patients with heart failure (HF) [4–8]. Most studies indicate that left BBB (LBBB) is an independent prognostic marker, whereas right BBB (RBBB) is a weaker marker or not associated with a worse prognosis. Conversely, two studies recently showed that RBBB but not LBBB is associated with an increased 1-year and 4-year mortality risk in hospitalized patients with HF [9, 10]. Patients with

* Correspondence: lixiaoping0119@163.com; drhua@aliyun.com
†Equal contributors
[1]Department of Cardiology, Sichuan Academy of Medical Sciences and Sichuan Provincial People's Hospital, Hospital of the University of Electronic Science and Technology of China, Chengdu, Sichuan 610072, China
[2]Cardiac Arrhythmia Center, State Key Laboratory of Cardiovascular Disease, Cardiovascular Institute and Fuwai Hospital, National Center for Cardiovascular Diseases, Chinese Academy of Medical Sciences and Peking Union Medical College, Beijing 100037, People's Republic of China
Full list of author information is available at the end of the article

intraventricular conduction delays (IVCDs) can also present with DCM, often without specifying the particular type of BBB. These patients also have worse clinical outcomes [1–3].

The prognostic implications of VCB in the long-term mortality of patients with DCM merit examination due to the lack of data on this issue. Therefore, in the present study, we evaluated the association of VCB patterns and all-cause mortality and compared the prognostic values of RBBB, LBBB, and IVCD in hospitalized patients with DCM.

Subjects and methods

Patients and follow-up

This study was a retrospective, observational cohort study of patients with DCM observed from November 2003 to September 2011. VCB (LBBB, RBBB, IVCD) were identified from records of individual 12-lead ECGs in 1317 patients (Fig. 1). The patients were admitted due to their decompensation symptoms and the physical signs of heart failure, and DCM was defined as systolic dysfunction with LV dilation in the absence of an apparent secondary cause of cardiomyopathy [11]. We measured the following DCM

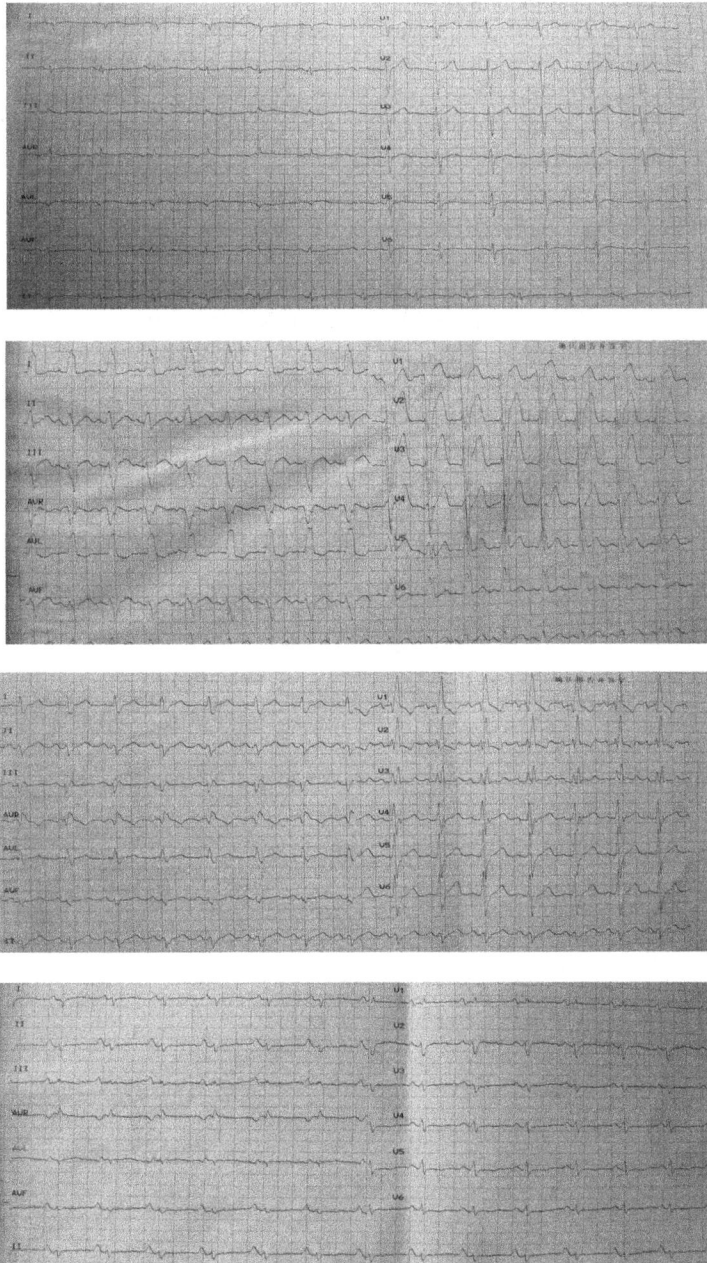

Fig. 1 An example figure of narrow QRS, LBBB, RBBB, and IVCD

exclusion criteria [12, 13]: systemic hypertension (>160/ 100 mmHg), coronary artery disease (>50 % in one or more major branches), chronic excess alcohol consumption (>40 g/day for females, > 80 g/day for males for more than five years after 6 months of abstinence), systemic diseases known to cause IDC, pericardial diseases, congenital heart disease, cor pulmonale, and rapid, sustained supraventricular tachycardia. Of the 1317 enrolled patients, 23 patients with missing electrocardiograph test results and 175 patients with various secondary cardiomyopathies were excluded from the study. The secondary cardiomyopathies included the following: 80 patients with ischemic heart disease by coronary angiography; 26 patients with overt hyper- and hypothyroidism thyroid disease; 24 patients with alcohol-induced cardiomyopathy; 16 patients with congenital heart disease; 16 patients with left ventricle noncompaction; 7 patients with chronic anemia (hemoglobin <60 g/L); 2 patients with peripartum cardiomyopathy; and 4 patients with rheumatic heart disease or systemic immune disease (Fig. 2). Thus, the final analysis included 1119 patients. The primary end point of the study was all-cause mortality, which was assessed for all patients through their medical records (patient's hospital records, periodically examining the patient in the outpatient clinic) and medical follow-up calls with trained personnel. Data from patients who underwent cardiac transplantation were censored at the time of transplantation. The median follow-up period was 34.3 (19.5–60.8) months, and the study protocol was approved by the Ethics Commission of Fuwai Hospital.

Echocardiography

The patients were imaged in the left lateral decubitus position using a commercially available system equipped with a 3.5 MHz transducer. Two-dimensional gray-scale, pulsed, continuous, color Doppler data were acquired from the parasternal and apical views. The left ventricular ejection fraction (LVEF) was calculated using the biplane Simpson's technique.

Because pulmonary artery systolic pressure (PASP) is equal to the right ventricular systolic pressure in the absence of pulmonary stenosis, PASP was estimated using Doppler echocardiography by calculating the right ventricular to right atrial pressure gradient during systole (approximated by the modified Bernoulli equation as $4v^2$, where v is the velocity of the tricuspid regurgitation jet in m/s). Right atrial pressure, estimated based on the echocardiographic characteristics of the inferior vena cava and assigned a standardized value, was then added to the calculated gradient to give PASP. According to the new guideline, presence of PASP ≥ 40 mmHg was likely to be pulmonary hypertension (PH) [14].

Statistical analyses

Continuous variables are expressed as the means ± SDs or medians and interquartile ranges. The categorical variables among groups were compared using chi-square (χ^2) tests. Analysis of variance was used to compare continuous variables among multiple groups. Hazard ratios with 95 % confidence intervals were used to estimate the adjusted relative risk of the VCB groups. The Kaplan-Meier

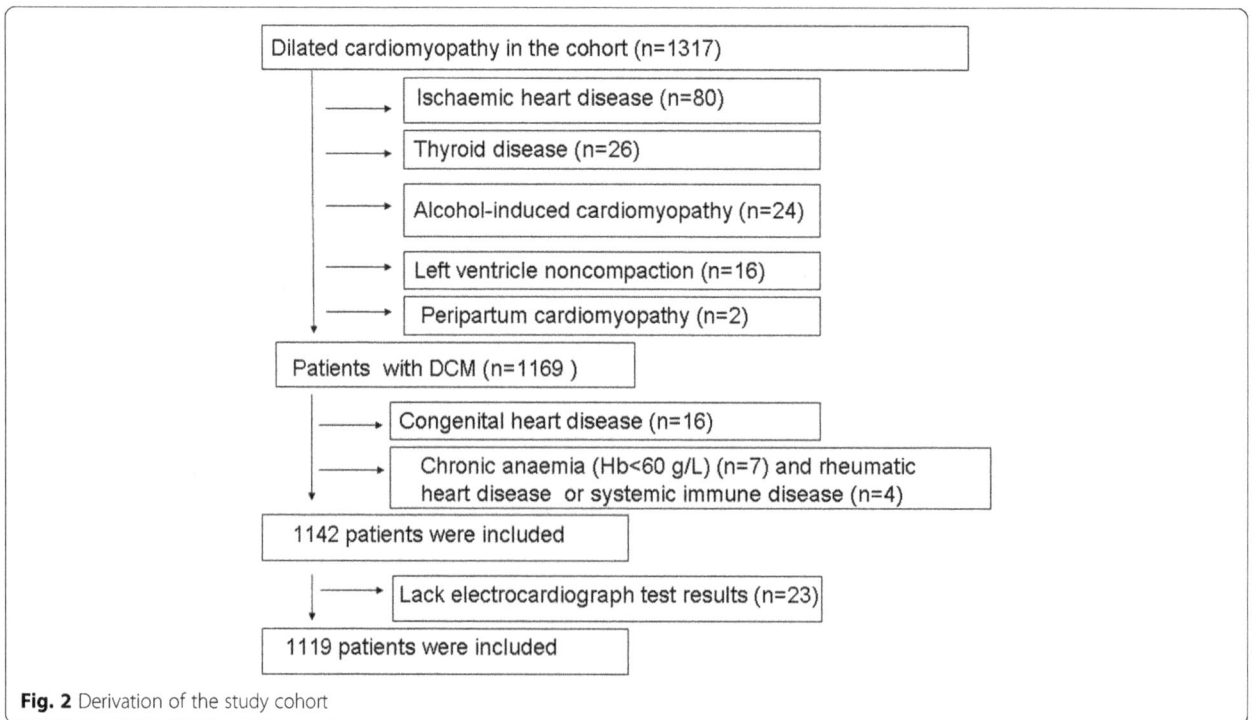

Fig. 2 Derivation of the study cohort

survival curves were compared using the log-rank test. Multivariate Cox proportional hazards regression models were used to adjust for any confounding variables among groups. First, the potential variables were evaluated by univariate analysis and were then selected based on their clinical and statistical significance. Second, a multivariate analysis was performed using Cox proportional hazards regression modelling adjusted for baseline variables. SPSS version 16.0 software (SPSS, Chicago, Illinois) was used for all statistical analyses. All of the tests were two-sided, and a p value < 0.05 was used to determine statistical significance.

Results

Characteristics of the study population

The cohort consisted of 1119 patients with DCM: 298 (26.6) women and 821 (73.4) men; 1076 (96.2) were from the Han population and 43 (3.8 %) were from other races: the mean age was 51.1 ± 14.7 years. Of those, 19.8 ($n = 221$) had LBBB, 7.3 ($n = 82$) had RBBB, 6.0 ($n = 67$) had IVCD, and 66.9 % ($n = 749$) had narrow QRS. Table 1 summarizes the baseline clinical characteristics of the cohort. Among the patients with VCBs (LBBB, RBBB and IVCD) and narrow QRS, the number of women with RBBB was lower, and there was a lower frequency of a history of hypertension but a greater frequency of PASP ≥ 40 mmHg in patients with RBBB. Patients with LBBB were older, were predominantly male, had more frequent essential hypertension and had longer QRS durations, QT intervals and larger LV diameters. The patients with IVCD had higher levels of circulating bilirubin, larger left atriums (LAs), larger right ventricle (RV) diameters, longer PR intervals, and less use of beta blockers, aspirin and spironolactone during admission.

Relation between VCB patterns and all-cause mortality

Among the 1119 patients studied, 268 died and 3 underwent heart transplantation during a median follow-up of 34.3 (19.5–60.8) months. The all-cause mortality rates were highest in patients with IVCD (47.8 %, $n = 32$); intermediate in patients with RBBB (32.9, $n = 27$) and LBBB (27.1 %, $n = 60$); and lowest in patients with narrow QRS (19.9 %, $n = 149$). Over the median of 34.3 month follow-up, there was a significant difference in all-cause mortality risk between the VCB and narrow QRS groups (log-rank $\chi^2 = 51.564$, $P < 0.001$) (Fig. 3).

Cox proportional hazard models

Table 2 summarizes the results of the Cox models in which each of the parameters were entered separately as the mortality explanatory variable. The univariate analysis indicated that age, history of essential hypertension and atrial fibrillation (AF), NYHA functional classes, disease duration, systolic blood pressure, diastolic blood pressure, LV, LA diameters, LVEF, PASP ≥ 40 mmHg, and the presence of LBBB, RBBB and IVCD were predictors of all-cause mortality in DCM patients. After adjustments for age, gender, history of essential hypertension and AF, smoking and drinking status, disease duration, blood pressure, heart rate, LV diameter and LVEF value, using either forward or backward selection, and the presence of RBBB, IVCD, PASP ≥ 40 mmHg, the NYHA functional class and LA diameter were the only variables that remained in the model and emerged as important predictors. However, unlike RBBB and IVCD, LBBB was not a predictor of death using the multivariate analysis.

Discussion

In this study, we investigated the associations among different patterns of VCB and all-cause mortality in patients with DCM. Our major new finding suggests that RBBB and IVCD upon admission, but not LBBB, were strong predictors of all-cause mortality in patients with DCM.

Several studies investigating the predictive value of QRS morphology in patients with HF yielded conflicting results regarding mortality risk associated with the BBB pattern [4–7]. Baldasseroni et al. [5, 6] reported that complete LBBB, but not RBBB, was associated with a higher adjusted 1-year mortality rate in 5,517 outpatients with HF. McCullough et al. [4] found higher 2-year mortality rates for RBBB and LBBB compared with patients with normal QRS, but a multivariate analysis demonstrated that RBBB was not as powerful a predictor of mortality as LBBB. Most recently, Mueller et al. [7] analyzed the impact of the BBB pattern on long-term mortality and found that the mortality was significantly higher in HF patients with RBBB. Two studies recently showed that RBBB, but not LBBB, is associated with increased mortality risk in HF patients [9, 10]. None of these studies, however, reported the relationship between RBBB and mortality risk in the patients with DCM. In the present study, we found that RBBB and IVCD patients with DCM had a higher all-cause mortality than patients with LBBB, and patients with any pattern of VCB had higher all-cause mortality rates than patients with a narrow QRS. A multivariate analysis demonstrated that RBBB and IVCD, but not LBBB, were the predictors of all-cause mortality in patients with DCM.

Approximately 30% of patients with heart failure or cardiomyopathy have VCBs, such as left or right bundle-branch blocks [5, 9]. Some studies have shown that in patients with HF, the prevalence of LBBB is higher than in patients with RBBB [4, 5, 7]. LBBB is associated with more severe HF characterized by an advanced NYHA functional class and decreased LVEF, whereas RBBB is more prevalent in men and is not associated with advanced HF symptoms or ventricular dysfunction [5, 6].

Table 1 Patient characteristics categorized by ventricular conduction block patterns

	All patients (n = 1119)	LBBB (n = 221)	RBBB (n = 82)	IVCD (n = 67)	Narrow QRS (n = 749)	P value
Age (years)	51.1 ± 14.7	57.2 ± 12.0	53.1 ± 14.7	52.3 ± 14.5	48.9 ± 14.9	**<0.001**[a]
Female gender, n (%)	298(26.6)	89(40.3)	16(19.5)	15(22.4)	178(23.8)	**<0.001**
History						
Disease duration (years)	2(0.5–6)	4(1–9)	4(1–8)	3(1.5–6)	2(0.35–5)	**0.001**
Essential hypertension, n (%)	294(26.3)	73(33.0)	15(18.3)	15(22.4)	191(25.5)	**0.034**
Diabetes mellitus, n (%)	160(14.3)	24(10.9)	15(18.3)	6(9.0)	115(15.4)	0.142
Atrial fibrillation, n (%)	257(23.0)	29(13.1)	20(24.4)	11(16.4)	197(26.3)	**<0.001**
Smoker, n (%)	517(46.2)	93(42.1)	33(40.2)	31(46.3)	360(48.1)	0.293
Drinker, n (%)	363(32.4)	59(26.7)	28(34.1)	22(32.8)	254(33.9)	0.243
NYHA class III and IV[c], n (%)	817(73.0)	162(73.3)	60(73.2)	54(80.6)	541(72.2)	0.532
Admission vital signs						
SBP (mm Hg)	113.0 ± 17.7	114.6 ± 17.3	110.2 ± 18.8	111.7 ± 19.8	113.0 ± 17.4	0.242
DBP(mm Hg)	72.5 ± 12.6	71.8 ± 12.4	71.8 ± 11.1	69.3 ± 12.4	73.0 + 12.8	0.099
Heart rate, beat/min	80.9 ± 17.4	78.3 ± 15.9	79.6 ± 15.5	78.6 ± 14.4	82.0 ± 18.2	**0.023**
Laboratory values at admission[b]						
TB (mmol/L)	26.2 ± 19.6	24.9 ± 19.1	25.3 ± 16.0	34.8 ± 26.7	26.0 ± 19.3	**0.004**
DB (mmol/L)	3.7(2.5–6.5)	3.2(2.15–6.05)	3.5(2.7–7.4)	4.9(3.2–9.2)	3.7(2.5–6.485)	**0.003**
Glucose (mmol/L)	5.62 ± 1.85	5.86 ± 1.94	5.50 ± 1.52	5.34 ± 1.44	5.59 ± 1.89	0.150
Triglyceride (mmol/L)	1.57 ± 1.02	1.63 ± 0.99	1.58 ± 0.94	1.38 ± 0.70	1.56 ± 1.06	0.410
Total cholesterol (mmol/L)	4.61 ± 1.13	4.75 ± 1.12	4.52 ± 0.98	4.39 ± 1.23	4.59 ± 1.14	0.125
Creatinine (μmol/L)	92.8 ± 35.2	91.0 ± 26.4	94.9 ± 25.9	97.9 ± 40.7	92.6 ± 37.8	0.526
BUN (μmol/L)	7.95 ± 3.97	7.88 ± 2.67	8.04 ± 2.69	8.89 ± 4.68	7.88 ± 4.32	0.262
CK-MB (IU/L)	13.5 ± 7.76	13.1 ± 6.77	12.0 ± 6.70	13.7 ± 7.59	13.8 ± 8.14	0.229
NT- Pro- BNP (fmol/mL)	2010.3 ± 1567.5	1998.0 ± 1595.8	2170.5 ± 1679.8	2358.4 ± 1638.4	1962.4 ± 1538.0	0.315
Electrocardiogram data						
QRS duration (ms)	119.6 ± 30.9	156.0 ± 24.4	153.3 ± 24.9	137.1 ± 23.1	103.6 ± 18.2	**<0.001**
QT (ms)	405.7 ± 54.2	434.4 ± 50.6	429.1 ± 51.1	421.3 ± 38.7	393.2 ± 52.4	**<0.001**
P (ms)	107.5 ± 21.6	102.7 ± 22.6	107.5 ± 23.6	108.2 ± 25.1	109.3 ± 20.3	**0.005**
PR (ms)	182.8 ± 32.9	184.9 ± 33.1	192.3 ± 42.0	193.6 ± 34.7	179.7 ± 30.7	**0.001**
Echocardiography data						
LV (mm)	68.0 ± 9.3	71.4 ± 11.4	68.7 ± 8.3	70.9 ± 13.1	66.7 ± 8.0	**<0.001**
LVEF (%)	31.9 ± 8.4	31.0 ± 8.2	31.8 ± 7.3	30.5 ± 9.0	32.3 ± 8.5	0.142
RV (mm)	23.6 ± 5.4	22.0 ± 5.0	24.1 ± 5.6	24.5 ± 5.5	24.0 ± 5.4	**<0.001**
LA (mm)	43.9 ± 7.7	43.1 ± 7.9	45.8 ± 8.4	46.6 ± 8.9	43.7 ± 7.5	**0.002**
PASP (>40 mmHg), n (%)	203(18.1)	35(15.8)	24(29.3)	15(22.4)	129(17.2)	**0.031**
Medicine during admission						
Diuretics, n (%)	1059(94.6)	205(92.8)	76(92.7)	63(94.0)	715(95.5)	0.362
ACEI/ARB, n (%)	951(85.0)	182(82.4)	70(85.4)	54(80.6)	645(86.1)	0.396
Beta-blockers, n (%)	1017(90.9)	195(88.2)	69(84.1)	56(83.6)	697(93.1)	**0.002**
Digoxin, n (%)	903(80.7)	168(76.0)	66(80.5)	59(88.1)	610(81.4)	0.127
Aspirin/anticoagulants n (%)	721(64.4)	131(59.3)	52(63.4)	34(50.7)	504(67.3)	**0.013**
Spironolactone, n (%)	1019(91.1)	191(86.4)	73(89.0)	57(85.1)	698(93.2)	**0.004**

[a]Data are expressed as the means ± SDs or medians (interquartile ranges) or as percentages, P values from an ANOVA or chi-square test for all four groups. Bold data indicated P <0.05

[b]Thirty-four patients lacked echocardiography data; 47 patients lacked data on PASP; 341 patients lacked NT-pro-BNP levels; 52 patients lacked fasting blood glucose levels; 46 patients lacked creatinine and BUN levels; 51 patients lacked CK-MB levels; and 89 patients lacked triglyceride and total cholesterol levels

[c]Abbreviations: NYHA New York Heart Association, SBP systolic blood pressure, DBP diastolic blood pressure, TB total bilirubin, DB direct bilirubin, BUN blood urea nitrogen, CK-MB heart-type creatine kinase isoenzyme, PASP pulmonary artery systolic pressure, NT-pro-BNP N-terminal fragment pro-brain natriuretic peptide, LV left ventricle, LA left atrium, LVEF left ventricular ejection fraction, ACEI angiotension-converting enzyme inhibitor, ARB angiotension receptor blocker

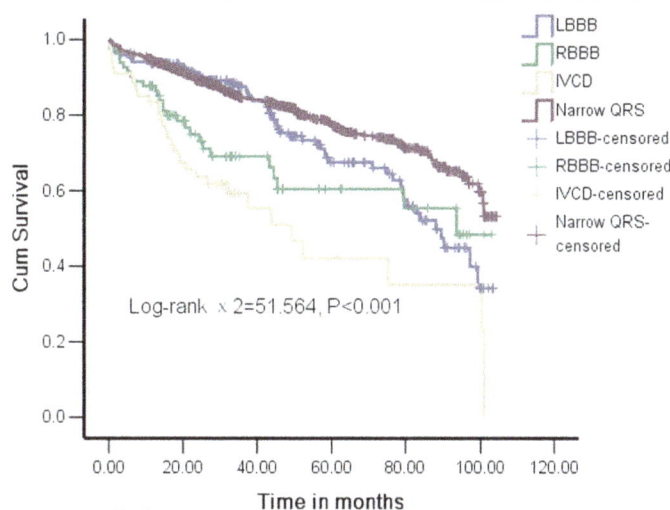

Fig. 3 Kaplan-Meier survival curves for patients with DCM: patients with LBBB, RBBB, IVCD and narrow QRS (log-rank $\chi^2 = 51.564$, $P < 0.001$). Abbreviations: DCM, dilated cardiomyopathy; VCB, Ventricular conduction block; LBBB, left bundle branch block; RBBB, right bundle branch block; IVCD, intraventricular conduction delay

In our study, the prevalence of VCB was 33.1 %; more patients had LBBB than RBBB or IVCD. Patients with LBBB had longer QRS durations, larger LV diameters and lower LVEF values than those with RBBB. However, patients with RBBB had more frequent of PASP ≥ 40 mmHg, along with larger RV diameters, than those with LBBB.

One of the reasons for a worse prognosis in patients with RBBB may be that they have an elevated pulmonary pressure compared with those with LBBB or a narrow QRS. Acquired RBBB is often associated with PH and right-sided cardiac failure, and PH complicated by heart failure is generally considered to be an indicator of a poor prognosis [11, 15]. In addition, right ventricular dysfunction has an additive predictive value in patients with left ventricular systolic dysfunction [16]. Furthermore, RBBB may be a marker not only of right ventricular dysfunction but also of severe intraventricular desynchronization of both ventricles. Recently, Fantoni et al. [17] reported that patients with RBBB had larger right ventricle electrical conduction delays compared with patients with LBBB using electromagnetic, catheter-based, 3-dimensional mapping. In the present study, compared with LBBB, patients with RBBB had more frequent of PASP ≥ 40 mmHg, larger RV diameters and higher all-cause mortality rates during follow-up.

Very limited data exists on patients with IVCD. Patients with myocardial infarction with IVCD had significantly greater interventricular asynchronies and higher BNP levels than post-myocardial infarction patients without IVCD [18]. In the Multicenter Unsustained Tachycardia Trial (MUSTT), patients with LBBB or IVCD had lower ejection fractions and a higher prevalence of congestive heart failure than those without these abnormalities. The presence of IVCD was associated with a 1.5-fold increased risk of cardiac arrest and total mortality in the patients treated with cardiac resynchronization therapy (CRT) [8]. In another study on heart failure with CRT, the all-cause mortality was also higher in patients with IVCD than LBBB or RBBB; the worst prognosis was seen in patients with IVCD [19]. The reason for the higher mortality rates in patients with IVCD is unclear, and further research is needed to confirm the role of IVCD in DCM.

The present study has several limitations. Like all hospital-based cohorts, this is a selected population of patients who have been referred for treatment. As with many studies of chronic diseases, the time of disease onset is not precisely known, and there may be variations in the length of the preclinical phase that influences the relationship between IVCD, PH and death. Because the N-terminal pro-brain natriuretic peptide (NT-pro-BNP) test was not commonly used until the later years of this study and was missing in 341 patients, we excluded NT-pro-BNP from the multivariate Cox analysis to avoid potential confounding variables in the statistical analyses.

Table 2 Cox-regression of all-cause mortality in patients with DCM

Variable	Univariate analysis			Multivariate analysis		
	HR	95 % CI	P-value	HR	95 % CI	P-value
Age	1.012	1.003–1.021	**0.007**	1.007	0.997–1.018	0.175
Gender	1.154	0.883–1.507	0.294	1.255	0.894–1.761	0.189
Essential hypertension	0.706	0.524–0.951	**0.022**	0.810	0.579–1.134	0.220
Atrial fibrillation	1.317	1.004–1.728	**0.047**	1.247	0.909–1.710	0.172
NYHA functional classes	1.619	1.376–1.905	**<0.001**	1.248	1.038–1.499	**0.018**
Disease duration	1.027	1.011–1.044	**0.001**	1.015	0.996–1.033	0.121
Smoker	0.973	0.850–1.114	0.691	0.972	0.819–1.154	0.746
Drinker	0.893	0.766–1.040	0.146	0.913	0.756–1.103	0.346
Heart rate	1.002	0.995–1.009	0.604	1.004	0.996–1.013	0.311
Systolic blood pressure	0.982	0.975–0.989	**<0.001**	0.992	0.981–1.003	0.148
Diastolic blood pressure	0.979	0.969–0.989	**<0.001**	0.989	0.974–1.004	0.136
Left ventricle	1.039	1.027–1.053	**<0.001**	1.016	0.998–1.016	0.078
Left atrium	1.055	1.040–1.071	**<0.001**	1.041	1.022–1.060	**<0.001**
LVEF	0.965	0.951–0.980	**<0.001**	0.984	0.966–1.003	0.093
LBBB	1.408	1.043–1.900	**0.025**	1.197	0.839–1.706	0.321
RBBB	2.091	1.387–3.154	**<0.001**	2.553	1.665–3.913	**<0.001**
IVCD	3.488	2.376–5.122	**<0.001**	3.726	2.417–5.745	**<0.001**
PASP ≥ 40 mmHg	1.992	1.529–2.596	**<0.001**	1.403	1.040–1.893	**0.027**

Note: The variables analyzed in the multivariate Cox mode included age, gender, the history of essential hypertension and atrial fibrillation, drinking and smoking status, disease duration, NYHA functional classes, systolic blood pressure, diastolic blood pressure, heart rate, left ventricle, right ventricle, left atrium diameter, LVEF, LBBB, RBBB, IVCD and PASP ≥ 40 mmHg. Bold data indicated P <0.05

Ideally, all patients with DCM should be confirmed to be free of coronary artery disease. In practice, however, coronary arteriography is not routinely performed in all patients with congestive heart failure. Because retrospective studies cannot control the conditions under which patients are recruited or investigated, aside the patients who were once undertaken coronary artery angiography, coronary CT scan or cardiac radionuclide imaging in the other hospitals, there were only 334 patients undertaken coronary artery angiography and 80 patients with positive results in the present study. In addition, to exclude the confusion with ventricular hypertrophy, we defined patients with VCB as QRS duration more than 120 ms. Finally, the patients who creceived ICDs (implantable cardiac defibrillators) or CRTs were not included, and the use of spironolactone and digoxin was higher in the present study.

Conclusions

The present study indicated that RBBB and IVCD at admission were independent predictors of all-cause mortality in patients with DCM.

Acknowledgments

This study was supported by grants from the National Natural Science Foundation of China (no. 81000104, 81160141, 81470521).

Authors' contributions

XL, RL, GN and WFconducted the patients' enrollment, data collection and follow-up work. XL, XY and XX participated in the data collection and performed the statistical analysis. WH, XW, XX and MF conceived of the study and participated in its design and coordination, and they helped to draft the manuscript. All of the authors read and approved of the final manuscript.

Competing interests

The authors declare that they have no competing interests.

Author details

[1]Department of Cardiology, Sichuan Academy of Medical Sciences and Sichuan Provincial People's Hospital, Hospital of the University of Electronic Science and Technology of China, Chengdu, Sichuan 610072, China. [2]Cardiac Arrhythmia Center, State Key Laboratory of Cardiovascular Disease, Cardiovascular Institute and Fuwai Hospital, National Center for Cardiovascular Diseases, Chinese Academy of Medical Sciences and Peking Union Medical College, Beijing 100037, People's Republic of China. [3]Temperature and Inflammation Research Center, Key Laboratory of Colleges and Universities in Sichuan Province, Chengdu Medical College, Chengdu 610500, People's Republic of China. [4]Division of Cardiovascular Diseases, Mayo Clinic College of Medicine, Rochester, MN 55905, USA. [5]Department of Cardiology, Lanzhou University Second Hospital, Lanzhou, Gansu 730030, People's Republic of China. [6]Department of Medicine, Sahlgrenska University hospital/Östra hospital, Gothenburg, Sweden. [7]The Center of Heart Development, Key Lab of MOE for Development Biology and Protein Chemistry, College of Life Science, Hunan Normal University, Changsha 410081, People's Republic of China.

References

1. Bristow MR, Feldman AM, Saxon LA. Heart failure management using implantable devices for ventricular resynchronization: Comparison of

Medical Therapy, Pacing, and Defibrillation in Chronic Heart Failure (COMPANION) trial. COMPANION Steering Committee and COMPANION Clinical Investigators. J Card Fail. 2000;6:276–85.

2. Kass DA, Chen CH, Curry C, Talbot M, Berger R, Fetics B, et al. Improved left ventricular mechanics from acute VDD pacing in patients with dilated cardiomyopathy and ventricular conduction delay. Circulation. 1999;99:1567–73.

3. Shamim W, Francis DP, Yousufuddin M, Varney S, Pieopli MF, Anker SD, et al. Intraventricular conduction delay: a prognostic marker in chronic heart failure. Int J Cardiol. 1999;70:171–8.

4. McCullough PA, Hassan SA, Pallekonda V, Sandberg KR, Nori DB, Soman SS, et al. Bundle branch block patterns, age, renal dysfunction, and heart failure mortality. Int J Cardiol. 2005;102:303–8.

5. Baldasseroni S, Gentile A, Gorini M, Marchionni N, Marini M, Masotti G, et al. Intraventricular conduction defects in patients with congestive heart failure: left but not right bundle branch block is an independent predictor of prognosis. A report from the Italian Network on Congestive Heart Failure (IN-CHF database). Ital Heart J. 2003;4:607–13.

6. Baldasseroni S, Opasich C, Gorini M, Lucci D, Marchionni N, Marini M, et al. Left bundle-branch block is associated with increased 1-year sudden and total mortality rate in 5517 outpatients with congestive heart failure: a report from the Italian network on congestive heart failure. Am Heart J. 2002;143:398–405.

7. Mueller C, Laule-Kilian K, Klima T, Breidthardt T, Hochholzer W, Perruchoud AP, et al. Right bundle branch block and long-term mortality in patients with acute congestive heart failure. J Intern Med. 2006;260:421–8.

8. Zimetbaum PJ, Buxton AE, Batsford W, Fisher JD, Hafley GE, Lee KL, et al. Electrocardiographic predictors of arrhythmic death and total mortality in the multicenter unsustained tachycardia trial. Circulation. 2004;110:766–9.

9. Barsheshet A, Leor J, Goldbourt U, Garty M, Schwartz R, Behar S, et al. Effect of bundle branch block patterns on mortality in hospitalized patients with heart failure. Am J Cardiol. 2008;101:1303–8.

10. Barsheshet A, Goldenberg I, Garty M, Gottlieb S, Sandach A, Laish-Farkash A, et al. Relation of bundle branch block to long-term (four-year) mortality in hospitalized patients with systolic heart failure. Am J Cardiol. 2011;107:540–4.

11. Maron BJ, Towbin JA, Thiene G, Antzelevitch C, Corrado D, Arnett D, et al. Contemporary definitions and classification of the cardiomyopathies: an American Heart Association Scientific Statement from the Council on Clinical Cardiology, Heart Failure and Transplantation Committee; Quality of Care and Outcomes Research and Functional Genomics and Translational Biology Interdisciplinary Working Groups; and Council on Epidemiology and Prevention. Circulation. 2006;113(14):1807–16.

12. Elliott P. Cardiomyopathy. Diagnosis and management of dilated cardiomyopathy. Heart. 2000;84(1):106–12.

13. Mohan SB, Parker M, Wehbi M, Douglass P. Idiopathic dilated cardiomyopathy: a common but mystifying cause of heart failure. Cleve Clin J Med. 2002;69(6):481–7.

14. Galiè N, Humbert M, Vachiery JL, Gibbs S, Lang I, Torbicki A, et al. 2015 ESC/ERS Guidelines for the diagnosis and treatment of pulmonary hypertension: The Joint Task Force for the Diagnosis and Treatment of Pulmonary Hypertension of the European Society of Cardiology (ESC) and the European Respiratory Society (ERS)Endorsed by: Association for European Paediatric and Congenital Cardiology (AEPC), International Society for Heart and Lung Transplantation (ISHLT). Eur Heart J. 2016;37(1):67–119.

15. Abd El Rahman MY, Abdul-Khaliq H, Vogel M, Alexi-Meskishvili V, Gutberlet M, Lange PE. Relation between right ventricular enlargement, QRS duration, and right ventricular function in patients with tetralogy of Fallot and pulmonary regurgitation after surgical repair. Heart. 2000;84:416–20.

16. de Groote P, Millaire A, Foucher-Hossein C, Nugue O, Marchandise X, Ducloux G, et al. Right ventricular ejection fraction is an independent predictor of survival in patients with moderate heart failure. J Am Coll Cardiol. 1998;32:948–54.

17. Fantoni C, Kawabata M, Massaro R, Regoli F, Raffa S, Arora V, et al. Right and left ventricular activation sequence in patients with heart failure and right bundle branch block: a detailed analysis using three-dimensional non-fluoroscopic electroanatomic mapping system. J Cardiovasc Electrophysiol. 2005;16:112–9.

18. Ciuraszkiewicz K, Janion M, Dudek D, Gawor Z. Plasma B-type natriuretic peptide as a marker of myocardial asynchrony. Cardiology. 2009;113:193–7.

19. Rickard J, Kumbhani DJ, Gorodeski EZ, Baranowski B, Wazni O, Martin DO, et al. Cardiac resynchronization therapy in non-left bundle branch block morphologies. Pacing Clin Electrophysiol. 2010;33:590–5.

10

Triptolide improves systolic function and myocardial energy metabolism of diabetic cardiomyopathy in streptozotocin-induced diabetic rats

Zhongshu Liang, Sunnar Leo, Helin Wen, Mao Ouyang, Weihong Jiang and Kan Yang[*]

Abstract

Background: Triptolide treatment leads to an improvement in Diabetic Cardiomyopathy (DCM) in streptozotocin-induced diabetic rat model. DCM is characterized by abnormal cardiac energy metabolism. We hypothesized that triptolide ameliorated cardiac metabolic abnormalities in DCM. We proposed ^{31}P nuclear magnetic resonance (^{31}P NMR) spectrometry method for assessing cardiac energy metabolism in vivo and evaluating the effect of triptolide treatment in DCM rats.

Methods: Six weeks triptolide treatment was conducted on streptozotocin-induced diabetic rats with dose of 100, 200 or 400 μg/kg/day respectively. Sex- and age-matched non-diabetic rats were used as control group. Cardiac chamber dimension and function were determined with echocardiography. Whole heart preparations were perfused with Krebs–Henseleit buffer and ^{31}P NMR spectroscopy was performed. Cardiac p38 Mitogen Activating Protein Kinase (MAPK) was measured using real time PCR and western blot analysis.

Results: In diabetic rats, cardiac mass index was significantly higher, where as cardiac EF was lower than control group. ^{31}P NMR spectroscopy showed that ATP and pCr concentrations in diabetic groups were also remarkably lower than control group. Compared to non-treated diabetic rats, triptolide-treated diabetic groups showed remarkable lower cardiac mass index and higher EF, ATP, pCr concentrations, and P38 MAPK expressions. Best improvement was seen in group treated with Triptolide with dose 200 μg/kg/day.

Conclusions: ^{31}P NMR spectroscopy enables assessment of cardiac energy metabolism in whole heart preparations. It detects energy metabolic abnormalities in DCM hearts. Triptolide therapy improves cardiac function and increases cardiac energy metabolism at least partly through upregulation of MAPK signaling transduction.

Keywords: Triptolide, Diabetic cardiomyopathy, ^{31}P NMR spectroscopy, Cardiac energy metabolism, MAPK

Background

Diabetic cardiomyopathy (DCM) is one of the most common diabetes-associated complications encountered in the clinical practice [1]. DCM has been known to impair the function of the cardiac muscle and has been associated with high morbidity and mortality rate [2–5]. DCM occurred independently of coronary artery disease and hypertension [2, 6, 7].

Numerous studies on DCM, either on animal or molecular study, have found that myocardial abnormal glucose utilization and the shift toward fatty acid oxidation are the major pathophysiological alterations that may lead to diabetes mellitus (DM)-associated myocardial remodeling and heart failure [2, 4, 5, 7–11].

In diabetic rat model, we previously demonstrated the significant improvement on myocardial remodeling following triptolide treatment [12]. The inhibition of inflammation process by triptolide was evident [12–14]. However, whether triptolide ameliorates cardiac metabolic abnormalities remains unclear [15]. Results from

* Correspondence: yangkanxy@gmail.com
Department of Cardiology, Third Xiangya Hospital, Central South University, Changsha, Hunan 410013, People's Republic China

limited studies has suggested that Mitogen Activated Protein Kinases (MAPK) may play an important role as MAPK has been known as an important factor that interacts with mitochondria in the production of ATP [16]. Evidence from previous study revealed that Triptolide treatment could strongly activate MAPK signal transduction pathways in cells. These findings can be really intriguing as one may speculate that Triptolide treatment may improve cardiac energy metabolism by upregulating MAPK signal transduction [17]. Therefore, we sought the alteration of MAPK signaling transduction in rat model following the induction of DCM and following triptolide treatment. Recently, nuclear magnetic resonance (NMR) spectroscopy has been applied extensively in biomedical field [18, 19]. As a non-invasive diagnostic method, NMR spectroscopy has advantage as it allows determination on dynamic changes of specific metabolites in intact organs or tissues [20, 21], such as phosphocreatine (pCr), adenosine triphosphate (ATP), inorganic phosphate (Pi), and intracellular pH (pHi) [22–24]. In addition, NMR spectroscopy allows real-time observations on physiological function and energy metabolism of certain organ (e.g. heart) in near-physiological condition [20].

In this study, ^{31}Phosphorus NMR (^{31}P NMR) spectroscopy was used to evaluate the effect of triptolide treatment on the cardiac energy metabolism in DCM rat model. To minimize interference [25], we decided to perform the measurement *in vitro*.

Methods

Animal model and treatment
The protocols used in this study were approved by the Committee of Animal Care and Use of Central South University. Eight weeks old male Sprague–Dawley (SD) rats (Animal Center of Central South University, China) were included in the study. Animals were placed in laminar flow cages on a 12 h dark and 12 h light cycle and were fed with standard chow and tap water ad libitum. DM was induced by injecting streptozocin (STZ, 70 mg/kg, dissolved in 0.1 M sodium citrate buffer, pH 4.5; Sigma, USA) intra-peritoneally after overnight fasting. Random blood glucose levels were measured at 3 days and 1 week following the injection using One Touch Sure Step

glucometer (LifeScan, USA). Tail vein bloods were used and only rats with blood glucose level > 16.7 mmol/l in both time points were finally used. All the diabetic animals were randomized into four groups (n = 12 each): three diabetic groups treated with triptolide (100, 200, or 400 µg/kg/day respectively) and one diabetic group treated with vehicle. 12 sex- and age-matched non-diabetic rats served as control group. In addition, to assess the side effects of triptolide treatment, 12 sex- and age-matched non-diabetic SD rats (intraperitoneal injection of sodium citrate buffer) were treated with triptolide 400 µg/kg/day. After dissolved in dimethylsulfoxide (DMSO), Triptolide (Chinese National Institute for the Control of Pharmaceutical and Biological Products, China) was administered via gastric irrigation once daily for 6 weeks. At the end of this study, cardiac function was assessed and animals were sacrificed. The hearts were quickly extirpated and subjected to biochemical analysis [12].

Cardiac function measurement
Echocardiography was performed using GE Vivid 7 (General Electric, USA) ultrasound system with a 10-MHz transducer. Prior to the examination [12, 26], rats were anesthetized with pentobarbital (50 mg/kg intraperitoneally) and fixed in the supine position. LV end-diastolic dimension (LVEDD) as well as LV end-systolic dimension (LVESD) were measured on the parasternal long axis view and were indexed to body weight. LV ejection fraction (LVEF) was also calculated. All measurements were performed in triplicate by an experienced investigator who was blinded to the study and the results were expressed as the average of obtained value.

^{13}P NMR spectroscopy
^{31}P NMR spectroscopy was performed in a whole heart as previously described [27]. Briefly, the heart was perfused with modified Krebs–Henseleit buffer (11 mmol/L glucose, 4.5 mmol/l pyruvate, and 0.5 mmol/l lactate, no phosphate) at constant flow rate (15 ml/min) and pressure (100 mmHg) [28]. The heart was put into 25 mm NMR tube and subjected to 400 MHz 9.4 T vertical wide bore superconducting magnet (BrukerBioSpec 9.4 T Animal MRI System, Switzerland). The temperature of the heart was kept at 37 °C during the procedure. Peak

Table 1 General data

	Control	TP	DM	DM + TP, L	DM + TP, M	DM + TP, H
Glucose (mmol/l)	6.7 ± 2.0	5.8 ± 1.5	34.3 ± 2.7*	33.3 ± 3.7	31.2 ± 3.3*	33.4 ± 2.9*
BW (g)	462.0 ± 21.5	470.0 ± 21.2	213.3 ± 20.1*	236.5 ± 38.4*	234.6 ± 33.1*	225.7 ± 30.3*
HW (mg)	1190.3 ± 15.3	1210.2 ± 13.4	756.5 ± 12.6*	763.5 ± 14.8*	779.4 ± 15.2*	736.5 ± 14.1*
HW/BW (mg/g)	2.37 ± 0.33	2.40 ± 0.31	3.92 ± 0.48*	3.40 ± 0.46*	3.10 ± 0.46*#	3.01 ± 0.54*#

BW body weight, HW heart weight, TP,L low-dose triptolide (100 µg/kg/day), TP,M medium-dose triptolide (200 µg/kg/day), TP,H high-dose triptolide (400 µg/kg/day).
*P < 0.05 versus Control; #P <0.05 versus DM

Table 2 Echocardiographic parameters

	Control	TP	DM	DM + TP, L	DM + TP, M	DM + TP, H
LVEDD, mm	6.4 ± 0.6	6.5 ± 0.7	5.9 ± 0.5	6.0 ± 0.6	5.6 ± 0.6	5.4 ± 0.8
LVEDD index, um/g	13.8 ± 1.6	13.7 ± 2.1	23.6 ± 3.0*	21.1 ± 1.9*	20.2 ± 1.5*#	19.0 ± 1.8*#
LVESD, mm	3.9 ± 0.4	3.8 ± 0.7	3.7 ± 0.6	3.8 ± 0.8	3.3 ± 0.5	3.2 ± 0.8
LVESD index, um/g	8.4 ± 0.8	8.3 ± 0.7	15.8 ± 1.9*	13.5 ± 1.7*	12.9 ± 1.3*#	12.5 ± 1.6*#
LVEF,%	76.4 ± 8.2	78.2 ± 6.3	66.6 ± 6.5*	72.8 ± 5.5	75.0 ± 5.8#	74.6 ± 6.4#
FS,%	44.7 ± 4.3	43.7 ± 5.1	35.8 ± 3.6*	38.9 ± 4.1	41.3 ± 4.9	42.4 ± 4.6

LVEDD left ventricular end-diastolic dimension, LVESD left ventricular end-systolic dimension, LVEF left ventricular ejection fraction, FS fractional shortening. TP,L low-dose triptolide (100 μg/kg/day), TP, M medium-dose triptolide (200 μg/kg/day); TP, H high-dose triptolide (400 μg/kg/day). *$P < 0.05$ versus Control; #$P < 0.05$versus DM

resolution was enhanced by shimming the proton signal to a line width between 20 and 35Hz. Using a spectrometer (Varian, Palo Alto, CA), consecutive 4 minutes of the spectra were acquired at 161.92 MHz.

Using a computer program (NMR1, Tripos, St. Louis, MO), the areas of the spectral peaks were fitted to sum of Lorentzian and Gaussian line shapes. After adjustment for spectral saturation, absolute ^{31}P concentrations were calculated by adding Atriptolide 10.6 mmol/l to the initial h-ATP peak area and calculating ATP and PCr peak areas relative to this area. pH was estimated from the chemical shift of the inorganic phosphate (P_i) peak (δ_{Pi}) relative to that of the PCr peak.

Solutions and ChemicalsA phosphate-free Tyrode solution was used in heart NMR which contained 136.3 mM NaCl, 5.4 mM KCl, 1.0 mM MgCl2, 0.9 mM CaCl2, 10.0 mM glucose, and 5.0 mM HEPES [16, 25]. The solution was pre-warmed to 40 °C and oxygenated with 100 % Oxygen. For a Na-free solution, Na + and Ca2+ were replaced with N-methyl-Dglucamine on an equimolar basis as follows: 137.2 mM N-methyl-D-glucamine, 5.4 mM KCl, 1.0 mM MgCl2, 10.0 mM glucose, and 5.0 mM HEPES. Phosphate-free KH solution contained 118 mM NaCl, 5.9 mM KCl, 2.5 mM CaCl2, 1.2 mM MgSO4, 25 mM NaHCO3, 12 mM glucose, and 0.5 mM Na2EDTA. The KH solution was oxygenated with 95 % O2-5 % CO2.

Real time polymerase chain reaction

Cardiac RNAs were extracted using TRIzol Reagent (Invitrogen, CA, USA) according to the company's protocol. After first strand cDNA synthesis, SYBR Green Real Time-PCR was performed using SBYR

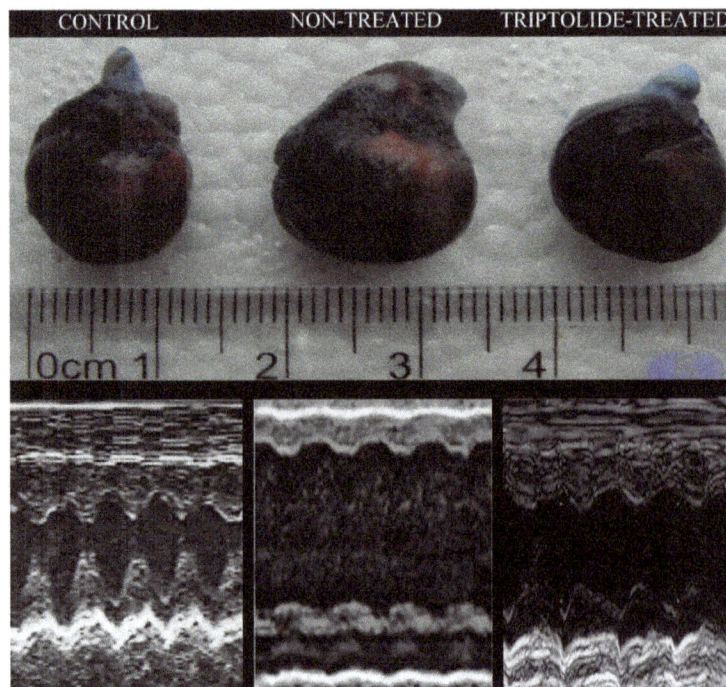

Fig. 1 Comparison of cardiac gross anatomy and systolic function between groups

Table 3 pHi values and concentrations of ATP and pCr in whole heart preparations treated at varying doses of triptolide

	Control	TP	DM	DM + TP, L	DM + TP, M	DM + TP, H
pHi	7.26 ± 0.12	7.24 ± 0.14	7.20 ± 0.12*	7.22 ± 0.12	7.24 ± 0.12#	7.23 ± 0.12
ATP (mmol/L)	0.17 ± 0.03	0.18 ± 0.01	0.07 ± 0.01*	0.10 ± 0.02*#	0.13 ± 0.02*#	0.14 ± 0.01*#
pCr (mmol/L)	21.3 ± 1.3	21.5 ± 2.8	13.7 ± 1.3*	16.6 ± 1.7*#	18.8 ± 2.3*#	18.9 ± 2.2*#

TP,L low-dose triptolide (100 µg/kg/day), TP,M medium-dose triptolide (200 µg/kg/day), TP,H high-dose triptolide (400 µg/kg/day). *P < 0.05 versus Control; #P < 0.05 versus DM

Premix Ex Taq (Takara Bio Inc., Japan). The sequences of the primers were p38: Forward Primer 5'-TCCAAGGGC TACACCAAATC-3', Reverse Primer 5'-TGTTCCAGG TAAGGGTGAGC-3'; β-actin Forward Primer 5'-GAGA GGGAAATCGTGCGTGAC-3',Reverse Primer 5'-CATCT GCTGGAAGGTGGACA-3'. The specificity of each PCR product was validated by the melting curve analysis. The expressions of mRNA were determined by constructing the differences between the cycle thresholds (Ct): $\Delta Ct = Ct$ gene of interest – Ct housekeeping gene. The conversion of ΔCt to relative gene expression is fold induction of $2^{-\Delta Ct}$.

Western blot analysis
Cardiac proteins were extracted using radio immune precipitation assay buffer. Protein concentration was determined using BCA Protein Assay Kit (CW0014, Beijing CoWin Bioscience Co. Ltd., China) according to the manufacturer's protocol. Denatured proteins were loaded into every single well and were separated by SDS-PAGE gel. Gels were transferred to an Immobilon-P membrane at 290 mA. The antibodies for phosphop38 MAPK and b-actin were purchased from Cell Signaling Technology (Beverly, MA). The expression of these proteins in the membrane was detected using an enhanced chemiluminescence kit (Western Bright, Advansta Co., U.S.A.).

Statistical analysis
All data were expressed as mean ± SD and compared by one way ANOVA with Tukey's post-hoc test using SPSS 16.0 (SPSS, Inc, Chicago, IL). The correlation between variables was calculated using linear regression analysis. Statistical significance was defined as p < 0.05.

Results
All mice treated with Streptozocin developed hyperglycemia. During the whole study, no evidence of ketoacidosis was observed in all diabetic mice. No significant change of blood pressure was observed in all animals. Compared to non-diabetic groups, all diabetic groups showed higher cardiac mass index (all p < 0.05). The increased mass indexes were mainly due to the significantly smaller body weight of the animals in these groups. Comparison of blood glucose level and cardiac mass index between control group and non-diabetic + Triptolide group showed no significant differences (Table 1).

Cardiac performance
When indexed to the body weight, both LVEDD and LVESD indexes were significantly higher in diabetic than in non-diabetic rats. LV systolic function, as evidenced by LVEF, was significantly higher in groups treated with Triptolide when compared to non-treated group. Moreover, FS in triptolide-treatment diabetic groups also showed the upward trend compared with the untreated diabetic group, but the difference did not reach statistical significance (Table 2). The comparison of cardiac size and function between groups is displayed on Fig. 1.

^{31}P NMR spectroscopy demonstrated that the values of pHi, ATP and pCr were significantly lower in the untreated diabetic rats as compared to non-diabetic rats (Table 3). A trend of increasing pHi, ATP, and pCr was observed following Triptolide treatment. Representative image of ^{31}P NMR spectroscopy is displayed in Fig. 2.

MAPK Signaling pathway
There was a two-fold decrease in p38 mRNA expression in diabetic rats when compared with control. p38 mRNA expression was found significantly higher in diabetic rats treated with Triptolide. Consistently, on Western blot analysis, both control and Triptolide-treated groups showed stronger bands for p38 protein expression than those of diabetic group (all p < 0.05, Table 4, Fig. 3).

Electron microscope
In diabetic rats, myocardial filaments were not intact. Mitochondria were disorganized with obvious vacuolar

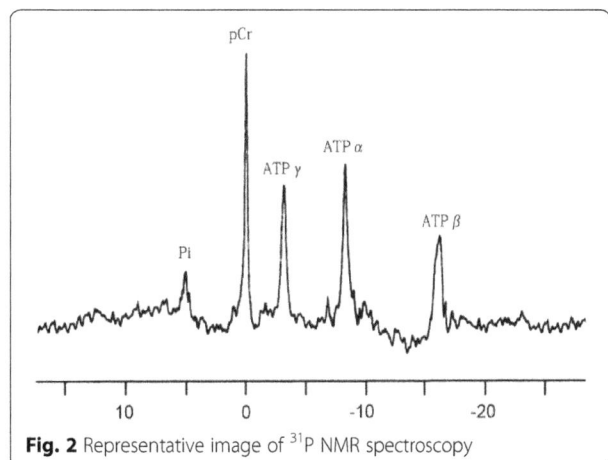

Fig. 2 Representative image of ^{31}P NMR spectroscopy

Table 4 p38 mRNA and protein expression (mean ± SD)

Parameter	Group		
	Control	DM	DM + TP
VEGF mRNA ($2^{-\Delta Ct}$)	0.116 ± 0.08	0.060 ± 0.03*	0.086 ± 0.03*#
PKG-1 protein expression (OD)	0.912 ± 0.18	0.413 ± 0.15*	0.704 ± 0.13*#

ΔCt, Ct gene of interest – Ct beta actin; OD, optical density as indexed to beta actin; DM, Diabetes Mellitus; TP, Triptolide. *$P < 0.05$ versus Control; #$P < 0.05$ versus DM

degeneration (Fig. 4). In Triptolide-treated diabetic group, myocardial filaments were relatively more intact with remarkable lesser vacuolar degeneration of mitochondria. In contrast, no evidence of vacuolar degeneration of mitochondria was found in control group.

Correlation analysis

The correlation between cardiac mass index and ATP as well as pCr was examined by linear regression analysis. Cardiac mass index was negatively correlated with ATP and pCr ($r = -0.75$ and $r = -0.73$ respectively, all $p < 0.01$, Fig. 5).

Discussion

Diabetes is the most common endocrine disease encountered in the clinical practice [29]. DM causes series of metabolic disorders, such as glucose, lipid and protein metabolism. Long term diabetes can lead to multisystem of organ damage [23]. Recent studies have associated mitochondrial dysfunction and DM [8, 29–31]. Mitochondria have been known asthe sites of energy metabolism. Mitochondrial dysfunction is one of the characteristics of DM and has occurred even in the early stage of the disease [5]. Increasing evidences have supported that mitochondrial energy metabolism dysfunction played a crucial role in the pathogenesis of DM [11, 26, 32]. Hence, we performed ^{31}P NMR spectroscopy in order to evaluate the energy metabolism in DCM rats. Secondarily, we sought to evaluate if Triptolide could improve myocardial energy metabolism.

Electron microscope is the common method used for evaluating the amount and structure of mitochondria. Cardiac muscle biopsy allows the measurement of ATP production [20–22]. However, all of these methods are invasive and can only be performed in vitro. In daily clinical setting, such kind of method is often found impractical. Therefore, a non invasive and reliable technique is needed. Japanese researchers found that both ^{31}P NMR detection and cardiac biopsy showed the similar result of myocardial energy metabolism [27]. This finding makes phosphorus NMR spectroscopy is more favorable providing that it is a non-invasive technique and can be performed in vivo. Since the chemical shift peak of pCr is stable and is not influenced by internal environment, it is often used as a standard to determine the remnant compounds of chemical shift such PME, Pi, PDE and ATP [22, 24]. Energy metabolism can be assessed by quantifying area calculation under the peak of each remnant compound, in which ATP is a direct energy supplier whereas pCr is energy storage [22, 24, 25]. When muscle contracts, pCr transmits high energy phosphate bond to ATP for energy supply, conversely, when muscle relaxes, the reaction of oxidative phosphorylation in mitochondrial membrane generates ATP and then the energy is transferred to pCr for storage [25, 27, 33]. Furthermore, phosphorus spectrum enables to calculate intracellular pH, assesses the degree of anaerobic glycolysis, and evaluates the efficiency of aerobic metabolism in cells [8, 34], which become an important indicator for assessment of mitochondrial function [25, 28].

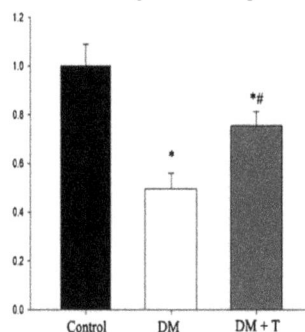

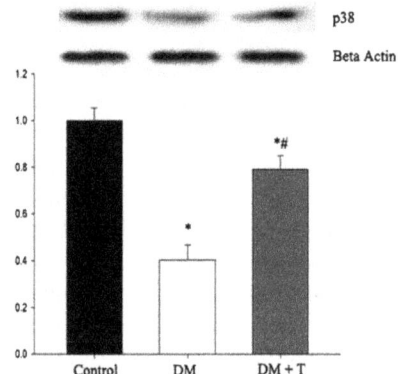

Fig 3 Relative mRNA and protein expression of cardiac p38 MAPK in different groups

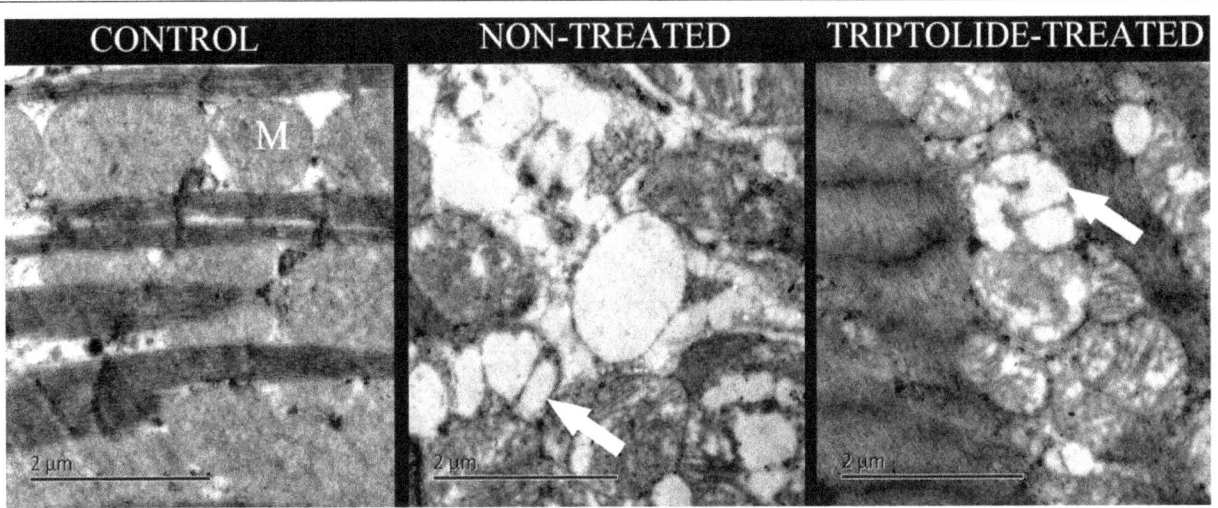

Fig. 4 Electron microscopic analysis of cardiomyocyte. M, Normal mitochondria; Arrow, Mitochondria with vacuolar degeneration

Our previous study has demonstrated that cardiac systolic function was impaired in diabetic rats and the cardiac index increased significantly [12]. Consistently, we observed the hemodynamic improvement following triptolide treatment. However, the exact mechanism involved in the hemodynamic improvement remains speculative. We believe the hemodynamic improvement following the treatment may be due to the anti-fibrotic property of Triptolide. Based on our previous findings, pro-fibrotic action of NF Kappa B in STZ mice were effectively suppressed by Triptolide [12]. Moreover, Triptolide treatment led to the inhibition of inflammatory cytokines such as Tumor Necrosis Alpha and Interleukin-1 which eventually attenuated the cardiac inflammation. We speculate that the Triptolide anti-fibrotic effect may lead to the improvement in ventricular remodeling and myocardial contraction. This, in turn, will ultimately improve the hemodynamic status of the failing hearts.

In this current study, we demonstrated that high-energy phosphate metabolism of the whole heart can be assessed

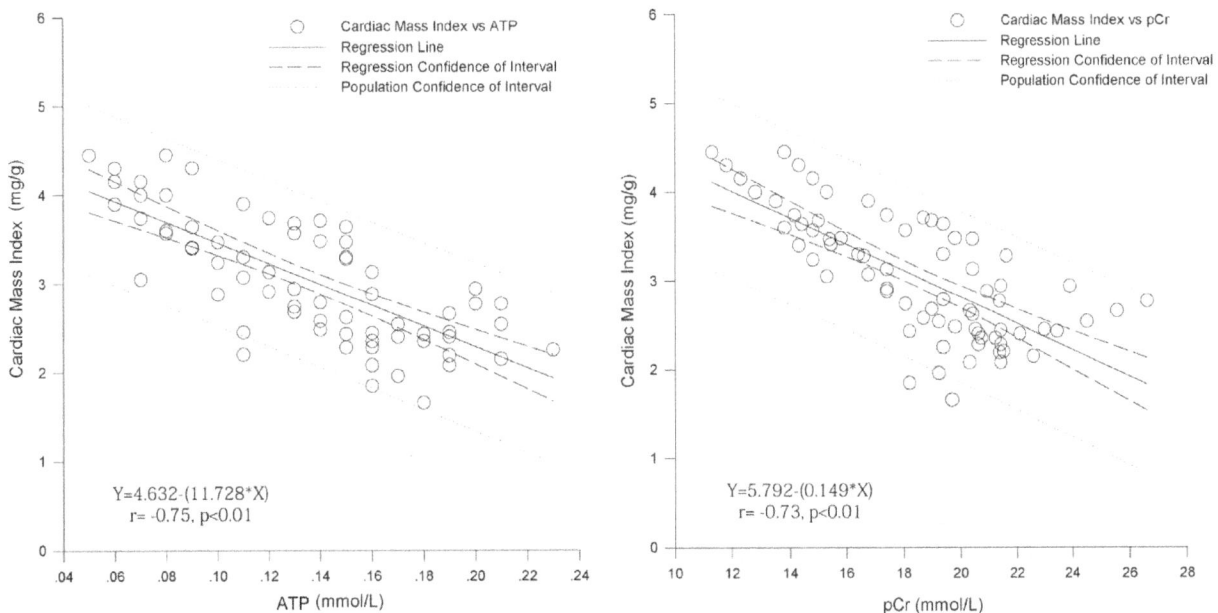

Fig. 5 Linear regression analysis between cardiac mass index and ATP as well as pCr

with NMR [20, 27], thereby evaluating the process of cardiac energy metabolism. As a non-invasive technique, NMR can be performed repeatedly as a continuous monitoring in clinical practice and therefore is important. In the setting of DM, it may aid especially in the detection and diagnosis of early stage DM [28].

Our study further confirmed that cardiac energy metabolism was impaired in DM. Cardiac index significantly increased while cardiac ATP and pCr concentration remarkably decreased. Triptolide probably inhibited cardiac remodeling through the immune and inflammatory suppression [12–14]. However, whether the improvement of cardiac energy metabolism was achieved via the same mechanism remains largely unclear. On one hand, it is possible that the inhibition of cardiac remodeling could improve left ventricular geometry and systolic function. This will increase cellular blood and oxygen supply which eventually improve the process of cardiac energy metabolism [3, 6]. On the other hand, our study revealed that MAPK signaling pathway may be involved in the process. MAPK mRNA and protein expression which significantly increased in Triptolide treated group suggested that Triptolide probably improve cardiac energy metabolism at least partly through MAPK signaling pathway. MAPK signaling pathway is known as the most important pathway that interacts with mitochondria in the production of ATP [16]. Mitochondria have been known as the main factory for ATP production. Interestingly, through electron microscopic analysis, we observed an increasing number of mitochondria following Triptolide treatment.

Despite significant improvement of LVEF, fractional shortening (FS) in triptolide-treatment diabetic groups only showed the upward trend compared with the untreated diabetic group. The difference did not reach statistical significance. This may due to sampling error as FS value itself is lower than EF value. We believe that by increasing sample size, the difference will reach the statistical significance.

Cardiac index and LVEDD were negatively correlated with cardiac ATP and pCr concentrations, suggesting that the cardiomyocyte high-energy phosphate bond decreased after cardiac remodeling induced by DM. The decrease of intra-mitochondrial energy production characterized the process and Triptolide can partially reverse the process. This further affirmed the potential value of Triptolide treatment in diabetic cardiomyopathy.

Conclusion

In the present study, we show that the abnormalities of cardiac energy metabolism in DCM rats could be improved partially by triptolide therapy. The improvement of cardiac energy metabolism following triptolide is at least

partly through the upregulation of MAPK signaling transduction. ^{31}P NMR spectroscopy enables the assessment of cardiac high-energy phosphates metabolism and therefore is able to evaluate the cardiac energy metabolism.

Competing interests
The authors declare that they have no competing interests.

Authors' contributions
ZL and SL made the original concept and study design; ZL, SL, and HW carried out the animal experiment, the acquisition, and the analysis of all data; ZL, MO, WJ, and KY made significant contribution in the interpretation of data and manuscript writing; KY gave the final approval of the version to be published. All authors read and approved the final manuscript.

Authors' information
Sunnar Leo contributed as co-first author.

References
1. Montaigne D, Marechal X, Coisne A, Debry N, Modine T, Fayad G, et al. Myocardial contractile dysfunction is associated with impaired mitochondrial function and dynamics in type 2 diabetic but not in obese patients. Circulation. 2014; in press.
2. Pham T, Loiselle D, Power A, Hickey AJ. Mitochondrial inefficiencies and anoxic ATP hydrolysis capacities in diabetic rat heart. Am J Physiol Cell Physiol. 2014; in press.
3. Mori J, Patel VB, Abo AO, Basu R, Altamimi T, Desaulniers J, et al. Angiotensin 1–7 ameliorates diabetic cardiomyopathy and diastolic dysfunction in db/db mice by reducing lipotoxicity and inflammation. Circ Heart Fail. 2014;7(2):327–39.
4. Ilkun O, Boudina S. Cardiac dysfunction and oxidative stress in the metabolic syndrome: an update on antioxidant therapies. Curr Pharm Des. 2013;19(27):4806–17.
5. Schilling JD, Mann DL. Diabetic cardiomyopathy: bench to bedside. Heart Fail Clin. 2012;8(4):619–31.
6. Anna Z, Angela S, Barbara B, Jana R, Tamara B, Csilla V, et al. Heart-protective effect of n-3 PUFA demonstrated in a rat model of diabetic cardiomyopathy. Mol Cell Biochem. 2014;389(1–2):219–27.
7. Dhalla NS, Takeda N, Rodriguez-Leyva D, Elimban V. Mechanisms of subcellular remodeling in heart failure due to diabetes. Heart Fail Rev. 2014;19(1):87–99.
8. Dhalla NS, Rangi S, Zieroth S, Xu YJ. Alterations in sarcoplasmic reticulum and mitochondrial functions in diabetic cardiomyopathy. Exp Clin Cardiol. 2012;17(3):115–20.
9. IS F a, Dick GM, Hollander JM. Diabetes mellitus reduces the function and expression of ATP-dependent K(+) channels in cardiac mitochondria. Life Sci. 2013;92(11):664–8.
10. Kok BP, Brindley DN. Myocardial fatty acid metabolism and lipotoxicity in the setting of insulin resistance. Heart Fail Clin. 2012;8(4):643–61.
11. Galloway CA, Yoon Y. Mitochondrial morphology in metabolic diseases. Antioxid Redox Signal. 2013;19(4):415–30.
12. Wen HL, Liang ZS, Zhang R, Yang K. Anti-inflammatory effects of triptolide improve left ventricular function in a rat model of diabetic cardiomyopathy. Cardiovasc Diabetol. 2013;12:50.
13. Wei D, Huang Z. Anti-inflammatory effects of triptolide in LPS-induced acute lung injury in mice. Inflammation. 2014; in press.
14. Sai K, Li WY, Chen YS, Wang J, Guan S, Yang QY, et al. Triptolide synergistically enhances temozolomide-induced apoptosis and potentiates inhibition of NF-kappaB signaling in glioma initiating cells. Am J Chin Med. 2014;42(2):485–503.
15. Li XJ, Jiang ZZ, Zhang LY. Triptolide: progress on research in pharmacodynamics and toxicology. J Ethnopharmacol. 2014; in press.
16. Javadov S, Jang S, Agostini B. Crosstalk between mitogen-activated protein kinases and mitochondria in cardiac diseases: Therapeutic perspectives. Pharmacol Ther. 2014;144(2):202–25.
17. Lu N, Liu J, Liu J, Zhang C, Jiang F, Wu H, et al. Antagonist effect of triptolide on AKT activation by truncated retinoid X receptor-alpha. Plos One. 2012;7(4), e35722.

18. Chmelik M, Považan M, Krššák M, Gruber S, Tkačov M, Trattnig S, et al. In vivo (31)P magnetic resonance spectroscopy of the human liver at 7 T: an initial experience. NMR Biomed. 2014;27(4):478–85.

19. Zhang CY, Zhang Q, Zhang HM, Yang HS. 3.0T 31P MR Spectroscopy in assessment of response to antiviral therapy for chronic hepatitis c. World J Gastroenterol. 2014;20(8):2107–12.

20. Banks L, Wells GD, McCrindle BW. Cardiac energy metabolism is positively associated with skeletal muscle energy metabolism in physically active adolescents and young adults. Appl Physiol Nutr Metab. 2014;39(3):363–8.

21. Lygate CA, Schneider JE, Neubauer S. Investigating cardiac energetics in heart failure. Exp Physiol. 2013;98(3):601–5.

22. Read EK, Ivancic M, Hanson P, Cade-Menun BJ, McMahon KD. Phosphorus speciation in a eutrophic lake by P NMR spectroscopy. Water Res. 2014;62C:229–40.

23. Willcocks RJ, Fulford J, Armstrong N, Barker AR, Williams CA. Muscle metabolism during fatiguing isometric quadriceps exercise in adolescents and adults. Appl Physiol Nutr Metab. 2014;39(4):439–45.

24. Cobert ML, Merritt ME, West LM, Ayers C, Jessen ME, et al. Metabolic characteristics of human hearts preserved for 12 hours by static storage, antegrade perfusion, or retrograde coronary sinus perfusion. J Thorac Cardiovasc Surg. 2014; in press.

25. Yaniv Y, Juhaszova M, Nuss HB, Wang S, Zorov DB, Lakatta EG, et al. Matching ATP supply and demand in mammalian heart: in vivo, in vitro, and in silico perspectives. Ann N Y Acad Sci. 2010;1188:133–42.

26. Gao Q, Wang XM, Ye HW, Yu Y, Kang PF, Wang HJ, et al. Changes in the expression of cardiac mitofusin-2 in different stages of diabetes in rats. Mol Med Rep. 2012;6(4):811–4.

27. Uetani T, Yamashita D, Shimizu J, Misawa H, Tatematsu Y, Hamaguchi Y, et al. Heart slice NMR. Am J Physiol Heart Circ Physiol. 2007;292(2):H1181–6.

28. Murray AJ, Lygate CA, Cole MA, Carr CA, Radda GK, Neubauer S, et al. Insulin resistance, abnormal energy metabolism and increased ischemic damage in the chronically infarcted rat heart. Cardiovasc Res. 2006;71(1):149–57.

29. Croston TL, Thapa D, Holden AA, Tveter KJ, Lewis SE, Shepherd DL, et al. Functional deficiencies of subsarcolemmal mitochondria in the type 2 diabetic human heart. Am J Physiol Heart Circ Physiol. 2014;307(1):H54–65.

30. Xu X, Kobayashi S, Chen K, Timm D, Volden P, Huang Y, et al. Diminished autophagy limits cardiac injury in mouse models of type 1 diabetes. J Biol Chem. 2013;288(25):18077–92.

31. Ritchie RH, Love JE, Huynh K, Bernardo BC, Henstridge DC, Kiriazis H, et al. Enhanced phosphoinositide 3-kinase(p110alpha) activity prevents diabetes-induced cardiomyopathy and superoxide generation in a mouse model of diabetes. Diabetologia. 2012;55(12):3369–81.

32. Muller AL, Freed D, Hryshko L, Dhalla NS. Implications of protease activation in cardiac dysfunction and development of genetic cardiomyopathy in hamsters. Can J Physiol Pharmacol. 2012;90(8):995–1004.

33. Angin Y, Steinbusch LK, Simons PJ, Greulich S, Hoebers NT, Douma K, et al. CD36 inhibition prevents lipid accumulation and contractile dysfunction in rat cardiomyocytes. Biochem J. 2012;448(1):43–53.

34. Atale N, Chakraborty M, Mohanty S, Bhattacharya S, Nigam D, Sharma M, et al. Cardioprotective role of Syzygium cumini against glucose-induced oxidative stress in H9C2 cardiac myocytes. Cardiovasc Toxicol. 2013;13(3):278–89.

11

Prevalence, associated factors and management implications of left ventricular outflow tract obstruction in takotsubo cardiomyopathy

Ole De Backer[1,2*], Philippe Debonnaire[2], Sofie Gevaert[1], Luc Missault[2], Peter Gheeraert[1] and Luc Muyldermans[2]

Abstract

Background: Some patients with Takotsubo cardiomyopathy (TTC) develop cardiogenic shock due to left ventricular outflow tract (LVOT) obstruction – there is, however, a paucity of data regarding this condition.

Methods: Prevalence, associated factors and management implications of LVOT obstruction in TTC was explored, based on two-year data from two Belgian heart centres.

Results: A total of 32 patients with TTC were identified out of 3,272 patients presenting with troponin-positive acute coronary syndrome. In six patients diagnosed with TTC (19%), a significant LVOT obstruction was detected by transthoracic echocardiography. Patients with LVOT obstruction were older and had more often septal bulging, and presented more frequently in cardiogenic shock as compared to those without LVOT obstruction ($P < 0.05$). Moreover, all patients with LVOT obstruction showed systolic anterior motion (SAM) of the anterior mitral valve leaflet, which was associated with a higher grade of mitral regurgitation (2.2 ± 0.7 vs. 1.0 ± 0.6, $P<0.001$). Adequate therapeutic management including fluid resuscitation, cessation of inotropic therapy, intravenous β-blocker, and the use of intra-aortic balloon pump resulted in non-inferior survival in TTC patients with LVOT obstruction as compared to those without LVOT obstruction.

Conclusions: TTC is complicated by LVOT obstruction in approximately 20% of cases. Older age, septal bulging, SAM-induced mitral regurgitation and hemodynamic instability are associated with this condition. Timely and accurate diagnosis of LVOT obstruction by echocardiography is key to successful management of these TTC patients with LVOT obstruction and results in a non-inferior outcome as compared to those patients without LVOT obstruction.

Keywords: Takotsubo cardiomyopathy, Apical ballooning, Outflow tract obstruction, Systolic anterior motion, Cardiogenic shock

Background

Takotsubo cardiomyopathy (TTC) – also called apical ballooning syndrome – is an increasingly reported clinical entity characterized by transient severe systolic heart failure that mimics an acute myocardial infarction in the absence of obstructive coronary artery disease [1,2]. This condition predominantly affects postmenopausal women and emotional/physical stress at onset is common, although a triggering event is not always present. Postulated pathogenic mechanisms include multivessel epicardial vasospasm, coronary microvascular dysfunction, and catecholamine-triggered myocyte injury. Other studies hypothesize that in the presence of increased catecholamine levels, a dynamic intraventricular pressure gradient develops, resulting in subendocardial 'stunning' of the left ventricular (LV) apical region [1-6].

Importantly, some patients with TTC develop cardiogenic shock due to severe systolic dysfunction or left

* Correspondence: ole.debacker@gmail.com
[1]Department of Cardiology, Ghent University Hospital, De Pintelaan 185, B-9000 Ghent, Belgium
[2]Department of Cardiology, AZ Sint-Jan Hospital, Bruges, Belgium

ventricular outflow tract (LVOT) obstruction. There is, however, a paucity of data regarding this latter condition. Accordingly, we explored the prevalence and characteristics of TTC in a population presenting with troponin-positive acute coronary syndrome (ACS) – with focus on LVOT obstruction and its management.

Methods

Study population

The study population consisted of all patients referred with troponin-positive ACS to two high-volume catheterisation laboratories (Ghent University Hospital, AZ Sint-Jan Bruges) in Belgium in a period of 24 consecutive months. The diagnosis of TTC was based on the Mayo-criteria [5]: (1) transient hypokinesia, akinesia, or dyskinesia of the LV mid segments with or without apical involvement – regional wall motion abnormalities extend beyond a single epicardial distribution; (2) absence of obstructive coronary artery disease or angiographic evidence of acute plaque rupture; (3) new electrocardiographic abnormalities (either ST-segment elevation and/or T-wave inversion) or elevated cardiac troponin; (4) absence of a pheochromocytoma, myocarditis or hypertrophic cardiomyopathy.

Clinical, biochemical, electrocardiographic, echocardiographic and angiographic data were retrospectively collected. Clinical data included demographics, cardiovascular risk factors, presenting symptoms and emotional or physical triggers. The peak Troponin-T (TnT)-value was measured as a marker of myocyte necrosis. Coronary and LV angiography were performed within 72 hours after onset of symptoms. LV angiograms were used to calculate LV ejection fraction (LVEF) and detect regional wall motion abnormalities. Based on review of the echocardiographic images, TTC patients were further dichotomized depending on the presence of significant LVOT obstruction. Due to the retrospective nature of this study, the choice of treatment was at the discretion of the treating physician. Approval for this study was provided by the local Ethical Committee of Ghent University Hospital (Ghent, Belgium) and all patients gave written informed consent for the use of anonymous clinical, procedural, and follow-up data.

Echocardiography

Within 24 hours of admission, all patients with suspected TTC underwent transthoracic echocardiography. A follow-up echocardiographic study was performed in most patients at random intervals, most often at day 4–14 (at discharge), at 4–8 weeks, and approximately one year after the acute phase. Standard gray-scale and color-Doppler images were acquired with ECG-triggering and in cine-loop format for on-line analysis. In particular, septal wall

thickness was measured at parasternal long axis view and septal bulging was defined as basal interventricular septum (IVS) thickness ≥12 mm. The same view was used for detection of systolic anterior motion (SAM) of the anterior mitral valve leaflet. LVEF was evaluated using Biplane Simpson method, as recommended [7]. In addition, regional wall motion abnormalities were assessed. Color Doppler was used to identify turbulent flow, suggesting increased pressure gradient in the LV. To further identify significant peak pressure gradients (defined as >20 mmHg), pulsed wave Doppler was used, set above the mitral leaflets tips (assessment of intraventricular pressure gradient) and into the LVOT (assessment of LVOT pressure gradient/obstruction). The final gradient was calculated using the modified Bernoulli equation based on maximal flow velocities derived from continuous wave Doppler imaging. As previously reported, mitral regurgitation (MR) severity (grade 0–4) was assessed using an integrative approach based on vena contracta width, color Doppler jet area, or by quantitative approach whenever possible (Doppler-volumetric/proximal isovelocity surface area) [8].

Statistical analysis

Continuous variables are reported as means ± standard deviation, unless otherwise specified. Categorical data are reported as absolute values and percentages. Continuous and categorical variables were compared by (un)paired t test, χ^2 test and Fisher test, as appropriate. All data were analysed using SPSS version 20.0 (SPSS Inc., Chicago, IL, USA). P values <0.05 were considered statistically significant.

Results

Overall study population

Out of 3,272 patients with troponin-positive ACS referred for coronary angiography, a total of 32 patients were identified with TTC – indicating an overall prevalence of 1.0% (Figure 1).

As shown in Table 1, TTC patients were predominantly older women (66 ± 15 years, 94% female). The overall cardiovascular risk profile was rather low, in line with the absence of significant coronary artery lesions on coronary angiography. The most common presenting symptoms were chest pain (n = 17; 53%), respiratory distress (n = 8; 25%), and cardiogenic shock (n = 5; 16%). Two other patients presented with ventricular tachycardia (VT) and fibrillation (VF), both were successfully resuscitated. In 22 patients, a stressful event preceding the acute phase of TTC could be identified. These events were considered emotionally mediated in 9 patients (28%) or alternatively due to a physical trigger in 13 other patients (41%) – these circumstances are detailed in Additional file 1: Table S1. On admission, ST-segment elevation mimicking acute

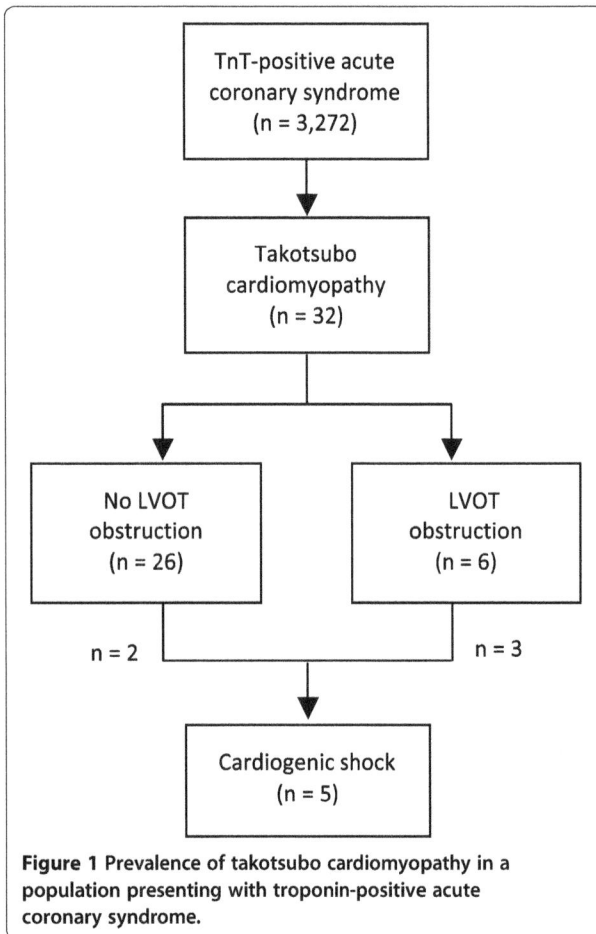

Figure 1 Prevalence of takotsubo cardiomyopathy in a population presenting with troponin-positive acute coronary syndrome.

anterior myocardial infarction was present in almost half of the patients (n = 15, 47%), while 16 patients (50%) presented with other ST/T abnormalities. On admission, TnT was elevated in 28 patients (88%) and peak in-hospital TnT was 0.93 ± 0.90 ng/mL (range 0.1 to 3.6 ng/mL). Echocardiography and LV angiography revealed a typical pattern of 'apical ballooning' with akinesia of the mid/apical LV segments and compensatory hyperkinesia of the basal segments in the majority of patients (n = 30). Only two patients presented with 'inverse' TTC or mid-ventricular ballooning, ie. akinesia of the mid LV segments. Per patient clinical, biochemical, electro-/echo-cardiographic and angiographic data are available in Additional file 1: Table S1.

Patients without vs. with LVOT obstruction
As shown in Table 1, a total of six patients (19%) were identified with significant LVOT obstruction and no patients were found to have a significant intraventricular pressure gradient. The TTC patient population was dichotomized based on the absence or presence of LVOT obstruction. The latter group was significantly older and presented more often with hemodynamic instability as compared to patients without LVOT obstruction (n = 26, 81%). In addition, a

higher basal IVS thickness leading to increased prevalence of septal bulging was found. Patients with LVOT obstruction all showed SAM and consequently more severe MR as compared to patients without LVOT obstruction (Table 1). Of note, none of these patients had a familial history of hypertrophic cardiomyopathy. Both patient groups without vs. with LVOT obstruction had similar peak TnT and mean LVEF at admission. No LVOT obstruction was found in the two patients that were resuscitated because of VT/VF.

LVOT obstruction and therapeutic management
Similar proportions of TTC patients without vs. with LVOT obstruction were initially treated with i.v. inotropics (27% vs. 33%, respectively; Table 1). However, inotropic therapy was immediately stopped in the two patients with LVOT obstruction from the moment of diagnosis by echocardiography. Patients without LVOT obstruction were given inotropic agents for a maximum duration of five days. In addition, an intra-aortic balloon pump (IABP) was used in 9 TTC patients (28%) because of severe systolic dysfunction (LVEF < 35%, n = 4), LVOT obstruction (n = 2), or non-specified reason(s) (n = 3). Only two patients received β-blocker i.v. – both patients were diagnosed with severe LVOT obstruction (pressure gradient ≥40 mmHg). Per patient therapeutical management data are available in Additional file 1: Table S1.

Patient outcome
A total of two TTC patients (32, 6%) without LVOT obstruction died in the acute setting due to refractory cardiogenic shock (n = 1) or acute respiratory distress syndrome (n = 1, see Additional file 1: Table S1). No mortality occurred in the group of patients diagnosed with LVOT obstruction. There was no residual dynamic LVOT pressure gradient detected at discharge in any of the patients initially presenting with LVOT obstruction. In accordance, there was no more SAM of the anterior mitral valve leaflet, resulting in an important reduction of MR severity (mean MR grade 1.2 ± 0.6 vs. 2.2 ± 0.7). Recovery of LV systolic function – defined as LVEF ≥55% – was observed within 19 ± 12 days (range 5 to 42 days – based on data obtained in 24 patients, see Additional file 1: Table S1). At medium to long-term follow-up, two patients experienced recurrence of TTC at 0.9 and 5.2 years after the first episode, while on oral β-blocker therapy. No evident relation was found between baseline clinical features, ECG pattern, TnT levels, and/or outcome (data not shown).

Discussion
The main findings of this study are: (1) LVOT obstruction is not uncommon in TTC, (2) patients with LVOT obstruction have a different clinical and echocardiographic baseline profile, and (3) an adequate and tailored therapy

Table 1 Baseline characteristics of patients with takotsubo cardiomyopathy

	Total (n = 32)	No LVOT obstruction (n = 26)	LVOT obstruction (n = 6)	P-value
Age (years), mean ± SD	66 ± 15	64 ± 15	77 ± 7	0.047*
Female, n (%)	30 (93.8)	24 (92.3)	6 (100)	1.000
Risk factors, n (%)				
Hypertension	18 (56.2)	13 (50.0)	5 (83.3)	0.196
Hypercholesterolemia	8 (25.0)	5 (19.2)	3 (50.0)	0.296
Diabetes mellitus	3 (9.4)	2 (7.7)	1 (16.7)	1.000
Trigger, n (%)				
Physical stress	13 (59.1)	12 (46.2)	1 (16.7)	0.387
Emotional stress	9 (40.9)	8 (30.8)	1 (16.7)	0.850
Presenting symptom, n (%)				
Chest pain	17 (53.1)	15 (57.7)	2 (33.3)	0.383
Respiratory distress	8 (25.0)	7 (26.9)	1 (16.7)	1.000
Cardiogenic shock	5 (15.6)	2 (7.7)	3 (50.0)	0.034*
VT/VF	2 (6.2)	2 (7.7)	0 (0.0)	1.000
ECG, n (%) or mean ± SD				
ST-elevation	17 (53.1)	13 (50.0)	4 (66.7)	0.659
ST-depression/negT	14 (43.8)	12 (46.2)	2 (33.3)	0.672
QRS (ms)	97 ± 10	98 ± 10	92 ± 7	0.179
QTc (ms)	421 ± 30	418 ± 27	435 ± 43	0.223
TnT (ng/mL), mean ± SD	0.93 ± 0.90	0.99 ± 0.96	0.68 ± 0.50	0.462
TTE, n (%) or mean ± SD				
LVEF (%)[#]	40.5 ± 10.3	41.1 ± 11.0	38.0 ± 5.8	0.512
IVS (mm)	10.8 ± 1.7	10.5 ± 1.4	12.0 ± 2.1	0.044*
Septal bulge	12 (37.5)	7 (26.9)	5 (83.3)	0.018*
SAM	6 (18.8)	0 (0.0)	6 (100)	< 0.001*
MR grade	1.25 ± 0.73	1.0 ± 0.6	2.2 ± 0.7	< 0.001*
Therapeutic options, n (%)				
Inotropics i.v.	9 (28.1)	7 (26.9)	2 (33.3)	1.000
Beta-blocker i.v.	2 (6.2)	0 (0.0)	2 (33.3)	0.030*
IABP	9 (28.1)	7 (26.9)	2 (33.3)	1.000
Recuperation, mean ± SD				
LVEF ≥55% (days)	19 ± 12	18 ± 11	23 ± 16	0.479

Continuous variables are reported as means ± SD.; categorical variables are reported as absolute values and percentages. Continuous and categorical variables were compared by use of (un)paired t test, χ^2 test and Fisher test, as appropriate. *Abbreviations*: *VT/VF* ventricular tachycardia/fibrillation, *TnT* troponin T, *TTE* transthoracic echocardiography, *LVEF* left ventricular ejection fraction, *IVS* interventricular septum thickness, *SAM*, systolic anterior motion, *MR*, mitral regurgitation, *IABP* intraaortic balloon pump. #LVEF as calculated on LV angiogram (and confirmed on transthoracic echocardiography).
*P-value < 0.05.

in TTC patients with LVOT obstruction results in a non-inferior outcome as compared to those without LVOT obstruction.

In line with previous findings [3-5,9], we report an overall prevalence of TTC of 1.0% in patients presenting with troponin-positive ACS – this prevalence is even higher when considering only female patients, as TTC predominantly occurs in postmenopausal women. TTC is not necessarily a benign disease, considering the occurence of cardiogenic shock, life-threatening arrhythmias, and sudden

cardiac death [10-12] as well as persistent wall motion abnormalities with delayed recovery [13,14]. Interestingly, we noted a co-incidence of LVOT obstruction in approximately one out of five subjects (19%) presenting with TTC – this is in line with other studies reporting a 5-25% prevalence of LVOT obstruction in TTC patients [6,15-18].

In addition, our study confirms the presence of a characteristic baseline profile in TTC patients with LVOT obstruction – as previously reported by El Mahmoud et al. [18] – and adds data regarding trigger, presenting

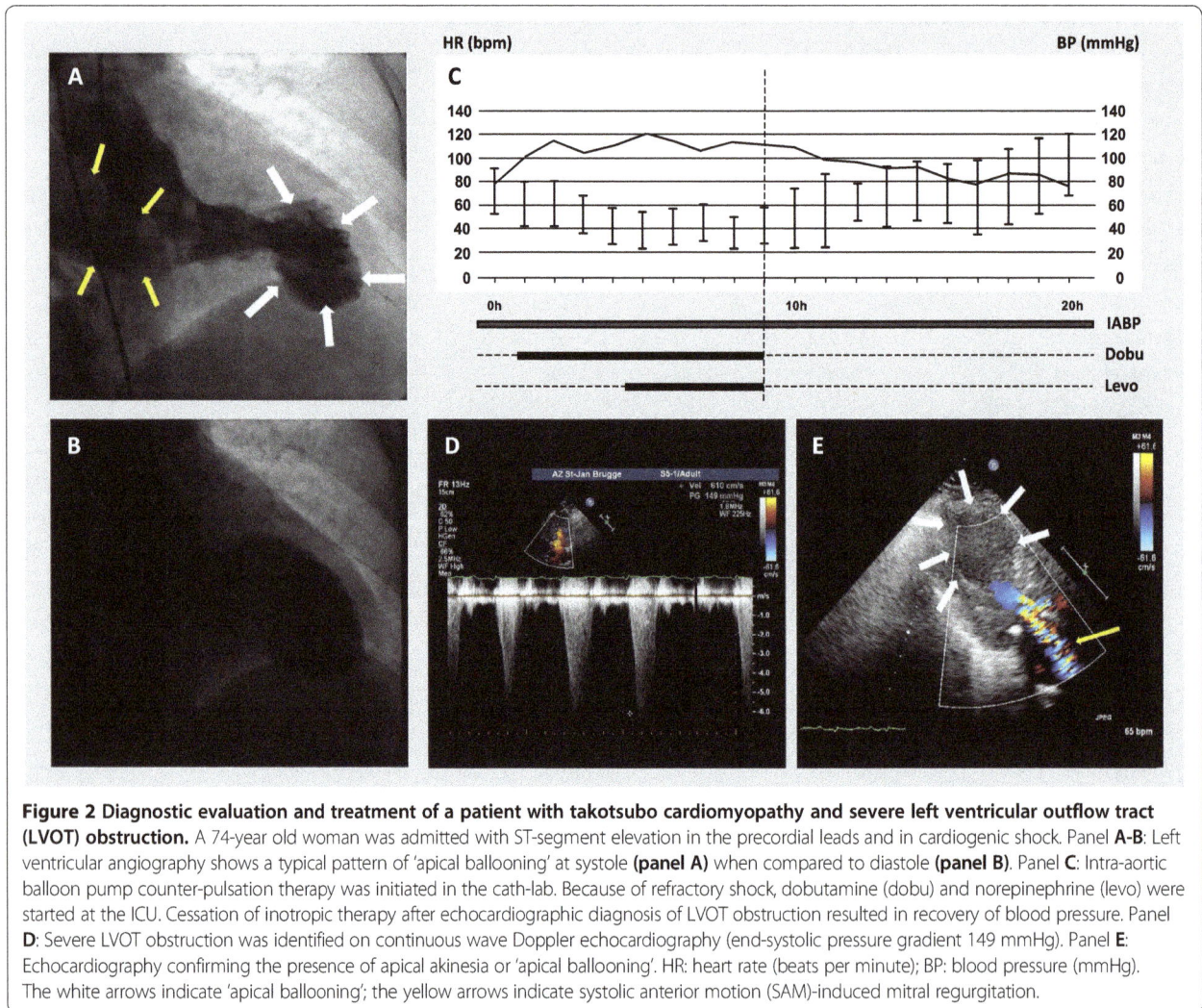

Figure 2 Diagnostic evaluation and treatment of a patient with takotsubo cardiomyopathy and severe left ventricular outflow tract (LVOT) obstruction. A 74-year old woman was admitted with ST-segment elevation in the precordial leads and in cardiogenic shock. Panel **A-B**: Left ventricular angiography shows a typical pattern of 'apical ballooning' at systole (**panel A**) when compared to diastole (**panel B**). Panel **C**: Intra-aortic balloon pump counter-pulsation therapy was initiated in the cath-lab. Because of refractory shock, dobutamine (dobu) and norepinephrine (levo) were started at the ICU. Cessation of inotropic therapy after echocardiographic diagnosis of LVOT obstruction resulted in recovery of blood pressure. Panel **D**: Severe LVOT obstruction was identified on continuous wave Doppler echocardiography (end-systolic pressure gradient 149 mmHg). Panel **E**: Echocardiography confirming the presence of apical akinesia or 'apical ballooning'. HR: heart rate (beats per minute); BP: blood pressure (mmHg). The white arrows indicate 'apical ballooning'; the yellow arrows indicate systolic anterior motion (SAM)-induced mitral regurgitation.

symptoms and therapeutic options. In particular, patients with LVOT obstruction were older and nearly all presented a septal bulge, associated with SAM of the mitral valve and significant MR. This morphological pattern of the IVS is mostly present in elderly patients with a medical history of hypertension and seems to be a predisposing and/or contributing factor to the development of LVOT obstruction in TTC patients, thereby mimicking a pattern of hypertrophic obstructive cardiomyopathy.

In 2001, Villareal et al. reported for the first time LVOT obstruction in three patients with TTC [19]. Other groups could confirm these pathologic findings, especially in women with a mid-ventricular septal thickening, suggesting that this could be an important factor in the development of this syndrome [20]. It was hypothesized that in the presence of increased concentrations of catecholamines – caused by a stressful event – this mid-ventricular septal thickening could lead to the development of a severe transient LV mid-cavity obstruction, resulting

in 'apical stunning' (unrelated to a specific coronary artery territory). Still, it remains unclear whether the observed LVOT pressure gradient is a 'consequence' rather than a 'cause' of TTC, also given the fact that LVOT obstruction does not occur in all TTC patients [21]. Remarkably, approximately half of our TTC patients with LVOT obstruction exhibited cardiogenic shock at admission, suggesting that this mechanism plays a detrimental role in the further clinical evolution of this disease. Of note, none of the TTC patients with LVOT obstruction died in our cohort and all patients had full LVEF recovery, which was accompanied by disappearance of the dynamic LVOT pressure gradient, disappearance of SAM and MR reduction.

Clinical implications
Identification of TTC patients at risk for LVOT obstruction is of critical importance as its presence has important therapeutical management implications. In particular, older age and presence of septal bulge are associated with LVOT

obstruction and may be considered potential risk factors. In addition, hemodynamic instability at presentation should raise suspicion of LVOT obstruction in these patients. In fact, the use of inotropic agents should be avoided in patients with LVOT obstruction, particularly when hemodynamic instability is present, as inotropic therapy may increase LVOT obstruction and worsen cardiogenic shock [22-25]. Administration of β-blockers has been shown not to be detrimental and potentially of benefit to alleviate LVOT obstruction in these patients [26]. However, patients without significant LVOT obstruction who are hypotensive due to severe LV dysfunction can be treated with inotropes such as dobutamine and dopamine, and in these cases, use of β-blockers is contraindicated [22]. Therefore, we suggest that transthoracic echocardiography should be systematically performed at admission in all patients presenting with TTC in order to identify presence of LVOT obstruction, especially when additional risk factors are present. The importance of echocardiography for the successful management of TTC patients in cardiogenic shock is illustrated by patient case #12, in which the detection of severe LVOT obstruction – evidenced by a peak end-systolic pressure gradient of 149 mmHg – led to cessation of all inotropic support and, ultimately, the survival of this patient who was admitted with profound cardiogenic shock (Figure 2).

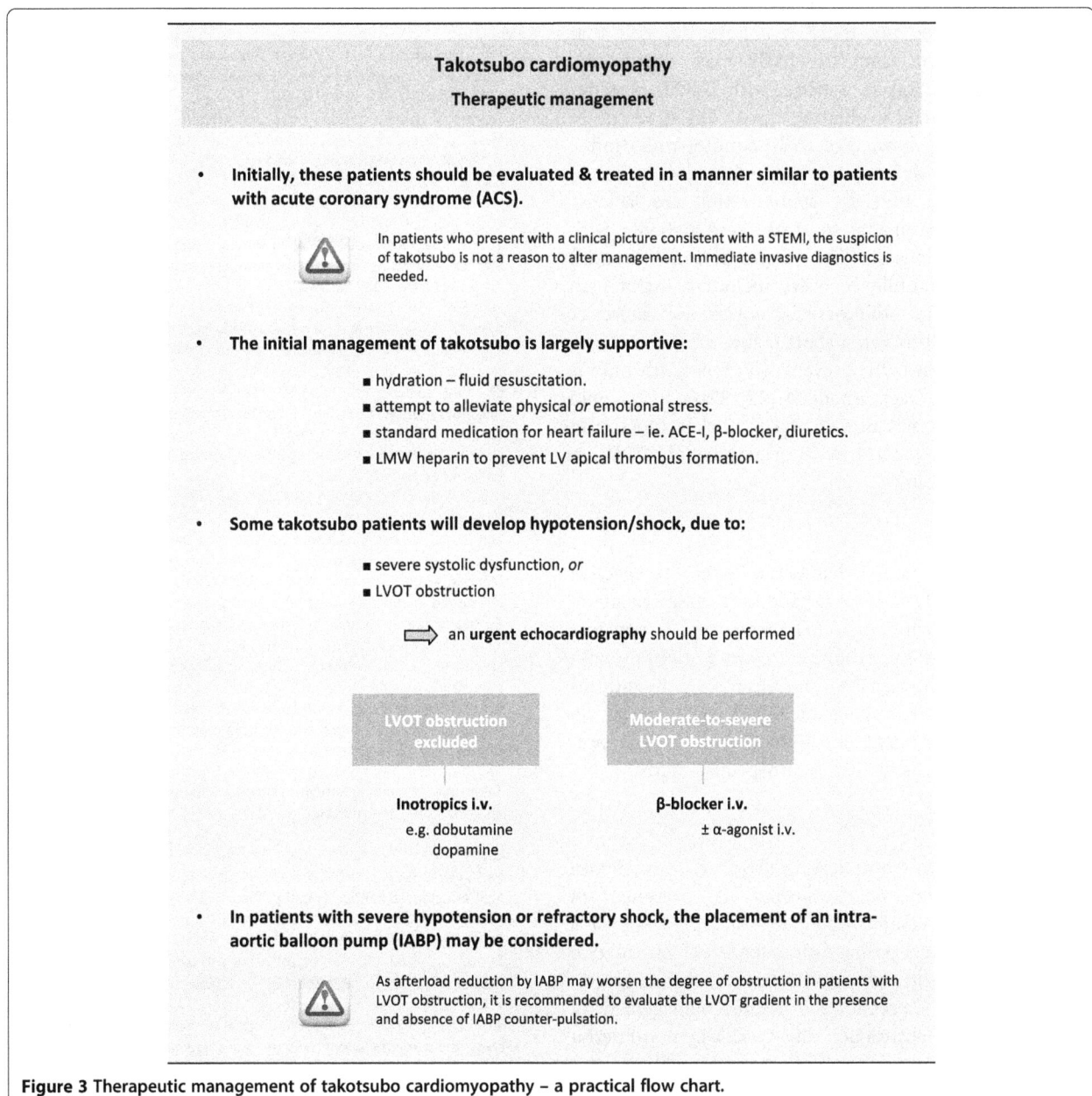

Takotsubo cardiomyopathy

Therapeutic management

- **Initially, these patients should be evaluated & treated in a manner similar to patients with acute coronary syndrome (ACS).**

  In patients who present with a clinical picture consistent with a STEMI, the suspicion of takotsubo is not a reason to alter management. Immediate invasive diagnostics is needed.

- **The initial management of takotsubo is largely supportive:**

  - hydration – fluid resuscitation.
  - attempt to alleviate physical *or* emotional stress.
  - standard medication for heart failure – ie. ACE-I, β-blocker, diuretics.
  - LMW heparin to prevent LV apical thrombus formation.

- **Some takotsubo patients will develop hypotension/shock, due to:**

  - severe systolic dysfunction, *or*
  - LVOT obstruction

    ⟹ an **urgent echocardiography** should be performed

LVOT obstruction excluded	Moderate-to-severe LVOT obstruction
Inotropics i.v.	**β-blocker i.v.**
e.g. dobutamine dopamine	± α-agonist i.v.

- **In patients with severe hypotension or refractory shock, the placement of an intra-aortic balloon pump (IABP) may be considered.**

  As afterload reduction by IABP may worsen the degree of obstruction in patients with LVOT obstruction, it is recommended to evaluate the LVOT gradient in the presence and absence of IABP counter-pulsation.

Figure 3 Therapeutic management of takotsubo cardiomyopathy – a practical flow chart.

Based on our findings and previous reports, we propose a practical flow chart for the management of patients with TTC in Figure 3. In general, the initial management of TTC should be largely supportive, including adequate hydration in non-acute heart failure patients and an attempt to alleviate the triggering physical or emotional stress. When confronted with TTC patients with hypotension/shock, urgent echocardiographic evaluation is indispensable in order to evaluate LV systolic function as well as the potential presence of LVOT obstruction. In patients with hypotension and moderate-to-severe LVOT obstruction, inotropic agents and vasodilators should be avoided and use of β-blockers warrants consideration. In patients with severe hypotension or refractory shock, the use of IABP may be considered. As there is a potential risk that afterload reduction from the IABP may worsen the degree of obstruction in patients with LVOT obstruction, we recommend evaluating the LVOT gradient in the presence and absence of IABP counter-pulsation

Controlled data defining the optimal medical regimen for TTC patients after the acute setting are lacking. However, it is reasonable to treat these patients with standard medications for LV systolic dysfunction until LV systolic function fully recovers, including angiotensin converting enzyme inhibitors, β-blockers and diuretics as appropriate. Moreover, a short course of low molecular weight heparins to prevent LV apical thrombus formation may be recommended [22]. Data that would support the persistent use of oral β-blocker therapy in order to prevent long-term re-occurence of TTC are currently not available.

Study limitations
We recognize this study is hampered by its retrospective and observational nature. In addition, assessment of independent predictors of LVOT obstruction is not possible, given the limited number of cases presenting with LVOT obstruction. However, our results are hypothesis generating and the impact of LVOT obstruction on therapeutic management and outcome of patients presenting with TTC needs further prospective study.

Conclusions
LVOT obstruction complicating TTC is a common transient phenomenon, suspected if presence of hemodynamic instability. Older age and presence of a septal bulge are predisposing factors for LVOT obstruction development. Timely and accurate diagnosis by echocardiography is key to successful and tailored management of TTC with LVOT obstruction and results in non-inferior outcome as compared to TTC patients without this condition.

Abbreviations
TTC: Takotsubo cardiomyopathy; LVOT: Left ventricular outflow tract; SAM: Systolic anterior motion; LV: Left ventricular; ACS: Acute coronary syndrome; TnT: Troponin-T; LVEF: Left ventricular ejection fraction; IVS: Interventricular septum; MR: Mitral regurgitation; VT: Ventricular tachycardia; VF: Ventricular fibrillation; IABP: Intra-aortic balloon pump.

Competing interests
The authors declare that they have no competing interests.

Authors' contributions
ODB collected and analysed all data and wrote the first draft of the manuscript. PD contributed essentially to the content of the manuscript. SG, LM, PG and LM revised the manuscript critically. All authors read and approved the final version of the manuscript.

References
1. Prasad A, Lerman A, Rihal CS: Apical ballooning syndrome (Tako-Tsubo or stress cardiomyopathy): a mimic of acute myocardial infarction. *Am Heart J* 2008, 155:408–417.
2. Sharkey SW, Windenburg DC, Lesser JR, Maron MS, Hauser RG, Lesser JN, Haas TS, Hodges JS, Maron BJ: Natural history and expansive clinical profile of stress (tako-tsubo) cardiomyopathy. *J Am Coll Cardiol* 2010, 55:333–341.
3. Tsuchihashi K, Ueshima K, Uchida T, Oh-mura N, Kimura K, Owa M, Yoshiyama M, Miyazaki S, Haze K, Ogawa H, Honda T, Hase M, Kai R, Morii I: Transient left ventricular apical ballooning without coronary artery stenosis: a novel heart syndrome mimicking acute myocardial infarction. *J Am Coll Cardiol* 2001, 38:11–18.
4. Bybee KA, Kara T, Prasad A, Lerman A, Barsness GW, Wright RS, Rihal CS: Systematic review: transient left ventricular apical ballooning: a syndrome that mimics ST-segment elevation myocardial infarction. *Ann Intern Med* 2004, 141:858–865.
5. Gianni M, Dentali F, Grandi AM, Sumner G, Hiralal R, Lonn E: Apical ballooning syndrome or takotsubo cardiomyopathy: a systematic review. *Eur Heart J* 2006, 27:1523–1529.
6. Nef HM, Möllmann H, Elsässer A: Tako-tsubo cardiomyopathy (apical ballooning). *Heart* 2007, 93:1309–1315.
7. Lang RM, Bierig M, Devereux RB, Flachskampf FA, Foster E, Pellikka PA, Picard MH, Roman MJ, Seward J, Shanewise JS, Solomon SD, Spencer KT, Sutton MS, Stewart WJ: Recommendations for chamber quantification: a report from the American Society of Echocardiography's Guidelines and Standards Committee and the Chamber Quantification Writing Group, developed in conjunction with the European Association of Echocardiography, a branch of the European Society of Cardiology. *J Am Soc Echocardiogr* 2005, 18:1440–1463.
8. Lancellotti P, Moura L, Pierard LA, Agricola E, Popescu BA, Tribouilloy C, Hagendorff A, Monin JL, Badano L, Zamorano JL: European Association of Echocardiography recommendations for the assessment of valvular regurgitation. Part 2: mitral and tricuspid regurgitation (native valve disease). *Eur J Echocardiogr* 2010, 11:307–332.
9. Sy F, Basraon J, Zheng H, Singh M, Richina J, Ambrose JA: Frequency of Takotsubo cardiomyopathy in postmenopausal women presenting with an acute coronary syndrome. *Am J Cardiol* 2013, 112:479–482.
10. Weihs V, Szücs D, Fellner B, Eber B, Weihs W, Lambert T, Metzler B, Titscher G, Hochmayer B, Dechant C, Eder V, Siostrzonek P, Leisch F, Pichler M, Pachinger O, Gaul G, Weber H, Podczeck-Schweighofer A, Nesser HJ, Huber K: Stress-induced cardiomyopathy (Tako-Tsubo syndrome) in Austria. *Eur Heart J Acute Cardiovasc Care* 2013, 2:137–146.
11. Pant S, Deshmukh A, Mehta K, Badheka AO, Tuliani T, Patel NJ, Dabhadkar K, Prasad A, Paydak H: Burden of arrhythmias in patients with Takotsubo Cardiomyopathy (apical ballooning syndrome). *Int J Cardiol* 2013, 170:64–68.
12. Brinjikji W, El-Sayed AM, Salka S: In-hospital mortality among patients with takotsubo cardiomyopathy: a study of the National Inpatient Sample 2008 to 2009. *Am Heart J* 2012, 164:215–221.

13. Medeiros K, O'Connor MJ, Baicu CF, Fitzgibbons TP, Shaw P, Tighe DA, Zile MR, Aurigemma GP: **Systolic and diastolic mechanisms in stress cardiomyopathy.** *Circulation* 2014, **129**:1659–1667.

14. Ahtarovski KA, Iversen KK, Christensen TE, Andersson H, Grande P, Holmvang L, Bang L, Hasbak P, Lonborg JT, Madsen PL, Engstrom T, Vejlstrup NG: **Takotsubo cardiomyopathy, a two-stage recovery of left ventricular systolic and diastolic function as determined by cardiac magnetic resonance imaging.** *Eur Heart J Cardiovasc Imaging* 2014, **15**:855–862.

15. De Backer O, Debonnaire P, Muyldermans L, Missault L: **Tako-tsubo cardiomyopathy with left ventricular outflow tract (LVOT) obstruction: case report and review of the literature.** *Acta Clin Belg* 2011, **66**:298–301.

16. Parodi G, Del Pace S, Salvadori C, Carabba N, Olivotto I, Gensini GF: **Left ventricular apical ballooning syndrome as a novel cause of acute mitral regurgitation.** *J Am Coll Cardiol* 2007, **50**:647–649.

17. Meimoun P, Malaquin D, Benali T, Boulanger J, Zemir H, Tribouilloy C: **Transient impairment of coronary flow reserve in tako-tsubo cardiomyopathy is related to left ventricular systolic parameters.** *Eur J Echocardiogr* 2009, **10**:265–270.

18. El Mahmoud R, Mansencal N, Pilliére R, Leyer F, Abbou N, Michaud P: **Prevalence and characteristics of LV outflow tract obstruction in Tako-Tsubo syndrome.** *Am Heart J* 2008, **156**:543–548.

19. Villareal RP, Achari A, Wilansky S, Wilson JM: **Anteroapical stunning and left ventricular outflow tract obstruction.** *Mayo Clin Proc* 2001, **76**:79–83.

20. Merli E, Sutcliffe S, Gori M, Sutherland GG: **Tako-Tsubo cardiomyopathy: new insights into the possible underlying pathophysiology.** *Eur J Echocardiogr* 2006, **7**:53–61.

21. Desmet W: **Dynamic LV obstruction in apical ballooning syndrome: the chicken or the egg.** *Eur J Echocardiogr* 2006, **7**:1–4.

22. Reeder GS, Prasad A: **Stress-induced cardiomyopathy.** In *UpToDate*. Edited by Post TW. Waltham, MA: UpToDate; 2013.

23. Yalcinkaya E, Bugan B, Celik M: **Refractory hypotension in Takotsubo cardio-myopathy: intuitive therapies could deteriorate hemodynamic stability.** *Am J Emerg Med* 2013, **31**:1619–1620.

24. Redfors B, Shao Y, Omerovic E: **Stress-induced cardiomyopathy in the critically ill – why inotropes fail to improve outcome.** *Int J Cardiol* 2013, **168**:4489–4490.

25. Vyas C, Shah S, Pancholy S, Patel T, Moussa I: **Consequences of misdiagnosis and mismanagement of Takotsubo cardiomyopathy.** *Acute Card Care* 2012, **14**:117–119.

26. Yoshioka T, Hashimoto A, Tsuchihashi K, Nagao K, Kyuma M, Ooiwa H, Nozawa A, Shimoshige S, Eguchi M, Wakabayashi T, Yuda S, Hase M, Nakata T, Shimamoto K: **Clinical implications of midventricular obstruction and intravenous propranolol use in transient left ventricular apical ballooning.** *Am Heart J* 2008, **155**:1–7.

12

Multiple focal and macroreentrant left atrial tachycardias originating from a spontaneous scar at the contiguous aorta-left atrium area in a patient with hypertrophic cardiomyopathy

Kyoichiro Yazaki* (ID), Yoichi Ajiro, Fumiaki Mori, Masahiro Watanabe, Kei Tsukamoto, Takashi Saito, Keiko Mizobuchi and Kazunori Iwade

Abstract

Background: Spontaneous scar-related left atrial tachycardia (AT) is a rare arrhythmia. We describe a patient with hypertrophic cardiomyopathy (HCM) who developed multiple, both focal and macroreentrant left ATs associated with a spontaneous scar located at the aorta-left atrium (LA) contiguous area.

Case presentation: A 65-year-old man with HCM complained of palpitations. Twelve-lead electrocardiogram showed narrow QRS tachycardia with 2:1 atrioventricular conduction. Two sessions of radiofrequency ablation (RFA) were required to eliminate all left ATs. In the first session, 3-dimensional electroanatomical mapping fused with the image constructed by multi-detector computed tomography showed a clockwise macroreentrant AT (AT1) associated with a low-voltage or dense scar area located along the aorta-LA contiguous area. AT1 was eliminated by RFA to the narrow isthmus with slow conduction velocity within the scar. Additional ATs (AT2-AT4) occurred 1 month after the first ablation. In the second session, AT2 and AT3 were identified as focal ATs with centrifugal propagation and few accompanying fragmentations, and AT4 as a macroreentrant AT with features similar to AT1. AT2 and AT3 were successfully eliminated by performing RFA to the earliest activation site, and AT4 was terminated by performing RFA to the narrow isthmus with slow conduction velocity. No ATs have recurred for 11 months after these RFAs. Interestingly, the substrate for all left ATs was associated with the aorta-LA contiguous area.

Conclusion: To our knowledge, this is the first case of multiple, both focal and macroreentrant left ATs associated with a contiguous aorta-LA spontaneous scar area in a patient with HCM.

Keywords: Case report, Atrial tachycardia, Contiguous aorta-left atrium area, Spontaneous scar, Hypertrophic cardiomyopathy, 3-D electroanatomical mapping

* Correspondence: kamisamakaranookurimono@gmail.com
Department of Cardiology, National Hospital Organization Yokohama Medical Center, 3-60-2 Harajuku, Totsuka-ku, Yokohama-shi, Kanagawa 245-8575, Japan

Background

The treatment of atrial tachycardia (AT) is important because, similar to atrial fibrillation [1], AT can lead to poor outcomes in patients with hypertrophic cardiomyopathy (HCM) [2]. While most ATs originating from the left atrium (LA) occur in association with a procedure-related scar due to cardiac surgery or catheter ablation [3–5], left ATs related to a non-procedure-related spontaneous scar have been reported in association with a substrate in the LA anterior wall [6]. A rigid aorta-LA connection exists, which may promote myocardial fibrosis [7, 8]. ATs are often classified according to their endocardial activation pattern as follows: (1) focal ATs, spreading centrifugally from the tachycardia origin based on microreentry, automaticity, or triggered activity, and (2) macroreentrant ATs with a continuous loop of the electrical wavelet based on macroreentry [9]. Scar-related ATs can be classified as either pattern. However, clinical reports particularly concerning spontaneous LA scars are limited.

Here, we describe a patient with HCM who had both focal and macroreentrant multiple ATs associated with a spontaneous scar at the contiguous aorta-LA region that were successfully ablated using 3-D electroanatomical mapping fused with the image constructed using multidetector computed tomography (MDCT).

Case presentation

A 65-year-old patient with HCM and a history of common atrial flutter ablation was referred to our clinic with complaints of recurrent shortness of breath and palpitations. Two years prior, echocardiogram showed HCM with a preserved left ventricular ejection fraction and a slightly enlarged LA; coronary angiogram showed intact coronary arteries, and results of a right ventricular myocardial biopsy showed mildly hypertrophic myocardium with mild fibrosis at the subendomyocardium and perivascular area. A concomitant cavotricuspid-isthmus-dependent atrial flutter was eliminated by performing linear ablation between the tricuspid annulus through the inferior vena cava during the same hospitalization.

Two years later, he again developed atrial arrhythmia. Twelve-lead electrocardiogram showed AT (AT1) with 2:1 atrioventricular conduction (Fig. 1a). An electrophysiological study was subsequently conducted. A 10-polar electrode catheter (Response™, St. Jude Medical Co., Ltd., Minnesota, USA) was placed in the coronary sinus (CS), and a 20-polar electrode catheter (LiveWire™, St. Jude Medical Co., Ltd.) was placed along the tricuspid annulus. Intracardiac electrograms were filtered at 50–500 Hz. Electroanatomical mapping was performed using a 3-D electroanatomical mapping system (Ensite NavX™, St. Jude Medical Co., Ltd.). AT1 persisted from the beginning of the first session with a tachycardia cycle length (TCL) of 248 ms. Because the atrial activation pattern in the CS

electrode was detected distal to the proximal sequence and the CS distal activation was earlier than the earliest activation site within the right atrium, we concluded that AT1 originated from the LA. A multipolar ring catheter (Reflection spiral™, St. Jude Medical Co., Ltd.) and a 4-mm open-irrigated-tip catheter (FlexAbility™, St. Jude Medical. Co., Ltd.) were inserted into the LA through a single transseptal puncture. Further activation mapping of the LA demonstrated that AT1 propagated in a figure-eight configuration around the mitral annulus clockwise, and the total activation time of AT1 accounted for almost the entire TCL (Additional file 1; Fig. 2a). 3-D electroanatomical voltage mapping fused with the constructed MDCT image showed a low-voltage (<0.5 mV), dense scar (<0.05 mV) area along the aorta-LA contiguous area from the mid-LA anterior wall through the anterior mitral annulus (Fig. 3); activation mapping indicated that this spontaneous scar area was related to the slow conduction zone for the AT1 circuit. We concluded that AT1 was a macroreentrant AT dependent on the isthmus located along the aorta-LA contiguous area; subsequent radiofrequency ablation (RFA) confirmed the existence of the circuit point-by-point in the entrainment study. AT1 was terminated by RFA at the site near the mitral annulus where a preceding local potential 110 ms before the P-wave onset and postpacing interval were equal to the TCL during the entrainment study. AT1 and the other ATs could not be provoked again during this session by burst pacing with or without isoproterenol infusion. Due to the severity of the patient's heart failure, a minimally invasive procedure was preferred; hence, additional RFA was not conducted during the first session.

One month later, another AT with a longer TCL of 286 ms (AT2) occurred (Fig. 1b), and the patient developed worsening heart failure. A second electrophysiological session was performed with the same system settings. AT2 was reproducibly provoked by atrial burst pacing without isoproterenol infusion. Activation mapping showed a centrifugal pattern with the origin located at the border of the aorta-LA contiguous, low-voltage area of the mid-anterior LA wall, different from the prior ablation points for AT1 (Additional file 2). Several entrainment studies could not demonstrate manifest entrainment, and there was no fragmented potential that accounted for almost the entire TCL around the earliest activation site. AT2 was terminated by performing RFA at the earliest atrial activation site (Fig. 2b). A third AT with a TCL of 330 ms (AT3) was easily and reproducibly provoked by burst pacing without isoproterenol infusion. AT3 also had centrifugal propagation similar to AT2 (Additional file 3). AT3 was successfully terminated by performing a single RFA at the earliest activation site near the AT2 ablation site (Fig. 2c). A fourth AT with a TCL of 350 ms (AT4) was also provoked by burst pacing

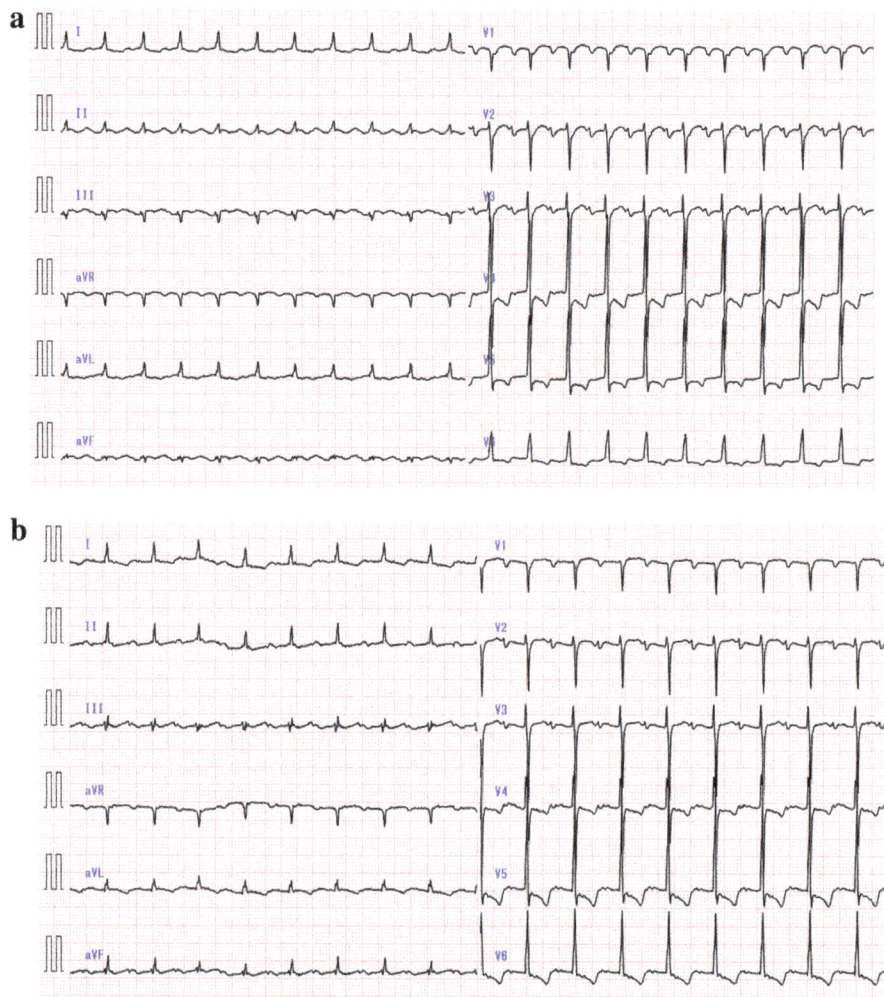

Fig. 1 a 12-lead electrocardiogram (ECG) showing narrow QRS tachycardia with 2:1 atrioventricular conduction. A saw-tooth wave was detected by the inferior lead, and the tachycardia cycle length (TCL) was 240 ms. **b** ECG showing narrow QRS tachycardia with 2:1 atrioventricular conduction. P-wave deflection was negative in V_1, and the TCL was 286 ms

without isoproterenol infusion; however, electroanatomical activation mapping of AT4 showed macroreentry in a clockwise fashion, mimicking peri-mitral flutter, similar to AT1 (Additional file 4; Fig. 2d). The critical isthmus of AT4 was located near the upper edge of the prior ablation area for AT1 where the long-duration, fractionated potential that accounted for about 70% of the TCL was recorded and the post-pacing interval was equal to the TCL during the entrainment study. This narrow isthmus was located between the dense scar and upper edge of a prior ablation area. A single RFA at this site terminated AT4, and AT4 was never provoked again by burst pacing with or without isoproterenol infusion. We aimed to achieve noninducibility of ATs, instead of creating a complete block line, because minimal procedures were required due to the severity of the patient's heart failure.

No ATs have recurred in this patient, up to 11 months after these interventions.

Discussion
The present case demonstrates two important issues: (1) a large spontaneous scar can exist along the aorto-LA contiguous region in the LA that can be arrhythmogenic; (2) multiple ATs with two different activation patterns - both focal and macroreentrant - can occur in association with a spontaneous scar in the LA.

In contrast to the right atrium, the LA has few anatomical obstacles [10]. However, a spontaneous scar can arise in the LA and can act as an arrhythmia substrate [11]. The most common region for a spontaneous scar to develop is the aorta-LA contiguous area; in this region, rigid contact between the aorta and LA exits, which can promote fibrosis and lead to scar formation [12, 13]. Hori Y. et al. demonstrated 68% of the LA very low voltage area (<0.2 mV) overlapped with areas of the LA that contact external anatomical structures, such as the aorta and vertebra, suggesting that contact with

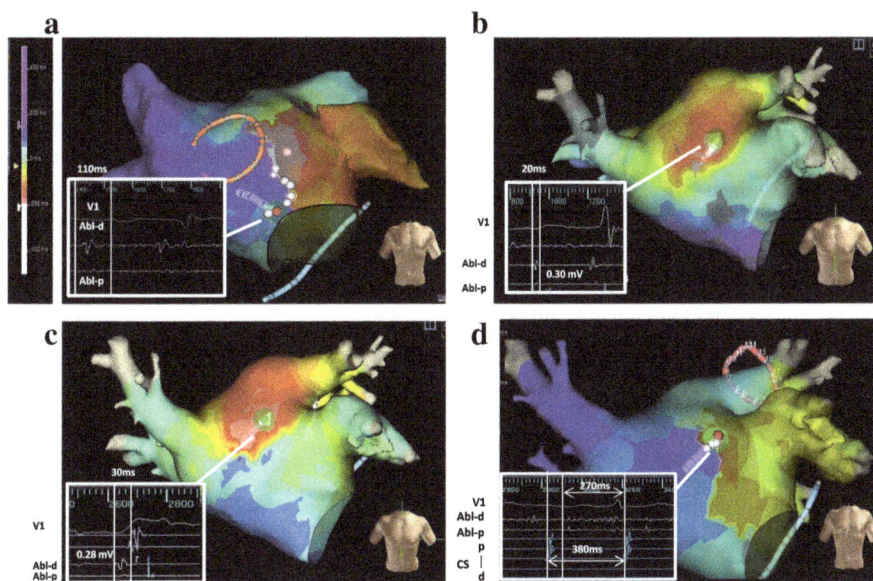

Fig. 2 Activation mapping during multiple atrial tachycardias: atrial tachycardia (AT)1 (**a**), AT2 (**b**), AT3 (**c**) and AT4 (**d**). The activation patterns of AT1 and AT4 showed macroreentry. AT1 and AT4 were terminated by performing radiofrequency ablation at the *red circle* where a long-duration, fractionated potential was recorded. The *white circles* represent the unsuccessful site for terminating AT. AT2 and AT3, which had a centrifugal pattern, were terminated at the early activation site where the local potentials preceded the P-wave onset. Abl-d = distal ablation electrode; Abl-p = proximal ablation electrode; CS-p = proximal coronary sinus electrode; CS-d = distal coronary sinus electrode

external anatomical structures may influence scar formation [13]. Wakabayashi Y. et al. reported a patient with HCM who had a spontaneous scar in the LA anterior wall in contact with the right pulmonary artery, implying that HCM-induced pressure overload might contribute to remodeling and fibrosis [6]. In the present case, heterogeneous myocardial damage, including a wide aorta-

LA contiguous scar area and electrically normal posterior LA wall, was observed, suggesting that mechanical stress due to the rigid connection played a more important role than pressure overload in fibrosis and scar formation of the LA. Interestingly, HCM itself plays a potential role in promoting myocardial fibrosis and scar formation. In addition to the genetic background of

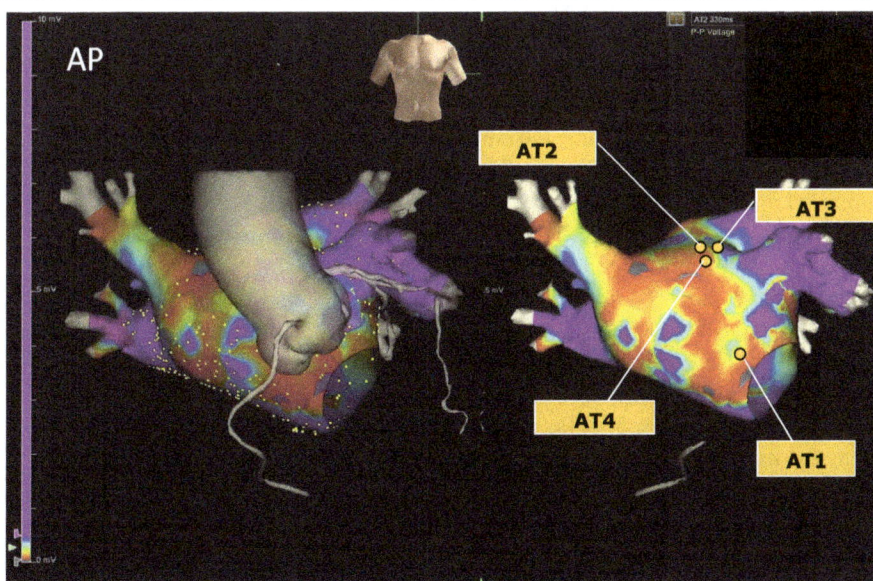

Fig. 3 Electroanatomical voltage mapping fused with MDCT. A low-voltage area existed along the aorta-left atrium contiguous region. Termination of the atrial tachycardias (AT1-4) was achieved at the points indicated by the *yellow circles*

HCM, it has been reported that transforming growth factor-β1, a potent stimulator of collagen-producing cardiac fibroblasts that also stimulates the differentiation of fibroblasts into more active myofibroblasts, is highly expressed in the myocardium of patients with HCM, implying that HCM increases the susceptibility to triggers that promote myocardial fibrosis [14–17]. Therefore, when cardiologists plan a therapeutic strategy for a patient with HCM who has various left ATs, they should consider the possibility of an existing spontaneous scar and its possible role as an arrhythmogenic substrate even if the patient has no history of surgical interventions to the LA.

Regarding the mechanism of AT from an electrophysiological aspect, macroreentry and microreentry have been reported in association with a spontaneous scar [7, 11]. In cases of spontaneous scar, the aorta-LA contiguous scar area has been reported to be involved in the reentry circuit of localized reentrant AT [12]. However, other mechanisms, such as automaticity and triggered activity, may also be involved in the arrhythmogenesis of ATs due to scar [18]. Furthermore, the mechanical stretch induced by LA enlargement itself may cause changes in cellular action potential and calcium current, which potentially alter the arrhythmogenicity of the tissue [19]. Considering the underlying mechanism of ATs in the present case, AT1 and AT4 (recurrence of AT1) were based on macroreentry, as depicted on activation mapping. AT2 and AT3 were focal ATs depicted as centrifugal propagation. After assessing the underlying mechanism of AT2 and AT3 in the present case, the following observations suggest the likelihood of triggered activity other than microreentry or automaticity: (1) AT2 and AT3 were easily provoked by burst pacing without isoproterenol; (2) no gradual acceleration and/or slowing, known as the warm up or cool down phenomenon, was observed; (3) no manifest entrainment was observed; and (4) no fractionated potential accounting for almost the entire TCL was observed around the earliest activation site of those ATs. While it is often difficult to identify the underlying mechanism of ATs in clinical practice [20, 21], we consider it important to assess the arrhythmia etiology and its mechanisms in order to provide appropriate comprehensive treatment. Because the present case implies the possible arrhythmogenesis of focal ATs, unlike microreentry from a spontaneous scar in the LA, we considered it important to remember that multiple ATs of various mechanisms can arise in association with a spontaneous scar.

The 3-D electroanatomical mapping fused with the image constructed by MDCT is the preferred modality for visualization of tachyarrhythmia propagation in relation to anatomical information. This modality is useful not only in planning the ablation strategy but also in understanding the relationship between anatomical obstacles and the injured myocardium, including low-voltage or silent areas as encountered in the present case. Therefore, we think it is best to use 3-D electroanatomical mapping fused with the image constructed by MDCT when planning ablation treatment for patients with multiple and various ATs associated with an atrial scar.

The case information presented here is beneficial to cardiologists, who should be aware of the possibility that focal and macroreentrant left ATs can occur in association with a spontaneous scar, especially in patients with HCM, even if they have no history of invasive intervention to the LA.

Conclusion

We have reported a case of multiple LA-AT associated with the aorta–LA contiguous low-voltage area and apparently involving various kinds of pathophysiology. Three-dimensional electroanatomical mapping fused with multi-detector computed tomography is useful for visualizing the relation between the aorta and the LA low-voltage area.

Abbreviations

AT: Atrial tachycardia; CS: Coronary sinus; ECG: Electrocardiogram; HCM: Hypertrophic cardiomyopathy; LA: Left atrium; MDCT: Multi-detector computed tomography; RFA: Radiofrequency application; RFCA: Radiofrequency catheter ablation; TCL: Tachycardia cycle length

Acknowledgement
We thank Editage (www.editage.jp) for English language editing.

Funding
The English editing and publishing fees were covered by the Clinical Research Division of Yokohama Medical Center.

Authors' contributions
Clinical data collection and interpretation: KY, YA, FM. Drafting: KY. Editing and revision: KY and YA. Final approval: KY, YA, FM, MW, KT, KM, TS, and KI. Funding: KI. All authors read and approved the final manuscript.

Competing interests
Yoichi Ajiro received rewards for supporting other research performed at St. Jude Medical, Co., Ltd. (Japan). The other authors declare that they have competing interests.

References
1. Olivotto I, Cecchi F, Casey SA, Dolara A, Traverse JH, Maron BJ. Impact of atrial fibrillation on the clinical course of hypertrophic cardiomyopathy. Circulation. 2001;104(21):2517–24.
2. Boolani H, Reddy YM, Ittaman S, Lakkireddy D. Recurrent unilateral pleural effusion in a hypertrophic cardiomyopathy patient secondary to atrial arrhythmias and the role of radiofrequency ablation. Europace. 2012;14(9):1371–2.
3. Duru F, Hindricks G, Kottkamp H. Atypical left atrial flutter after intraoperative radiofrequency ablation of chronic atrial fibrillation: successful ablation using three-dimensional electroanatomic mapping. J Cardiovasc Electrophysiol. 2001;12(5):602–5.

4. Kalman JM, VanHare GF, Olgin JE, Saxon LA, Stark SI, Lesh MD. Ablation of 'incisional' reentrant atrial tachycardia complicating surgery for congenital heart disease. Use of entrainment to define a critical isthmus of conduction. Circulation. 1996;93(3):502–12.

5. Ejima K, Shoda M, Miyazaki S, Yashiro B, Wakisaka O, Manaka T, Hagiwara N. Localized reentrant tachycardia in the aorta contiguity region mimicking perimitral atrial flutter in the context of atrial fibrillation ablation. Heart Vessel. 2013;28(4):546–9.

6. Wakabayashi Y, Hayashi T, Mitsuhashi T, Momomura S-I. Localized reentrant atrial tachycardia without a history of catheter ablation in a patient with apical hypertrophic cardiomyopathy. Circ J. 2014;78(12):2990–2.

7. Fukamizu S, Sakurada H, Hayashi T, Hojo R, Komiyama K, Tanabe Y, Tejima T, Nishizaki M, Kobayashi Y, Hiraoka M. Macroreentrant atrial tachycardia in patients without previous atrial surgery or catheter ablation: clinical and electrophysiological characteristics of scar-related left atrial anterior wall reentry. J Cardiovasc Electrophysiol. 2013;24(4):404–12.

8. Pak HN, Oh YS, Lim HE, Kim YH, Hwang C. Comparison of voltage map-guided left atrial anterior wall ablation versus left lateral mitral isthmus ablation in patients with persistent atrial fibrillation. Heart Rhythm. 2011;8(2):199–206.

9. Zhou G-B, Hu J-Q, Guo X-G, Liu X, Yang J-D, Sun Q, Ma J, Ouyang F-F, Zhang S. Very long-term outcome of catheter ablation of post-incisional atrial tachycardia: Role of incisional and non-incisional scar. Int J Cardiol. 2016;205:72–80.

10. Feld GK, Shahandeh-Rad F. Activation patterns in experimental canine atrial flutter produced by right atrial crush injury. J Am Coll Cardiol. 1992;20(2):441–51.

11. Verma A, Wazni OM, Marrouche NF, Martin DO, Kilicaslan F, Minor S, Schweikert RA, Saliba W, Cummings J, Burkhardt JD, et al. Pre-existent left atrial scarring in patients undergoing pulmonary vein antrum isolation: an independent predictor of procedural failure. J Am Coll Cardiol. 2005;45(2):285–92.

12. Maeda S, Yamauchi Y, Tao S, Okada H, Obayashi T, Hirao K. Small reentrant atrial tachycardia adjacent to left aortic sinus of Valsalva. Circ J. 2013;77(12):3054–5.

13. Hori Y, Nakahara S, Kamijima T, Tsukada N, Hayashi A, Kobayashi S, Sakai Y, Taguchi I. Influence of left atrium anatomical contact area in persistent atrial fibrillation. Circ J. 2014;78(8):1851–7.

14. Li G, Li RK, Mickle DA, Weisel RD, Merante F, Ball WT, Christakis GT, Cusimano RJ, Williams WG. Elevated insulin-like growth factor-I and transforming growth factor-beta 1 and their receptors in patients with idiopathic hypertrophic obstructive cardiomyopathy. A possible mechanism. Circulation. 1998;98(19 Suppl):II144–9. discussion II149-50.

15. Ayca B, Sahin I, Kucuk SH, Akin F, Kafadar D, Avsar M, Avci II, Gungor B, Okuyan E, Dinckal MH. Increased transforming growth factor-beta levels associated with cardiac adverse events in hypertrophic cardiomyopathy. Clin Cardiol. 2015;38(6):371–7.

16. Lijnen P, Petrov V. Transforming growth factor-beta 1-induced collagen production in cultures of cardiac fibroblasts is the result of the appearance of myofibroblasts. Methods Find Exp Clin Pharmacol. 2002;24(6):333–44.

17. Li G, Borger MA, Williams WG, Weisel RD, Mickle DAG, Wigle ED, Li R-K. Regional overexpression of insulin-like growth factor-I and transforming growth factor-β1 in the myocardium of patients with hypertrophic obstructive cardiomyopathy. J Thorac Cardiovasc Surg. 2002;123(1):89–95.

18. Mary-Rabine L, Hordof AJ, Danilo P, Malm JR, Rosen MR. Mechanisms for impulse initiation in isolated human atrial fibers. Circ Res. 1980;47(2):267–77.

19. Deroubaix E, Folliguet T, Rucker-Martin C, Dinanian S, Boixel C, Validire P, Daniel P, Capderou A, Hatem SN. Moderate and chronic hemodynamic overload of sheep atria induces reversible cellular electrophysiologic abnormalities and atrial vulnerability. J Am Coll Cardiol. 2004;44(9):1918–26.

20. Higa S, Chen S-A. Focal atrial tachycardia. J Arrhythm. 2006;22(3):132–48.

21. Higa S, Tai CT, Lin YJ, Liu TY, Lee PC, Huang JL, Hsieh MH, Yuniadi Y, Huang BH, Lee SH, et al. Focal atrial tachycardia: new insight from noncontact mapping and catheter ablation. Circulation. 2004;109(1):84–91.

13

Differentiation of infiltrative cardiomyopathy from hypertrophic cardiomyopathy using high-sensitivity cardiac troponin T

Toru Kubo[1*], Yuichi Baba[1], Takayoshi Hirota[1], Katsutoshi Tanioka[1], Naohito Yamasaki[1], Shigeo Yamanaka[2], Tatsuo Iiyama[3], Naoko Kumagai[3], Takashi Furuno[1], Tetsuro Sugiura[2] and Hiroaki Kitaoka[1]

Abstract

Background: Because infiltrative cardiomyopathy and hypertrophic cardiomyopathy (HCM) share clinical and hemodynamic features of left ventricular (LV) hypertrophy and abnormal diastolic function, it is often difficult to distinguish these entities.

Methods: We investigated the potential role of high-sensitivity cardiac troponin T (hs-cTnT) for differentiation of infiltrative cardiomyopathy from HCM.

Results: The study group consisted of 46 consecutive patients with infiltrative cardiomyopathies or HCM in whom sarcomere protein gene mutations were identified at Kochi Medical School Hospital; of these, there were 11 patients with infiltrative cardiomyopathy (cardiac amyloidosis in 8 patients and Fabry disease in 3 patients) and 35 HCM patients. Serum hs-cTnT level was significantly higher in patients who had infiltrative cardiomyopathy than in those who had HCM (0.083 ± 0.057 ng/ml versus 0.027 ± 0.034 ng/ml, $p < 0.001$), whereas brain natriuretic peptide levels did not differ between the two groups. In two age-matched the 2 cohorts (patients evaluated at > 40 years at age), hs-cTnT level, maximum LV wall thickness, posterior wall thickness, peak early (E) transmitral filling velocity, peak early diastolic (Ea) velocity of tissue Doppler imaging at the lateral corner and E/Ea ratios at both the septal and lateral corners were significantly different between the two groups. As for diagnostic accuracy to differentiate the two groups by using receiver operating characteristic analysis, hs-cTnT was the highest value of area under the curve (0.939) and E/Ea (lateral) was second highest value (0.914).

Conclusions: Serum hs-cTnT is a helpful diagnostic indicator for accurate differentiation between infiltrative cardiomyopathy and HCM.

Keywords: Infiltrative cardiomyopathy, Hypertrophic cardiomyopathy, High-sensitivity cardiac troponin T

Background

Infiltrative cardiomyopathies such as cardiac amyloidosis and Fabry disease are difficult to differentiate from hypertrophic cardiomyopathy (HCM) because these cardiomyopathies share clinical and hemodynamic features of left ventricular (LV) hypertrophy and abnormal diastolic function [1–13]. Amyloidosis is a systemic and progressive disease and frequently involves more than one organ. Cardiac involvement in amyloidosis is the most important prognostic factor, and when cardiac amyloidosis is the first or main manifestation of the disease, correct diagnosis is sometimes difficult [1–5]. Fabry disease is a relatively prevalent cause of LV hypertrophy and is associated with significant morbidity and early death due to heart failure or ventricular arrhythmias [6–9, 14]. Since disease-specific enzyme replacement therapy is now available for Fabry disease, correct diagnosis is important [15, 16]. Although cardiac amyloidosis and cardiac involvement in Fabry disease show concentric LV hypertrophy, LV hypertrophy is usually asymmetric and predominantly septal in HCM, and there is often a considerable phenotypic overlap in infiltrative and hypertrophic cardiomyopathies (Fig. 1) [17].

* Correspondence: jm-kubotoru@kochi-u.ac.jp
[1]Department of Cardiology, Neurology and Aging Science, Kochi Medical School, Oko-cho, Nankoku-shi 783-8505 Kochi, Japan
Full list of author information is available at the end of the article

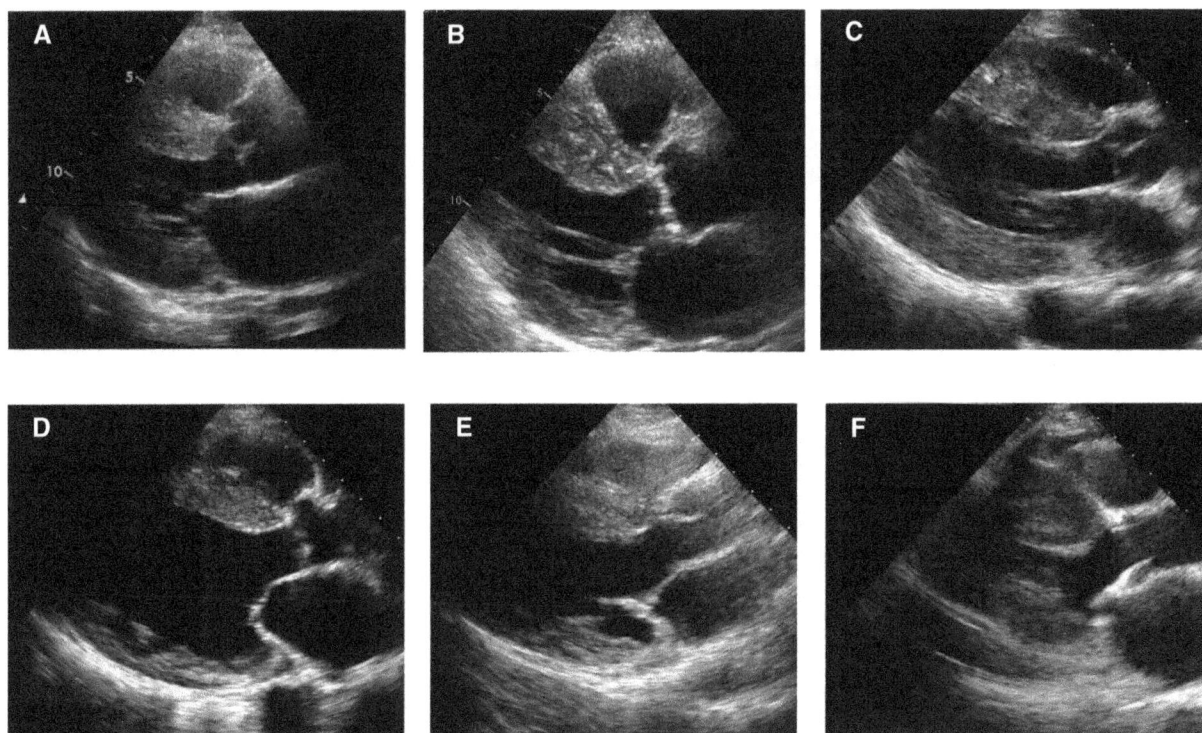

Fig. 1 Long-axis two-dimensional echocardiograms (diastole phase) of patients with cardiomyopathies. **a**: a cardiac amyloidosis patient with concentric left ventricular (LV) hypertrophy, **b**: a cardiac amyloidosis patient with asymmetric septal hypertrophy (ASH) at first glance (but actually concentric hypertrophy rather than ASH if moderator band is removed), **c**: a cardiac Fabry patient with concentric LV hypertrophy, **d**: a cardiac Fabry patient with ASH (in a terminal stage patient with Fabry disease, LV systolic dysfunction with localized thinning of the base of the LV posterior wall is seen.), **e**: a hypertrophic cardiomyopathy (HCM) patient with ASH, **f**: a HCM patient with concentric LV hypertrophy at first glance

Recently, a new generation of high-sensitivity assays for cardiac troponins has been developed to identify minimal cardiac damage in the setting of acute coronary syndromes [18, 19]. Elevations of cardiac troponin levels in high-sensitivity assays have been reported to be associated with poor outcome in not only ischemic heart disease but also non-ischemic heart failure [20, 21]. Although high-sensitivity troponin levels seem to be different among various cardiomyopathies, there has been no detailed comparison of these biomarkers' values [22–27]. In the present study, we investigated the potential role of high-sensitivity cardiac troponin T (hs-cTnT) for differentiation of infiltrative cardiomyopathy from HCM.

Methods

Subjects

The study group consisted of 46 consecutive patients with infiltrative cardiomyopathies or HCM in whom sarcomere protein gene mutations were identified at Kochi Medical School Hospital; of these, there were 11 patients with infiltrative cardiomyopathy (cardiac amyloidosis in 8 patients and Fabry disease in 3 patients) and 35 HCM patients. In this study, we excluded patients with evidence of coronary artery disease and patients

with renal failure (estimated glomerular filtration rate (eGFR) < 30 ml/min per 1.73 m^2). Informed consent was obtained from all patients or their parents in accordance with the guidelines of the Ethics Committee on Medical Research of Kochi Medical School.

Clinical evaluation

The diagnosis of amyloidosis was made by biopsy study of an involved organ that demonstrated typical Congo red birefringence when viewed under polarized light. Of the 8 patients with cardiac amyloidosis, 2 had AL amyloidosis and 6 were considered to have senile amyloidosis with transthyretin. The diagnosis of Fabry disease was based on low plasma alfa-galactosidase A activity, family surveys, and tissue confirmation. The diagnosis of HCM was based on echocardiographic demonstration of a hypertrophied, nondilated LV (maximum LV wall thickness ≥ 15 mm) in the absence of systemic hypertension or other cardiac disease (e.g. aortic stenosis) capable of producing clinically evident hypertrophy at some point of clinical course. In this study, all HCM patients with sarcomere gene mutations in whom serum hs-cTnT was measured were enrolled. Sarcomere gene mutations in our current study were S297X, V593fs, V762D, R945fs

Table 1 Clinical characteristics in 46 patients with cardiomyopathy

	Infiltrative cardiomyopathy ($n = 11$)	HCM ($n = 35$)	p value
Age*, years	68 ± 11	57 ± 16	0.015
Gender: men, n (%)	8 (73 %)	16 (46 %)	0.118
Hs-cTnT*, ng/ml	0.083 ± 0.057	0.027 ± 0.034	<0.001
BNP*, pg/ml	349 ± 341	288 ± 378	0.322
eGFR, ml/min per 1.73 m²	61 ± 17	73 ± 21	0.090
NYHA functional class, n (%)			0.071
I	2 (18 %)	20 (57 %)	
II	8 (73 %)	14 (40 %)	
III	1 (9 %)	1 (3 %)	
Hx. of heart failure admission, n (%)	5 (45 %)	6 (17 %)	0.100
Atrial fibrillation, n (%)	1 (9 %)	4 (11 %)	1.00

Data are shown as mean ± SD or number (percent)
A mark of * is the results of Wilcoxon rank sum test
HCM hypertrophic cardiomyopathy, *Hs-cTnT* High-sensitivity cardiac troponin T, *BNP* Brain natriuretic peptide, *eGFR* estimated glomerular filtration rate, *NYHA* New York Heart Association functional class

and R1138C in cardiac myosin-binding protein C gene, R663C and N562K in cardiac beta-myosin heavy chain gene, D46V in cardiac troponin T gene and R162W in cardiac troponin I gene. These were not found in at least 200 chromosomes from healthy Japanese individuals. There were 7 patients with dilated phase of HCM defined as LV systolic dysfunction of global ejection fraction (EF) < 50 %.

Evaluation of patients included medical history, clinical examination, 12-lead electrocardiography, and conventional and Doppler echocardiography. Maximum LV wall thickness was defined as the greatest thickness in any single segment. Left ventricular end-diastolic diameter (LVEDD) and end-systolic diameter (LVESD) were measured from M-mode and 2-D images obtained from parasternal long-axis views. Global EF was determined from apical two- and four-chamber views. Mitral inflow velocities were determined using pulsed-wave Doppler with the sample volume positioned at the tips of the mitral leaflets in the four-chamber view. Peak early (E) and late (A) transmitral filling velocities were measured. Tissue Doppler imaging was performed in the pulse-Doppler mode to allow for a spectral display and recording of mitral annulus velocities at septal and lateral corners. Peak early diastolic (Ea) velocity was measured, and the E/Ea ratio was calculated. LV outflow tract gradient was calculated form continuous-wave Doppler using the simplified Bernoulli equation. LV outflow tract obstruction was defined as the presence of basal LV outflow gradient ≥ 30 mmHg at rest. Right ventricular hypertrophy was defined as thickness of right ventricular free wall > 5 mm.

Peripheral venous blood samples were collected for measurements of serum hs-cTnT and plasma brain natriuretic peptide (BNP) at the same time in clinically stable condition. Blood was taken at a random time mainly in our outpatient clinic. Serum hs-cTnT was measured by Elecsys Troponin T - High Sensitive immunoassay (Roche Diagnostics Ltd., Rotkreuz, Switzerland). The normal range of this troponin marker in an apparently healthy adult population is less than or equal to 0.014 ng/ml (99 percentile). Plasma BNP was measured using an enzyme immunoassay (TOSOH II; TOSOH, Tokyo, Japan).

Statistical analysis

All data are expressed as mean ± SD or frequency (percentage). Differences between clinical variables of the

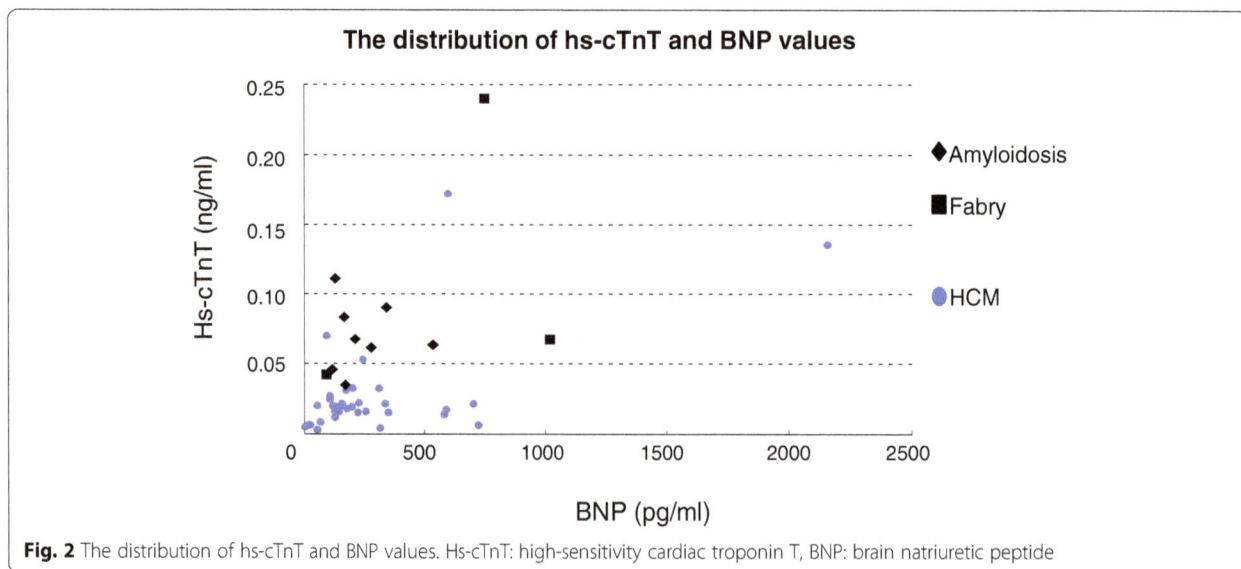

Fig. 2 The distribution of hs-cTnT and BNP values. Hs-cTnT: high-sensitivity cardiac troponin T, BNP: brain natriuretic peptide

infiltrative cardiomyopathy group and HCM group were examined with univariate analysis. For analysis of continuous variables, a *t*-test or Wilcoxon rank sum test was used, and a chi-square test or Fisher's exact test was used for analysis of categorical variables. The diagnostic accuracies of parameters including biomarkers and echocardiographic indices were compared by receiver operating characteristic (ROC) analysis. Age, New York Heart Association functional class, eGFR, E/Ea (lateral), and hs-cTnT were included in a multivariate logistic regression model to identify independent correlations of the differentiation between the two types of cardiomyopathies. Statistical analysis was performed using SPSS (version 14.0 J) statistical software (SPSS Japan Inc., Tokyo).

Results

Patients characteristics

Clinical characteristics of the patients in the present study are summarized in Table 1. Patients who had infiltrative cardiomyopathy were older than patients who had HCM. Patients with infiltrative cardiomyopathy were more symptomatic than patients with HCM. Figure 2 shows the distribution of hs-cTnT and BNP values in all patients. There was less overlap of hs-cTnT values than BNP values between the two groups. Serum

hs-cTnT level was significantly higher in patients who had infiltrative cardiomyopathy than in those who had HCM, while BNP levels did not differ between the two groups (Table 1). Table 2 shows the echocardiographic measurements in the two groups. Maximum LV wall thickness was smaller and posterior wall thickness was greater in patients with infiltrative cardiomyopathy than in those with HCM, although interventricular septal wall thickness was not different. There was no significant difference in the LV or left atrial sizes between the two groups. In Doppler echocardiographic measurements, E wave velocity was higher in patients who had infiltrative

Table 2 Echocardiographic findings in 46 patients with cardiomyopathy

	Infiltrative cardiomyopathy (n = 11)	HCM (n = 35)	p value
Maximum LV wall thickness, mm	17 ± 3	20 ± 4	0.021
Interventricular wall thickness, mm	16 ± 3	16 ± 4	0.628
Posterior wall thickness*, mm	15 ± 3	11 ± 2	<0.001
LV end-diastolic diameter*, mm	44 ± 5	44 ± 6	0.836
LV end-systolic diameter*, mm	32 ± 7	28 ± 7	0.118
Ejection fraction*, %	54 ± 13	62 ± 13	0.104
Left atrial diameter, mm	44 ± 6	43 ± 8	0.723
E*, cm/s	89 ± 23	69 ± 21	0.012
A, cm/s	67 ± 33	64 ± 19	0.704
E/A*	1.7 ± 1.0	1.1 ± 0.5	0.141
Dct*, msec	208 ± 81	200 ± 68	0.857
Ea septal*, cm/s	3.9 ± 1.1	5.2 ± 2.3	0.116
Ea lateral*, cm/s	4.8 ± 1.3	8.1 ± 3.5	<0.001
E/Ea septal	24 ± 7	15 ± 7	<0.001
E/Ea lateral*	20 ± 8	10 ± 4	<0.001
Presence of LVOTO, n (%)	1 (9 %)	7 (20 %)	0.658
Presence of RVH, n (%)	6 (55 %)	18 (51 %)	0.857

Data are shown as mean ± SD or number (percent)
A mark of * is the results of Wilcoxon rank sum test
HCM Hypertrophic cardiomyopathy, LV Left ventricular, LVOTO Left ventricular outflow tract obstruction, RVH Right ventricular hypertrophy

Table 3 Clinical findings in 41 patients with cardiomyopathy evaluated at > 40 years

	Infiltrative cardiomyopathy (n = 11)	HCM (n = 30)	p value
Age*, years	68 ± 11	62 ± 11	0.059
Gender: men, n (%)	8 (73 %)	13 (43 %)	0.095
Hs-cTnT*, ng/ml	0.083 ± 0.057	0.025 ± 0.031	<0.001
BNP*, pg/ml	349 ± 301	248 ± 203	0.332
eGFR, ml/min per 1.73 m²	61 ± 17	69 ± 19	0.220
NYHA functional class, n (%)			0.124
I	2 (18 %)	16 (53 %)	
II	8 (73 %)	13 (43 %)	
III	1 (9 %)	1 (3 %)	
Hx. of heart failure admission, n (%)	5 (45 %)	6 (20 %)	0.111
Maximum LV wall thickness, mm	17 ± 3	20 ± 4	0.029
Interventricular wall thickness, mm	16 ± 3	16 ± 4	0.562
Posterior wall thickness*, mm	15 ± 3	10 ± 2	<0.001
LV end-diastolic diameter, mm	44 ± 5	45 ± 6	0.877
LV end-systolic diameter*, mm	32 ± 7	28 ± 8	0.161
Ejection fraction, %	54 ± 13	61 ± 13	0.147
Left atrial diameter, mm	44 ± 6	44 ± 9	0.950
E*, cm/s	89 ± 23	69 ± 21	0.019
A, cm/s	67 ± 33	67 ± 19	0.985
E/A*	1.7 ± 1.0	1.1 ± 0.5	0.069
Dct*, msec	208 ± 81	198 ± 70	0.825
Ea septal*, cm/s	3.9 ± 1.1	5.0 ± 2.3	0.226
Ea lateral*, cm/s	4.8 ± 1.3	7.9 ± 3.3	<0.001
E/Ea septal	24 ± 7	16 ± 7	0.002
E/Ea lateral*	20 ± 8	10 ± 4	<0.001
Presence of LVOTO, n (%)	1 (9 %)	5 (17 %)	1.000
Presence of RVH, n (%)	6 (55 %)	14 (47 %)	0.655

Data are shown as mean ± SD or number (percent)
A mark of * is the results of Wilcoxon rank sum test
HCM Hypertrophic cardiomyopathy, Hs-cTnT High-sensitivity cardiac troponin T, BNP Brain natriuretic peptide, eGFR estimated glomerular filtration rate, NYHA, New York Heart Association functional class, LV Left ventricular, LVOTO Left ventricular outflow tract obstruction, RVH Right ventricular hypertrophy

Table 4 Diagnostic accuracy to differentiate the 2 groups. ROC analysis

	AUC value
Hs-cTnT	0.939
E/Ea (lateral)	0.914
Posterior wall thickness	0.906
Ea (lateral)	0.845
E/Ea (septal)	0.806
E	0.742
Maximum LV wall thickness	0.739

ROC receiver operating characteristic, *AUC* area under the curve, *Hs-cTnT* high-sensitivity cardiac troponin T, *LV* left ventricular

cardiomyopathy than in patients who had HCM. Ea at the lateral corner was significantly lower and E/Ea ratios at both the septal and lateral corners were significantly higher in patients who had infiltrative cardiomyopathy than in patients who had HCM.

Differentiation of the two groups in patients evaluated at > 40 years of age

In clinical practice, phenotypic expression in infiltrative cardiomyopathies is usually after middle-age. We therefore focused on patients evaluated at > 40 years of age in order to clarify the usefulness of hs-cTnT for differentiation of infiltrative cardiomyopathy from HCM. Table 3 shows the clinical characteristics of the two groups of patients evaluated at > 40 years of age. Hs-cTnT level, maximum LV wall thickness, posterior wall thickness, early filling velocity, Ea (lateral) and E/Ea ratios at both the septal and lateral corners were significantly different between the two groups. Area under the curve values in ROC curves are shown in Table 4. Hs-cTnT was highest and E/Ea (lateral) was

second highest to differentiate the two groups. The multivariate logistic regression analysis showed that the independent determinants of the differentiation between the two types of cardiomyopathies were hs-cTnT ($p = 0.047$) and E/Ea (lateral) ($p = 0.028$). When the cut-off levels were defined as hs-cTnT of 0.035 ng/ml and E/Ea (lateral) of 11, combined measurements of these parameters resulted in 100 % sensitivity and 95 % specificity for the diagnosis of infiltrative cardiomyopathy (Fig. 3).

Discussion

To the best of knowledge, this is the first report that a new generation of assays, hs-cTnT, is able to differentiate accurately between infiltrative cardiomyopathy, including cardiac amyloidosis and cardiac involvement of Fabry disease, and HCM. Serum hs-cTnT is a helpful diagnostic indicator and should be measured in the evaluation of patients with thickening of the LV wall.

Although the underlying cause is different, infiltrative cardiomyopathy and HCM share clinical and hemodynamic features of LV hypertrophy and abnormal diastolic function [1–13]. It is often difficult to distinguish these entities by routine clinical examinations. Diagnosis of cardiac amyloidosis based on conventional modalities is often only possible once the disease is in a relatively advanced stage [1–5]. In hemodynamic parameters on echocardiography, a restrictive pattern of transmitral flow velocity, which is considered to be characteristic for cardiac amyloidosis, is not always observed in patients with this disease: cardiac amyloidosis can present as an abnormal relaxation pattern, depending on the left atrial or LV end-diastolic pressure. In Fabry disease, cardiac involvement occurs in the majority of patients and is mainly manifested as LV hypertrophy. There have been several reports of Fabry disease sometimes being

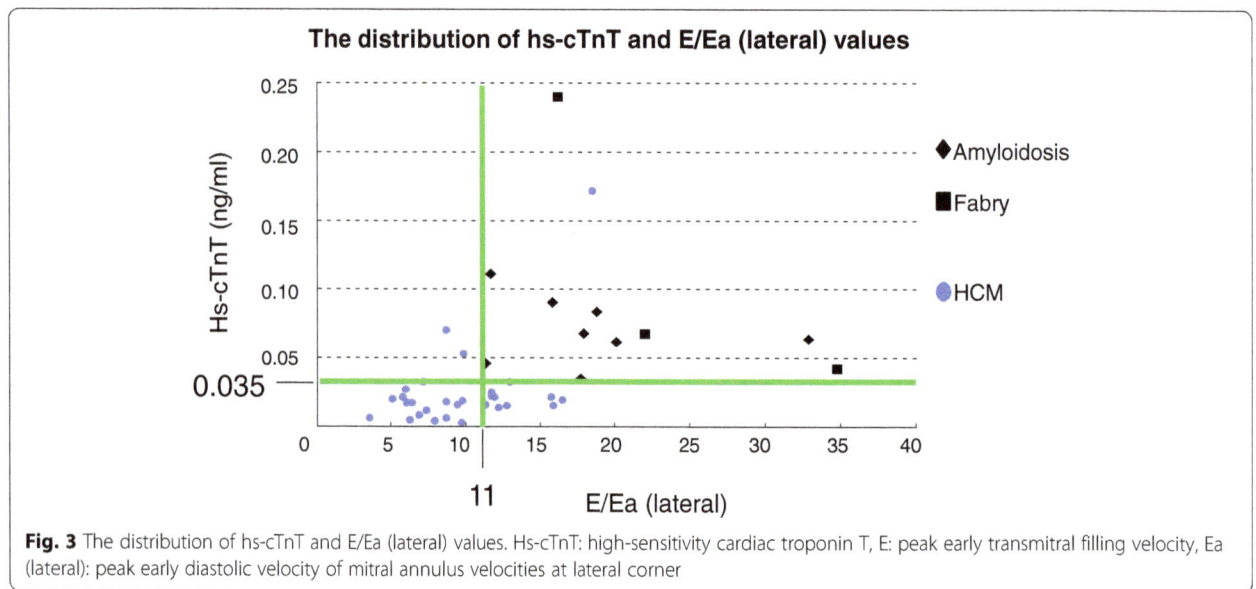

Fig. 3 The distribution of hs-cTnT and E/Ea (lateral) values. Hs-cTnT: high-sensitivity cardiac troponin T, E: peak early transmitral filling velocity, Ea (lateral): peak early diastolic velocity of mitral annulus velocities at lateral corner

undiagnosed in HCM cohorts [6–9]. On the other hand, clinical management differs among these cardiomyopathies in terms of prognosis and treatment. Compared with HCM, cardiac amyloidosis and Fabry disease are more progressive and show a poorer prognosis. Furthermore, there are several effective treatments available for these infiltrative cardiomyopathies: high-dose chemotherapy and stem-cell transplantation for AL amyloidosis and enzyme replacement therapy for Fabry disease [15, 16, 28]. To optimize survival in patients with these infiltrative cardiomyopathies, early diagnosis and institution of therapy are essential.

In the present study, we evaluated the value of hs-cTnT to distinguish between infiltrative cardiomyopathies and HCM. Serum hs-cTnT level is a useful marker to differentiate two groups. The mechanisms of myocyte injury and release of cardiac troponins in patients with non-ischemic heart failure or cardiomyopathies remain unresolved. Various reasons have been proposed for high troponin levels, including increased wall stress, myocyte damage from inflammatory cytokines or oxidative stress, altered calcium handling, and coronary microvascular dysfunction [29]. For the hypertrophied myocardium, coronary microvascular dysfunction is considered to be the most plausible mechanism for elevation of cardiac troponins. In fact, microvascular dysfunction has been reported in cardiac amyloidosis, Fabry disease, and HCM [30–32]. Microvascular dysfunction and subsequent ischemia may be important components of the disease progression in patients with cardiac hypertrophy. Although the reason is unclear why hs-cTnT level is higher in patients who had infiltrative cardiomyopathy than in those who had HCM, we speculate that apoptotic or necrotic injury may be induced by the toxic effect of accumulated substances themselves in infiltrative cardiomyopathy.

In the present study, E/Ea at lateral corner (not septal corner) was second highest in area under the curve values in ROC curves to differentiate the two groups. This may result from the findings that amyloid deposition in cardiac amyloidosis is diffuse, whereas LV hypertrophy is usually asymmetric and predominantly septal in HCM.

Limitations

There are several limitations to be acknowledged in the present study. First, the number of subjects was small and some of the statistical analyses might have been affected. We need to have more data on hs-cTnT levels in various clinical severities in each disease entity. A diagnostic challenge remains in patients with infiltrative cardiomyopathies who have relatively mild abnormalities on echocardiography. Second, due to the retrospective design of the study, it is possible that there is a selection

bias, although the study population consisted of consecutive patients with cardiomyopathies. Third, we could not distinguish between cardiac amyloidosis and cardiac involvement of Fabry disease within infiltrative cardiomyopathies by using hs-cTnT measurements. This biomarker has not been fully evaluated in Fabry disease.

Conclusions

Measurement of serum hs-cTnT enables accurate discrimination between infiltrative cardiomyopathy and HCM. The combination of this biomarker and conventional echocardiographic parameters helps to differentiate these cardiomyopathies.

Competing interests
The authors declare that they have no competing interests.

Authors' contributions
TK, TS, and HK conceived the idea for the study and planned the investigations. TK, YB, TH, KT, NY, TF, and HK undertook clinical investigations of patients. SY measured serum high-sensitivity cardiac troponin T. NK performed statistical analysis and TI supervised statistical analysis for this paper. All authors read and approved the final manuscript.

Author details
[1]Department of Cardiology, Neurology and Aging Science, Kochi Medical School, Oko-cho, Nankoku-shi 783-8505Kochi, Japan. [2]Department of Laboratory Medicine, Kochi Medical School, Kochi, Japan. [3]Clinical Trial Center, Kochi Medical School, Kochi, Japan.

References
1. Falk RH, Comenzo RL, Skinner M. The systemic amyloidosis. N Engl J Med. 1997;337:898–909.
2. Cueto-Garcia L, Reeder GS, Kyle RA, Wood DL, Seward JB, Naessens J, et al. Echocardiographic findings in systemic amyloidosis: spectrum of cardiac involvement and relation to survival. J Am Coll Cardiol. 1985;6:737–43.
3. Falk RH, Plehn JF, Deering T, Schick Jr EC, Boinay P, Rubinow A, et al. Sensitivity and specificity of the echocardiographic features of cardiac amyloidosis. Am J Cardiol. 1987;59:418–22.
4. Palka P, Lange A, Donnelly JE, Scalia G, Burstow DJ, Nihoyannopoulos P. Doppler tissue echocardiographic features of cardiac amyloidosis. J Am Soc Echocardiogr. 2002;15:1353–60.
5. Oki T, Tanaka H, Yamada H, Tabata T, Oishi Y, Ishimoto T, et al. Diagnosis of cardiac amyloidosis based on the myocardial velocity profile in the hypertrophied left ventricular wall. Am J Cardiol. 2004;93:864–9.
6. Nakao S, Takenaka T, Maeda M, Kodama C, Tanaka A, Tahara M, et al. An atypical variant of Fabry's disease in men with left ventricular hypertrophy. N Engl J Med. 1995;333:288–93.
7. Sachdev B, Takenaka T, Teraguchi H, Tei C, Lee P, McKenna WJ, et al. Prevalence of Anderson-Fabry disease in male patients with late onset hypertrophic cardiomyopathy. Circulation. 2002;105:1407–11.
8. Monserrat L, Gimeno-Blanes JR, Marin F, Hermida-Prieto M, Garcia-Honrubia A, Perez I, et al. Prevalence of Fabry disease in a cohort of 508 unrelated patients with hypertrophic cardiomyopathy. J Am Coll Cardiol. 2007;50:2399–403.
9. Elliott P, Baker R, Pasquale F, Quarta G, Ebrahim H, Mehta AB. Hughes DA, and ACES study group: Prevalence of Anderson-Fabry disease in patients with hypertrophic cardiomyopathy: the European Anderson-Fabry Disease Survey. Heart. 2011;97:1957–60.
10. Weidmann F, Strotmann JM. Use of tissue Doppler imaging to identify and manage systemic diseases. Clin Res Cardiol. 2008;97:65–73.
11. Spirito P, Seidman CE, McKenna WJ, Maron BJ. The management of hypertrophic cardiomyopathy. N Engl J Med. 1997;336:775–85.
12. Maron BJ, McKenna WJ, Danielson GK, Kappenberger LJ, Kuhn HJ, Seidman CE, et al. American College of Cardiology/European Society of Cardiology

clinical expert consensus document on hypertrophic cardiomyopathy. A report of the American College of Cardiology Foundation Task Force on Clinical Expert Consensus Documents and the European Society of Cardiology Committee for Practice Guidelines. J Am Coll Cardiol. 2003;42:1687–713.

13. Maron BJ, Maron MS. Hypertrophic cardiomyopathy. Lancet. 2013;381:242–55.

14. Takenaka T, Teraguchi H, Yoshida A, Taguchi S, Ninomiya K, Umekita Y, et al. Terminal stage cardiac findings in patients with cardiac Fabry disease: an electrocardiographic, echocardiographic, and autopsy study. J Cardiol. 2008;51:50–9.

15. Eng CM, Guffon N, Wilcox WR, Germain DP, Lee P, Waldek S, et al. Safety and efficacy of recombinant human alpha-galactosidase A: replacement therapy in Fabry's disease. N Engl J Med. 2001;345:9–16.

16. Weidemann F, Niemann M, Breunig F, Herrmann S, Beer M, Stork S, et al. Long-term effects of enzyme replacement therapy on Fabry cardiomyopathy: evidence for a better outcome with early treatment. Circulation. 2009;119:524–9.

17. Ochi Y, Kubo T, Kitaoka H. Repeated heart failure in a 74-year-old man with left ventricular hypertrophy. Heart. 2014;100:710.

18. Reichlin T, Hochholzer W, Bassetti S, Steuer S, Stelzig C, Hartwiger S, et al. Early diagnosis of myocardial infarction with sensitive cardiac troponin assays. N Engl J Med. 2009;361:858–67.

19. Keller T, Zeller T, Peetz D, Tzikas S, Roth A, Czyz E, et al. Sensitive troponin assay in early diagnosis of acute myocardial infarction. N Engl J Med. 2009;361:868–77.

20. Sato Y, Fujiwara H, Takatsu Y. Cardiac troponin and heart failure in the era of high-sensitivity assays. J Cardiol. 2012;60:160–7.

21. Latini R, Masson S, Anand IS, Missov E, Carlson M, Vago T, et al. Nal-HeFT Investigators: Prognostic value of very low plasma concentrations of troponin T in patients with stable chronic heart failure. Circulation. 2007;116:1242–9.

22. Kristen AV, Giannitsis E, Lehrke S, Hegenbart U, Konstandin M, Lindenmaier D, et al. Assessment of disease severity and outcome in patients with systemic light-chain amyloidosis by the high-sensitivity troponin T assay. Blood. 2010;116:2455–61.

23. Apridonidze T, Steingart RM, Comenzo RL, Hoffman J, Goldsmith Y, Bella JN, et al. Clinical and echocardiographic correlates of elevated troponin in amyloid light-chain cardiac amyloidosis. Am J Cardiol. 2012;110:1180–4.

24. Dispenzieri A, Gertz MA, Kumar SK, Lacy MQ, Kyle RA, Saenger AK, et al. High sensitivity cardiac troponin T in patients with immunoglobulin light chain amyloidosis. Heart. 2014;100:383–8.

25. Qian G, Wu C, Zhang Y, Chen YD, Dong W, Ren YH. Prognostic value of high-sensitivity cardiac troponin T in patients with endomyocardial-biopsy proven cardiac amyloidosis. J Geriatr Cardiol. 2014;11:136–40.

26. Kubo T, Kitaoka H, Yamanaka S, Hirota T, Baba Y, Hayashi K, et al. Significance of high-sensitivity cardiac troponin T in hypertrophic cardiomyopathy. J Am Coll Cardiol. 2013;62:1252–9.

27. Jenab Y, Pourjafari M, Darabi F, Boroumand MA, Zoroufian A, Jalali A. Prevalence and determinants of elevated high-sensitivity cardiac troponin T in hypertrophic cardiomyopathy. J Cardiol. 2014;63:140–4.

28. Skinner M, Sanchorawala V, Seldin DC, Dember LM, Falk RH, Berk JL, et al. High-dose melphalan and autologous stem cell transplantation in patietns with AL amyloidosis: an 8-year study. Ann Intern Med. 2004;140:85–93.

29. Takashio S, Yamamuro M, Izumiya Y, Sugiyama S, Kojima S, Yamamoto E, et al. Coronary microvascular dysfunction and diastolic load correlate with cardiac troponin T release measured by a highly sensitive assay in patients with nonischemic heart failure. J Am Coll Cardiol. 2013;62:632–40.

30. Abdelmoneim SS, Bernier M, Bellavia D, Syed IS, Mankad SV, Chandrasekaran K, et al. Myocardial contrast echocardiography in biopsy-proven primary cardiac amyloidosis. Eur J Echocardiogr. 2008;9:338–41.

31. Elliott PM, Kindler H, Shah JS, Sachdev B, Rimoldi OE, Thaman R, et al. Coronary microvascular dysfunction in male patients with Anderson-Fabry disease and the effect of treatment with alpha galactosidase A. Heart. 2006;92:357–60.

32. Timmer SA, Germans T, Gotte MJ, Russel IK, Lubberink M, Ten Berg JM, et al. Relation of coronary microvascular dysfunction in hypertrophic cardiomyopathy to contractile dysfunction independent from myocardial injury. Am J Cardiol. 2011;107:1522–8.

14

Noncompaction cardiomyopathy: a substrate for a thromboembolic event

Marcelo Dantas Tavares de Melo*, José Arimateia Batista de Araújo Filho, Jose Rodrigues Parga Filho, Camila Rocon de Lima, Charles Mady, Roberto Kalil-Filho and Vera Maria Cury Salemi

Abstract

Background: Noncompaction cardiomyopathy (NCC) is a rare genetic cardiomyopathy characterized by a thin, compacted epicardial layer and an extensive noncompacted endocardial layer. The clinical manifestations of this disease include ventricular arrhythmia, heart failure, and systemic thromboembolism.

Case presentation: A 43-year-old male was anticoagulated by pulmonary thromboembolism for 1 year when he developed progressive dyspnea. Cardiovascular magnetic resonance imaging showed severe biventricular trabeculation with an ejection fraction of 15%, ratio of maximum noncompacted/compacted diastolic myocardial thickness of 3.2 and the presence of exuberant biventricular apical thrombus.

Conclusion: Still under discussion is the issue of which patients and when they should be anticoagulated. It is generally recommended to those presenting ventricular systolic dysfunction, antecedent of systemic embolism, presence of cardiac thrombus and atrial fibrillation. In clinical practice the patients with NCC and ventricular dysfunction have been given oral anticoagulation, although there are no clinical trials showing the real safety and benefit of this treatment.

Keywords: Cardiomyopathy, Echocardiography, Magnetic resonance, Noncompaction, Thromboembolism

Background

According to the American Heart Association, noncompaction cardiomyopathy (NCC) is a genetic disorder [1] characterized by intrauterine arrest of the process of myocardial compaction that starts at the 8th week of gestation. Clinical manifestations include ventricular arrhythmia, heart failure, and systemic thromboembolism, especially encephalic. Ventricular hypertrabeculation is believed to be an anatomical substrate for the formation of thrombi. The literature shows an important variation in the incidence of embolic events in NCC between 0% and 38%, with few references to pulmonary thromboembolism [2]. Yousef et al. found it in 7% of patients [3]. The main limitation of these findings is the small number of patients in the studies.

Case presentation

A 43-year-old male, obese, former-smoker patient was suffering from gout and had been anticoagulated by pulmonary thromboembolism for 1 year when he developed progressive dyspnea without anginal complaints. He was directed to a tertiary hospital for investigation of heart failure. Through echocardiographic evaluation, severe biventricular diffuse systolic dysfunction with suspicion of noncompacted cardiomyopathy was identified, even though such a hypothesis could not be confirmed [Figure 1]. Cardiovascular magnetic resonance imaging (CMRI) showed severe biventricular trabeculation with an ejection fraction of 15%, ratio of maximum noncompacted/compacted diastolic myocardial thickness of 3.2 and the presence of exuberant biventricular apical thrombus [Figure 2, Additional file 1]. CMRI disclosed transmural late

* Correspondence: marcelo_dtm@yahoo.com.br
Heart Institute (InCor) do Hospital das Clínicas da Faculdade de Medicina da Universidade de São Paulo, São Paulo, Brazil

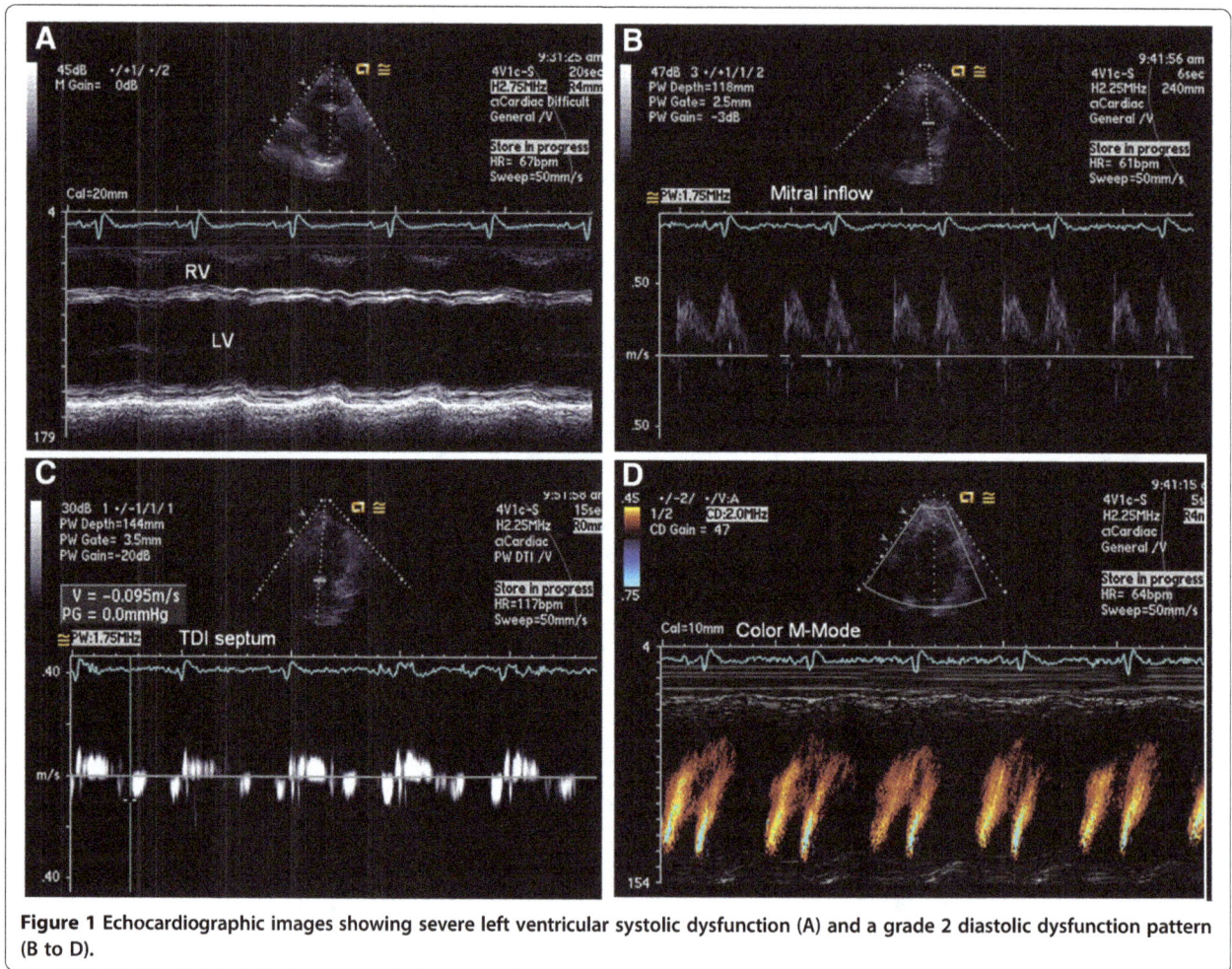

Figure 1 Echocardiographic images showing severe left ventricular systolic dysfunction (A) and a grade 2 diastolic dysfunction pattern (B to D).

gadolinium enhancement at 2/17 segments (mid-anteroseptal and apical septal). Coronary computed tomography angiogram showed a calcified nonobstructive plaque in the proximal left anterior descending coronary artery [Figure 3].

In 2008, according to Fazio et al., NCC does not present thromboembolic risk and there is no indication for anticoagulation [4]. On the other hand, nowadays, the indication for anticoagulation treatment in NCC is still debatable. Almeida et al. recommended anticoagulation only in cases of left ventricular dilation and dysfunction or with previous embolic events [5]. Recently, Stöllberger and Finsterer stated that thrombi may also develop in patients with NCC even with preserved systolic function [6]. It is generally recommended to those presenting ventricular systolic dysfunction, antecedent of systemic embolism, presence of cardiac thrombus and atrial fibrillation [7]. CMRI plays a crucial role in the diagnosis of left ventricular noncompaction, especially for its accuracy in detecting ventricular thrombi. No prospective study

demonstrates the benefits of anticoagulation in NCC patients, which generates uncertainty and insecurity, because there are reports of patients without ventricular dysfunction or atrial fibrillation who have suffered a systemic thromboembolism.

Conclusion

This case report presents a patient with severe biventricular dysfunction in sinus rhythm, with previous pulmonary thromboembolism and biventricular thrombi. He presents a formal indication for anticoagulation. On the other hand, more studies are necessary to clarify this approach for patients presenting NCC with ventricular dysfunction in sinus rhythm.

Consent

Written informed consent was obtained from the patient for publication of this Case report and any accompanying images. A copy of the written consent is available for review by the Editor of this journal.

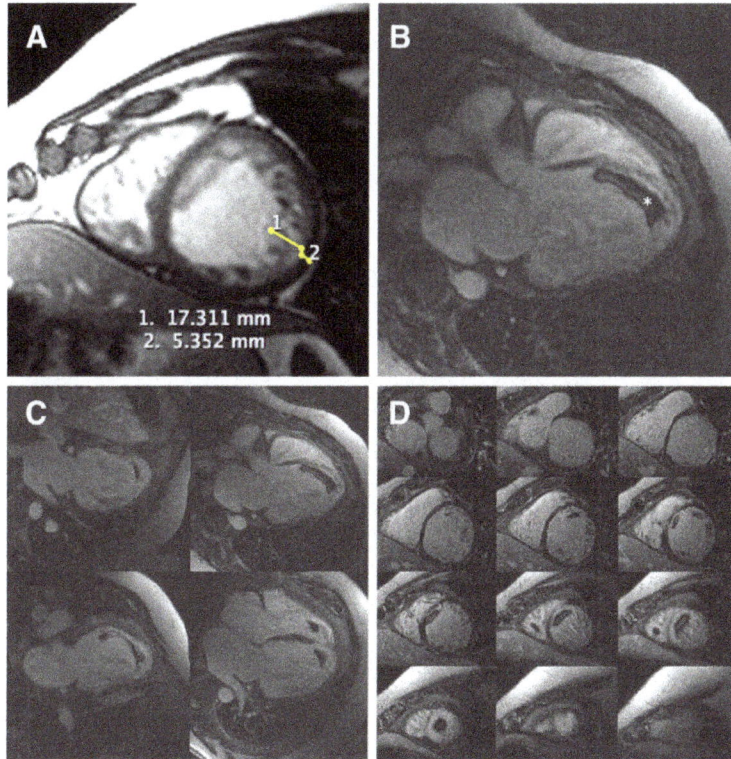

Figure 2 Cardiovascular magnetic resonance short axis cine images showing left ventricular wall and trabeculation, with maximum non-compacted to compacted thickness ratio of 3.2 (normal < 2.3) (A); delayed enhancement long-axis five-chamber view showing left ventricular apical thrombus (B); multiple long-axis four-chambers disclosing biventricular thrombus (C); multiple short-axis two-chambers illustrating the same biventricular thrombus (D). LV (left ventricle).

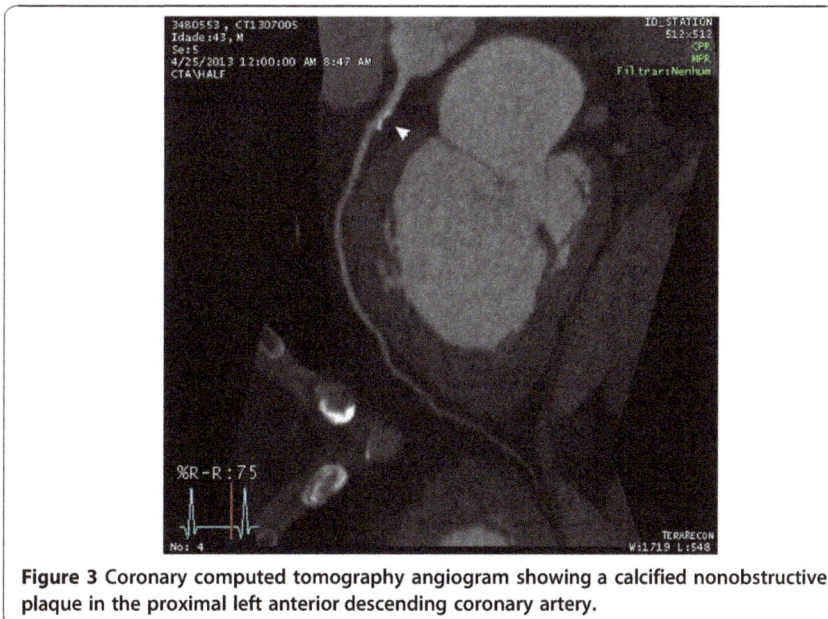

Figure 3 Coronary computed tomography angiogram showing a calcified nonobstructive plaque in the proximal left anterior descending coronary artery.

Abbreviations

CMRI: Cardiovascular magnetic resonance imaging; NCC: Noncompaction cardiomyopathy.

Competing interests

The authors declare that they have no competing interests.

Authors' contributions

MDTM: diagnosed and wrote the paper. JABAF: performed and analyzed the resonance magnetic imaging examination. JRPF: discussed the MRI diagnosis and reviewed the paper. CRL: wrote the paper. CM: reviewed the paper. RKF: reviewed the paper. VMCS: performed the echocardiographic exam and wrote the paper. All authors read and approved the final manuscript.

References

1. Maron BJ, Towbin JA, Thiene G, Antzelevitch C, Corrado D, Arnett D, et al. American Heart Association; Council on Clinical Cardiology, Heart Failure and Transplantation Committee; Quality of Care and Outcomes Research and Functional Genomics and Translational Biology Interdisciplinary Working Groups; Council on Epidemiology and Prevention. Contemporary definitions and classification of the cardiomyopathies: an American Heart Association Scientific Statement from the Council on Clinical Cardiology, Heart Failure and Transplantation Committee; Quality of Care and Outcomes Research and Functional Genomics and Translational Biology Interdisciplinary Working Groups; and Council on Epidemiology and Prevention. Circulation. 2006;113(14):1807–16.
2. Oechslin E, Jenni R. Left ventricular non-compaction revisited: a distinct phenotype with genetic heterogeneity. Eur Heart J. 2011;32(12):1446–56.
3. Yousef ZR, Foley PW, Khadjooi K, Chalil S, Sandman H, Mohammed NU, et al. Left ventricular non-compaction: clinical features and cardiovascular magnetic resonance imaging. BMC Cardiovasc Disord. 2009;9:37.
4. Fazio G, Corrado G, Zachara E, Rapezzi C, Sulafa AK, Sutera L, et al. Anticoagulant drugs in noncompaction: a mandatory therapy? J Cardiovasc Med (Hagerstown). 2008;9(11):1095–7.5.
5. Almeida AG, Pinto FJ. Non-compaction cardiomyopathy. Heart. 2013;99 (20):1535–42.
6. Stöllberger C, Finsterer J. Ischemic stroke in left ventricular noncompaction and celiac disease. Int J Cardiol. 2014;176(2):534–6.
7. Udeoji DU, Philip KJ, Morrissey RP, Phan A, Schwarz ER. Left ventricular noncompaction cardiomyopathy: updated review. Ther Adv Cardiovasc Dis. 2013;7(5):260–73.

15

Severe reversible cardiomyopathy associated with systemic inflammatory response syndrome in the setting of diabetic hyperosmolar hyperglycemic non-ketotic syndrome

Justin Berk[*] ⓘ, Raymond Wade, Hatice Duygu Baser and Joaquin Lado

Abstract

Background: This case study features a woman who presented with clinical and laboratory findings consistent with hyperosmolar hyperglycemic non-ketotic syndrome (HHNS), systemic inflammatory response syndrome (SIRS), and non-thyroidal illness syndrome (NTIS) who was noted to have a transient decrease in myocardial function. To our knowledge, this is the first case discussing the overlapping pathophysiological mechanisms could increase susceptibility to SIRS-induced cardiomyopathy. It is imperative that this clinical question be investigated further as such a relationship may have significant clinical implications for prevention and future treatments, particularly in patients similar to the one presented in this clinical case.

Case presentation: A 53-year old Caucasian female presented to the Emergency Department for cough, nausea, vomiting and "feeling sick for 3 weeks." Labs were indicative of diabetic ketoacidosis. Initial electrocardiograms were suggestive of possible myocardial infarction and follow-up echocardiogram showed severely depressed left ventricular systolic function which resolved upon treatment of ketoacidosis.

Conclusion: We suggest that her cardiomyopathy could have three synergistic sources: SIRS, HHNS and NTIS. Overlapping mechanisms suggest uncontrolled diabetes mellitus and NTIS could increase susceptibility to SIRS-induced cardiomyopathy as seen in this case. HHNS and SIRS cause cardiac tissue injury through mechanisms including impairment of fatty acid oxidation and formation of reactive oxygen species, as well as modifying the function of membrane calcium channels. As a result, it is conceivable that diabetes may amplify the deleterious effects of inflammatory stressors on cardiac myocytes. This novel case report offers a path for future research into prevention and treatment of SIRS-induced cardiomyopathy in, but not exclusive to, the setting of diabetes.

Keywords: Cardiomyopathy, Diabetes, Systemic inflammatory response syndrome, Non-thyroidal illness syndrome, Hyperosmolar hyperglycemic non-ketotic syndrome

* Correspondence: justin.berk@ttuhsc.edu
Department of Internal Medicine, Texas Tech University Health Sciences
Center, School of Medicine, 3601 4th St Stop 9410, Lubbock, TX 79416, USA

Background

This case study features a woman who presented with clinical and laboratory findings consistent with hyperosmolar hyperglycemic non-ketotic syndrome (HHNS), systemic inflammatory response syndrome (SIRS), and non-thyroidal illness syndrome (NTIS) who was noted to have a transient decrease in myocardial function. We suggest that her cardiomyopathy could have three synergistic sources: SIRS, HHNS and NTIS. Overlapping mechanisms suggest uncontrolled diabetes mellitus and NTIS could increase susceptibility to SIRS-induced cardiomyopathy as seen in this case.

Case presentation

A 53-year old female presented to the Emergency Department for cough, nausea, vomiting and "feeling sick for 3 weeks." She reported an allergy to penicillin but no other significant past medical history. On initial assessment, patient was afebrile, tachycardic (125 beats/minute), tachypneic (22 breaths/minute), with blood pressure of 109/74 mmHg, and oxygen saturation of 72 % on room air. Physical exam showed no other abnormalities.

Initial laboratories showed leukocytosis (WBC 22,000 k/mcgl), hyperglycemia (glucose 796 mg/dl), hyponatremia (Na 120 mEq/L; corrected 131 mEq/L), a hemoglobin A1c of 17.2 %, and an elevated troponin T (0.19 ng/mL) and BNP (2137 pg/mL). Measured osmolarity was 349 mOsm/L with only small ketones in the blood and an arterial lactate of 5.62 mmol/L. Arterial blood gas suggested metabolic acidosis (pH = 7.264 | PCO2 = 25.9 mmHg | Bicarbonate = 13 mmol/L). Calculated anion gap was 30 mEq/l. Chest X-ray showed bilateral reticular opacities without cardiomegaly (Fig. 1). The patient was also found to have an abnormal thyroid hormone profile suggesting NTIS: TSH 1.35 mcgUI/mL (nr: 0.27–4.20), free T4 0.88 ng/dL (nr: 0.93–1.70), free T3 0.95 pg/ml (nr:2.30–

4.20), mixed hyperlipidemia, mild elevation of lipase and amylase, and transaminitis.

Intravenous fluids, insulin and levofloxacin were started; the patient's clinical condition improved in 24 hours, although she continued to complain of shortness of breath and remained hypotensive. Blood and urine cultures were ultimately negative. Initial EKG changes suggested previous myocardial infarction (Fig. 2). A transthoracic echocardiogram demonstrated a severely depressed LV systolic function (ejection fraction = 26 %), grade 2 diastolic dysfunction, and multiple regional wall motion abnormalities (Fig. 3a-3b). However, on Day 4 after admission, a Myoview stress test showed no stress-induced ischemia, normal LV function, no regional wall motion abnormalities, and an estimated ejection fraction of 50 %. A repeat transthoracic echocardiogram performed on Day 7 demonstrated an ejection fraction of 50–55 % (Fig. 3c-3d). A follow-up EKG on Day 4 showed no significant changes (Fig. 4).

On 6-month follow-up, the patient's A1c remained elevated but the NTIS and cardiomyopathy had resolved. Her HgA1c was 9.4 %, TSH 1.86 mcgUI/mL (nr: 0.27–4.20), free T4 1.01 ng/dl (nr: 0.93–1.70), free T3 2.89 pg/ml (nr:2.30–4.20). BNP was 42 pg/ml (normal).

Discussion

Our patient presented a case of severe reversible myocardial dysfunction with HHNS as debut of diabetes mellitus, NTIS, and meeting SIRS criteria. Although sepsis of pulmonary origin was initially suspected, the clinical course (normal body temperature, normalization in blood leukocytes count in less than 24 and negative cultures) suggest that SIRS was secondary to HHNS [1]. The observed NTIS was also likely secondary to HHNS and SIRS.

Myocardial dysfunction is a common complication in patients with SIRS secondary to sepsis and is associated with an increased risk of mortality of up to 70–90 % [2, 3]. Systolic and diastolic myocardial dysfunction has been described in other situations of SIRS such as severe trauma and burns [4].

A common mechanism among these clinical situations is a high level of pro-inflammatory cytokines such as tumor necrosis alpha (TNF-alpha) and interleukin 6 (IL-6). Bacterial products and pro-inflammatory cytokines increase production of nitric oxide [5–7] and reactive oxygen species (ROS) [8, 9] that inhibit the function of proteins involved in myocardial contraction and relaxation [9, 10].

The sarcoendoplasmic reticulum adenosine triphosphatase 2a (SERCA2a) and sarcolemmal voltage-gated L-type calcium channels are often affected. As a consequence, Ca^{2+} entry into cells and release from sarcoplasmic reticulum (SR) decreases and sarcomere shortening is

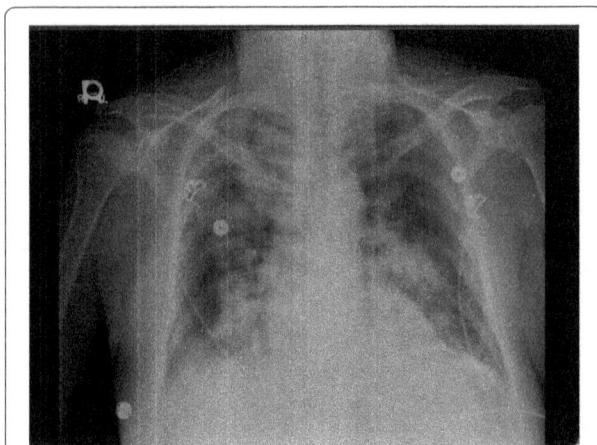

Fig. 1 Chest X-ray, Portable film notable for bilateral, patchy hilar infiltrates consistent with pulmonary edema in the setting of depressed ejection fraction

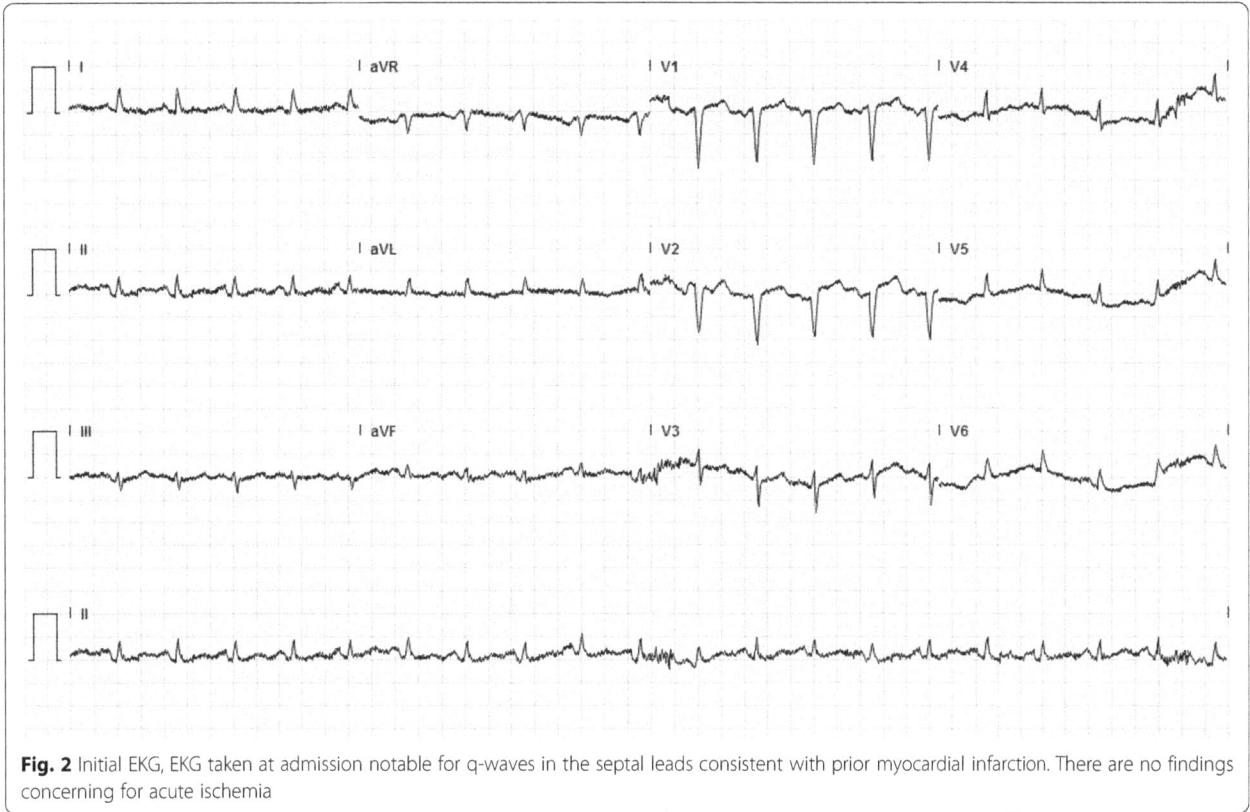

Fig. 2 Initial EKG, EKG taken at admission notable for q-waves in the septal leads consistent with prior myocardial infarction. There are no findings concerning for acute ischemia

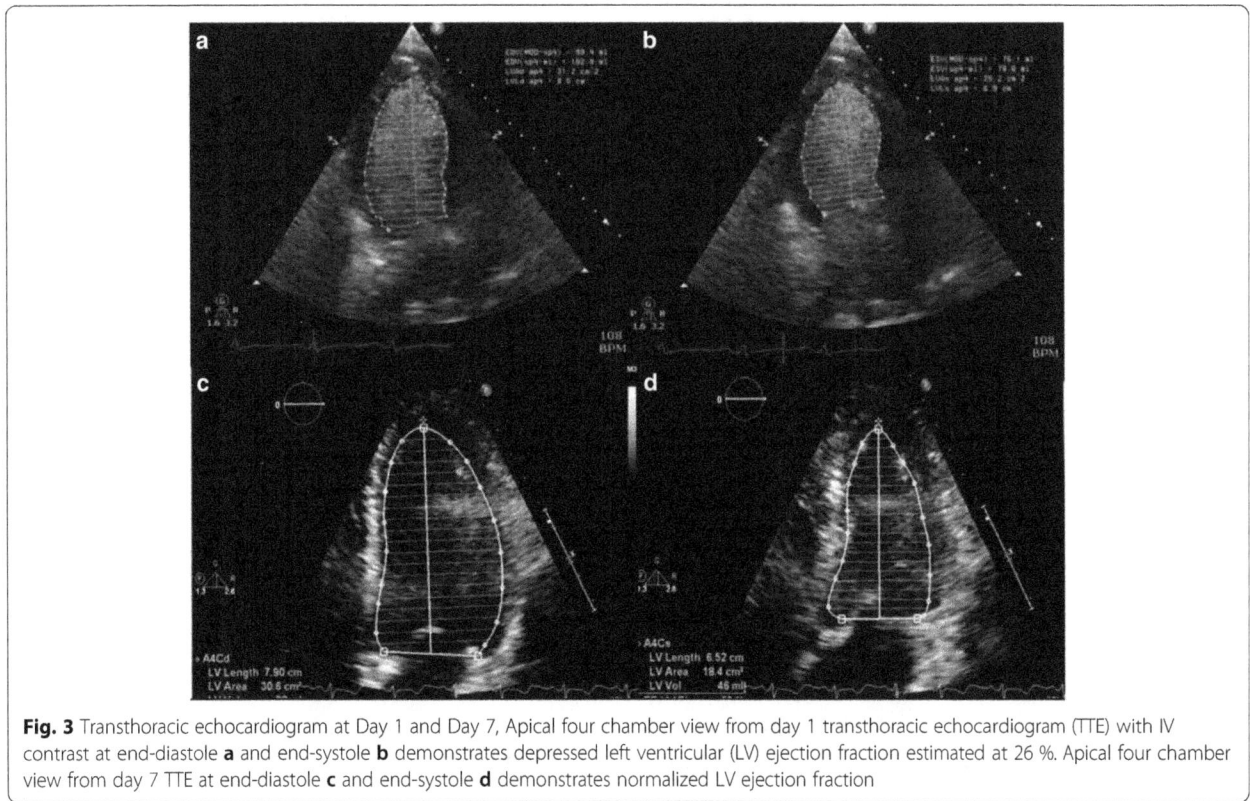

Fig. 3 Transthoracic echocardiogram at Day 1 and Day 7, Apical four chamber view from day 1 transthoracic echocardiogram (TTE) with IV contrast at end-diastole **a** and end-systole **b** demonstrates depressed left ventricular (LV) ejection fraction estimated at 26 %. Apical four chamber view from day 7 TTE at end-diastole **c** and end-systole **d** demonstrates normalized LV ejection fraction

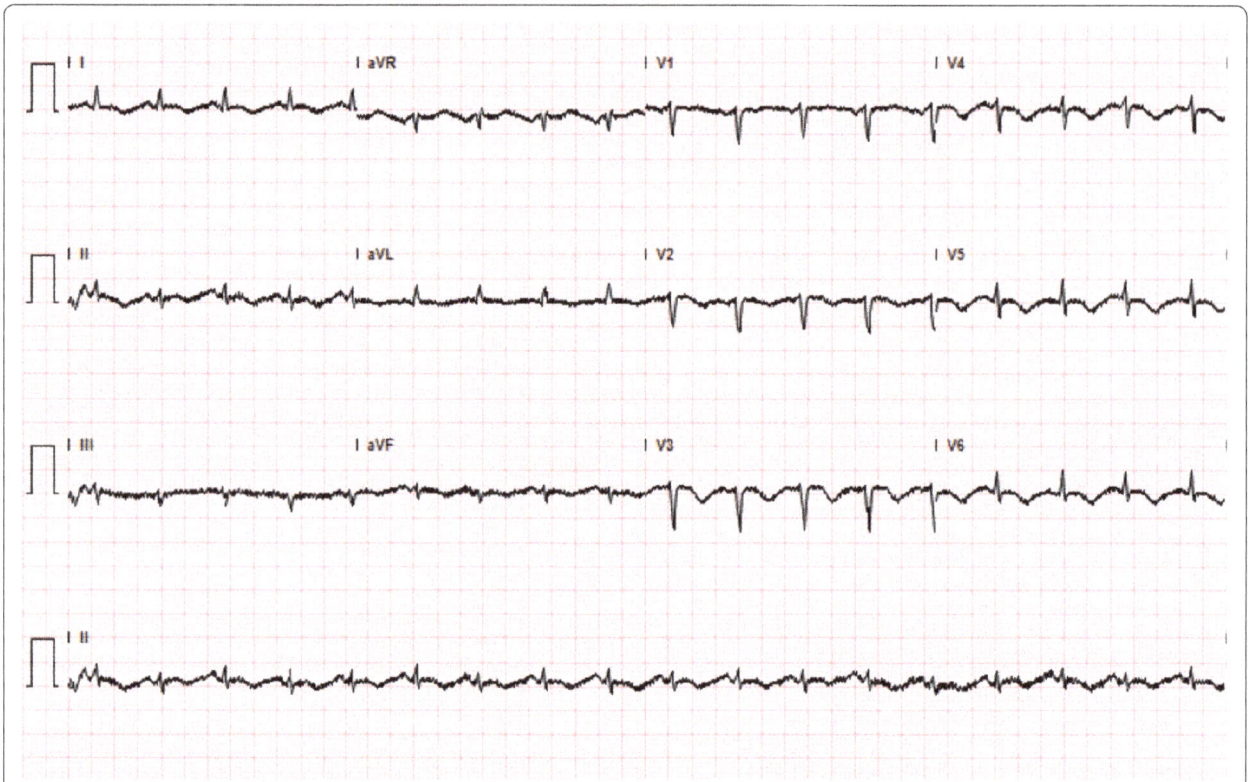

Fig. 4 Follow-up EKG on Day 4 of hospitalization

reduced [11, 12]. Bacterial products and pro-inflammatory cytokines also inhibit *SERCA2a* gene expression [13], reduce myofilament sensitivity to Ca^{2+} [14], and downregulate and desensitize beta-adrenergic receptors [15, 16].

SIRS can cause myocardial energy deficiency. Low ATP levels and a decrease in the phosphocreatine/ATP ratio have been found in deadly cases of septic shock [17–19]. Both glucose oxidation and fatty acid oxidation (FAO), the main sources of myocardial ATP, decrease in non-surviving humans with septic shock [20]. Pyruvate dehydrogenase complex [21] and phosphofructokinase activities [22] decrease during septic shock leading to dissociation of glycolysis from glucose oxidation.

Factors responsible for FAO inhibition during septic shock are a decrease in mitochondrial membrane carnitine shuttle activity and a decrease in peroxisome proliferator-activated receptor alpha and peroxisome proliferator-activated receptor gamma co-activator-1α gene expression [23, 24]. Also, mitochondrial complexes I, II and III activities decrease in cases of prolonged septic shock [25, 26]. Multiple reviews have been published to discuss these and other possible mechanisms of sepsis-induced cardiomyopathy [8, 27–30].

Acute hyperglycemic crisis can cause SIRS, and both hyperosmolar hyperglycemic non-ketotic syndrome and diabetic ketoacidosis are associated with a severe inflammatory state [31]. However, other features of hyperglycemic

crisis, such as dehydration and electrolyte imbalance, likely exacerbated the patient's cardiomyopathy.

Diabetic cardiomyopathy refers to ventricular dysfunction in the absence of coronary artery disease and hypertension [32]. Diastolic and systolic dysfunction can be seen as early functional alteration of diabetic cardiomyopathy [32]. The pathogenic mechanisms involved are complex, interrelated and not all well characterized, although inflammation seems to play a significant role [32]. Under normal circumstances, the heart obtains energy mostly from FAO. In diabetic hearts, glucose uptake, glycolysis and glucose oxidation are reduced [32] and FA uptake increased. An increase in FA uptake is associated with increased triglycerides synthesis that causes myocardial lipotoxicity and cell death. Also, higher FAO rates increase oxygen consumption at the expense of mitochondrial uncoupling and increased oxidative stress. Our patient had elevated troponin T levels indicating cellular death or myocardial cell membrane alterations. Additionally, the hyperosmolar state may cause dehydration, which would decrease preload and further lower left ventricular systolic function.

Our patient also presented with low thyroid hormone levels with normal TSH, a condition known as NTIS or sick euthyroid syndrome. Although NTIS is probably the most common cause of hypothyroidism, the current consensus advises against the administration of thyroid hormones to patients with NTIS as thyroid hormones increase respiratory rate, oxygen consumption, energy expenditure and heat production, NTIS is considered an adaptive response to counteract catabolism during illness [33], and this is the primary reasoning against administration of thyroid hormone to patients with NTIS [34]. However, SIRS is associated with myocardial hypothyroidism in large animal models of septic shock [35] and hypothyroidism can cause systolic and diastolic myocardial dysfunction. In this context, thyroid hormone administration, in attempt to normalize thyroid hormone levels inside the myocardium, could have been beneficial and devoid of harmful effects. In fact, hypothyroidism increases serum levels of troponin T and creatine kinase CK-MB isoenzymes that are markers of myocardial damage. Patients with heart failure and low serum T3 have poor hemodynamics and a higher probability of death [36]. Finally, thyroid hormone administration to patients with advanced congestive heart failure was well tolerated and increased cardiac output without an appreciable increase in ischemia or arrhythmias [36–38].

Conclusion

As we have explained, both HHNS and SIRS cause cardiac tissue injury through similar mechanisms including impairment of fatty acid oxidation and formation of reactive oxygen species, as well as modifying the function of membrane calcium channels. As a result, it is conceivable that diabetes may amplify the deleterious effects of inflammatory stressors on cardiac myocytes. It is imperative that this clinical question be investigated further as such a relationship may have significant clinical implications for prevention and future treatments, particularly in patients similar to the one presented in this clinical case.

Consent

Written informed consent was obtained from the patient for publication of this Case Report and any accompanying images through standard institutional protocol. A copy of the written consent is available for review by the Editor-in-Chief of this journal.

Abbreviations
SIRS: Systemic Inflammatory Response Syndrome; HHNS: Hyperosmolar Hyperglycemic Non-Ketotic Syndrome; NTIS: Non-thyroidal Illness Syndrome; FAO: Fatty Acid Oxidation.

Competing interests
The authors declare that they have no competing interests, financial or non-financial.

Author's contributions
JB and RW drafted the manuscript and performed initial literature review. HB provided cardiology consultation, interpreted cardiology images, and edited the manuscript. JL conceived the study, participated in the design and coordination of the manuscript, provided resources for literature review,

and conducted final edits of the manuscript. All authors read and approved the final manuscript.

Authors' information
Not applicable.

Acknowledgements
Substantial contributions were made by all attributed authors. We gratefully acknowledge the providers and ancillary staff that provided compassionate care to the patient.

References
1. Gogos CA, Giali S, Paliogianni F, Dimitracopoulos G, Bassaris HP, Vagenakis AG. Interleukin-6 and C-reactive protein as early markers of sepsis in patients with diabetic ketoacidosis or hyperosmosis. Diabetologia. 2001;44:1011–4.
2. Poelaert J, Declerck C, Vogelaers D, Colardyn F, Visser CA. Left ventricular systolic and diastolic function in septic shock. Intensive Care Med. 1997;23:553–60.
3. Landesberg G, Gilon D, Meroz Y, Georgieva M, Levin PD, Goodman S, et al. Diastolic dysfunction and mortality in severe sepsis and septic shock. Eur Heart J. 2012;33:895–903.
4. Ren J, Wu S. A burning issue: do sepsis and systemic inflammatory response syndrome (SIRS) directly contribute to cardiac dysfunction? Front Biosci J Virtual Libr. 2006;11:15–22.
5. Finkel MS, Oddis CV, Jacob TD, Watkins SC, Hattler BG, Simmons RL. Negative inotropic effects of cytokines on the heart mediated by nitric oxide. Science. 1992;257:387–9.
6. Schulz R, Nava E, Moncada S. Induction and potential biological relevance of a Ca2 + −independent nitric oxide synthase in the myocardium. Br J Pharmacol. 1992;105:575–80.
7. Ziolo MT, Kohr MJ, Wang H. Nitric oxide signaling and the regulation of myocardial function. J Mol Cell Cardiol. 2008;45:625–32.
8. Rudiger A, Singer M. Mechanisms of sepsis-induced cardiac dysfunction. Crit Care Med. 2007;35:1599–608.
9. Werdan K, Schmidt H, Ebelt H, Zorn-Pauly K, Koidl B, Hoke RS, et al. Impaired regulation of cardiac function in sepsis, SIRS, and MODS. Can J Physiol Pharmacol. 2009;87:266–74.
10. Pagani FD, Baker LS, Hsi C, Knox M, Fink MP, Visner MS. Left ventricular systolic and diastolic dysfunction after infusion of tumor necrosis factor-alpha in conscious dogs. J Clin Invest. 1992;90:389–98.
11. Yokoyama T, Vaca L, Rossen RD, Durante W, Hazarika P, Mann DL. Cellular basis for the negative inotropic effects of tumor necrosis factor-alpha in the adult mammalian heart. J Clin Invest. 1993;92:2303–12.
12. Hobai IA, Buys ES, Morse JC, Edgecomb J, Weiss EH, Armoundas AA, et al. SERCA Cys674 sulphonylation and inhibition of L-type Ca2+ influx contribute to cardiac dysfunction in endotoxemic mice, independent of cGMP synthesis. Am J Physiol Heart Circ Physiol. 2013;305:H1189–1200.
13. Kao Y-H, Chen Y-C, Cheng C-C, Lee T-I, Chen Y-J, Chen S-A. Tumor necrosis factor-alpha decreases sarcoplasmic reticulum Ca2 + −ATPase expressions via the promoter methylation in cardiomyocytes. Crit Care Med. 2010;38:217–22.
14. Goldhaber JI, Kim KH, Natterson PD, Lawrence T, Yang P, Weiss JN. Effects of TNF-alpha on [Ca2+] i and contractility in isolated adult rabbit ventricular myocytes. Am J Physiol. 1996;271(4 Pt 2):H1449–1455.
15. Gulick T, Chung MK, Pieper SJ, Lange LG, Schreiner GF. Interleukin 1 and tumor necrosis factor inhibit cardiac myocyte beta-adrenergic responsiveness. Proc Natl Acad Sci U S A. 1989;86:6753–7.
16. Balligand JL, Ungureanu D, Kelly RA, Kobzik L, Pimental D, Michel T, et al. Abnormal contractile function due to induction of nitric oxide synthesis in rat cardiac myocytes follows exposure to activated macrophage-conditioned medium. J Clin Invest. 1993;91:2314–9.
17. Raymond RM. When does the heart fail during shock? Circ Shock. 1990;30:27–41.
18. Solomon MA, Correa R, Alexander HR, Koev LA, Cobb JP, Kim DK, et al. Myocardial energy metabolism and morphology in a canine model of sepsis. Am J Physiol. 1994;266(2 Pt 2):H757–768.

19. Brealey D, Brand M, Hargreaves I, Heales S, Land J, Smolenski R, et al. Association between mitochondrial dysfunction and severity and outcome of septic shock. Lancet. 2002;360:219–23.
20. Langley RJ, Tsalik EL, Velkinburgh JC V, Glickman SW, Rice BJ, Wang C, et al. An Integrated Clinico-Metabolomic Model Improves Prediction of Death in Sepsis. Sci Transl Med. 2013;5:195ra95.
21. Crossland H, Constantin-Teodosiu D, Gardiner SM, Constantin D, Greenhaff PL. A potential role for Akt/FOXO signalling in both protein loss and the impairment of muscle carbohydrate oxidation during sepsis in rodent skeletal muscle. J Physiol. 2008;586(Pt 22):5589–600.
22. Gellerich FN, Trumbeckaite S, Hertel K, Zierz S, Müller-Werdan U, Werdan K, et al. Impaired energy metabolism in hearts of septic baboons: diminished activities of Complex I and Complex II of the mitochondrial respiratory chain. Shock Augusta Ga. 1999;11:336–41.
23. Drosatos K, Drosatos-Tampakaki Z, Khan R, Homma S, Schulze PC, Zannis VI, et al. Inhibition of c-Jun-N-terminal kinase increases cardiac peroxisome proliferator-activated receptor alpha expression and fatty acid oxidation and prevents lipopolysaccharide-induced heart dysfunction. J Biol Chem. 2011;286:36331–9.
24. Feingold K, Kim MS, Shigenaga J, Moser A, Grunfeld C. Altered expression of nuclear hormone receptors and coactivators in mouse heart during the acute-phase response. Am J Physiol Endocrinol Metab. 2004;286:E201–207.
25. Singer M. The role of mitochondrial dysfunction in sepsis-induced multi-organ failure. Virulence. 2014;5:66–72.
26. Carré JE, Singer M. Cellular energetic metabolism in sepsis: the need for a systems approach. Biochim Biophys Acta. 2008;1777:763–71.
27. Levy RJ, Deutschman CS. Evaluating myocardial depression in sepsis. Shock Augusta Ga. 2004;22:1–10.
28. Merx MW, Weber C. Sepsis and the Heart. Circulation. 2007;116:793–802.
29. Zanotti-Cavazzoni SL, Hollenberg SM. Cardiac dysfunction in severe sepsis and septic shock. Curr Opin Crit Care. 2009;15:392–7.
30. Fernandes Jr CJ, de Assuncao MSC. Myocardial dysfunction in sepsis: a large. Unsolved Puzzle Crit Care Res Pract. 2012;2012:1–9.
31. Stentz FB, Umpierrez GE, Cuervo R, Kitabchi AE. Proinflammatory cytokines, markers of cardiovascular risks, oxidative stress, and lipid peroxidation in patients with hyperglycemic crises. Diabetes. 2004;53:2079–86.
32. Bugger H, Abel ED. Molecular mechanisms of diabetic cardiomyopathy. Diabetologia. 2014;57:660–71.
33. Wartofsky L, Burman KD. Alterations in thyroid function in patients with systemic illness: the "euthyroid sick syndrome.". Endocr Rev. 1982;3:164–217.
34. Kaptein EM, Beale E, Chan LS. Thyroid hormone therapy for obesity and nonthyroidal illnesses: a systematic review. J Clin Endocrinol Metab. 2009;94:3663–75.
35. Castro I, Quisenberry L, Calvo R-M, Obregon M-J, Lado-Abeal J. Septic shock non-thyroidal illness syndrome causes hypothyroidism and conditions for reduced sensitivity to thyroid hormone. J Mol Endocrinol. 2013;50:255–66.
36. Iervasi G, Pingitore A, Landi P, Raciti M, Ripoli A, Scarlattini M, et al. Low-T3 syndrome: a strong prognostic predictor of death in patients with heart disease. Circulation. 2003;107:708–13.
37. Ladenson PW, Sherman SI, Baughman KL, Ray PE, Feldman AM. Reversible alterations in myocardial gene expression in a young man with dilated cardiomyopathy and hypothyroidism. Proc Natl Acad Sci U S A. 1992;89:5251–5.
38. Hamilton MA, Stevenson LW, Fonarow GC, Steimle A, Goldhaber JI, Child JS, et al. Safety and hemodynamic effects of intravenous triiodothyronine in advanced congestive heart failure. Am J Cardiol. 1998;81:443–7.

16

Arrhythmogenic substrate at the interventricular septum as a target site for radiofrequency catheter ablation of recurrent ventricular tachycardia in left dominant arrhythmogenic cardiomyopathy

Stepan Havranek[1*], Tomas Palecek[1], Tomas Kovarnik[1], Ivana Vitkova[2], Miroslav Psenicka[1], Ales Linhart[1] and Dan Wichterle[3]

Abstract

Background: Left dominant arrhythmogenic cardiomyopathy (LDAC) is a rare condition characterised by progressive fibrofatty replacement of the myocardium of the left ventricle (LV) in combination with ventricular arrhythmias of LV origin.

Case presentation: A thirty-five-year-old male was referred for evaluation of recurrent sustained monomorphic ventricular tachycardia (VT) of 200 bpm and right bundle branch block (RBBB) morphology. Cardiac magnetic resonance imaging showed late gadolinium enhancement distributed circumferentially in the epicardial layer of the LV free wall myocardium including the rightward portion of the interventricular septum (IVS). The clinical RBBB VT was reproduced during the EP study. Ablation at an LV septum site with absence of abnormal electrograms and a suboptimum pacemap rendered the VT of clinical morphology noninducible. Three other VTs, all of left bundle branch block (LBBB) pattern, were induced by programmed electrical stimulation. The regions corresponding to abnormal electrograms were identified and ablated at the mid-to-apical RV septum and the anteroseptal portion of the right ventricular outflow tract. No abnormalities were found at the RV free wall including the inferolateral peritricuspid annulus region. Histological examination confirmed the presence of abnormal fibrous and adipose tissue with myocyte reduction in endomyocardial samples taken from both the left and right aspects of the IVS.

Conclusion: LDAC rarely manifests with sustained monomorphic ventricular tachycardia. In this case, several VTs of both RBBB and LBBB morphology were amenable to endocardial radiofrequency catheter ablation.

Keywords: Left dominant arrhythmogenic cardiomyopathy, Ventricular tachycardia, Magnetic resonance imaging, Endomyocardial biopsy, Catheter ablation

* Correspondence: stepan.havranek@lf1.cuni.cz
[1]2nd Department of Medicine – Department of Cardiovascular Medicine,
First Faculty of Medicine, Charles University and General University Hospital
in Prague, U Nemocnice 2, Prague 128 08, Czech Republic
Full list of author information is available at the end of the article

Background

Left dominant arrhythmogenic cardiomyopathy (LDAC) has been recently introduced as a rare condition characterised by progressive fibrofatty replacement exclusive to the myocardium of the left ventricle (LV) in combination with ventricular arrhythmias of LV origin [1-9]. Sustained ventricular tachycardia (VT) has been observed rarely and catheter ablation for VT in an LDAC patient has never been reported.

Case presentation

A thirty-five-year-old male was referred for evaluation of recurrent hemodynamically tolerated sustained monomorphic ventricular tachycardia of 200 bpm, which had right bundle branch block (RBBB) morphology with leftward axis deviation (Figure 1). He suffered from nonsyncopal palpitations in the past 3 months. He was in functional class NYHA I and had no symptoms suggestive of ischemic heart disease. His medical history was unremarkable. There was no family history of cardiomyopathies or sudden unexplained death. His 12-lead ECG in sinus rhythm was clearly abnormal with borderline Q-waves in the inferior leads, mid-QRS notching and slurring of narrow QRS complexes (QRSd of 98 ms) in limb and right precordial leads, respectively, and flattened biphasic or negative T waves in the inferolateral leads (Figure 1).

Echocardiography detected slight LV dilatation (end-diastolic diameter of 63 mm) with mild global hypokinesia (ejection fraction of 42%). CT coronary angiography excluded coronary artery disease. Cardiac magnetic resonance imaging (CMR) showed late gadolinium enhancement (LGE), which was distributed circumferentially in the epicardial layer of the LV free wall myocardium (approximately one-third of the LV wall thickness) including the rightward portion of the interventricular septum (IVS) (Figure 2). The LGE spread also to a small adjacent region of the mid-anterior free wall of right ventricle (RV). Moreover, T1-weighted and SPIR magnetic resonance sequences visualised adipose infiltration of myocardium in the anterior right IVS and an adjacent portion of the anterior RV free wall in the zone of positive LGE. The LV was slightly dilated (end-diastolic diameter of 62 mm, end-diastolic volume of 287 mL) with mild global hypokinesia (ejection fraction of 50%). There were no wall motion abnormalities of the RV. The typical scar distribution together with ECG abnormalities and VT of RBBB morphology suggested the diagnosis of LDAC. Treatment with bisoprolol 2.5 mg and trandolapril 4 mg daily was initiated.

Because of recurrent VT despite medical therapy, an electrophysiological study, 3D electroanatomical mapping, and ablation were indicated. The procedure was performed under local anesthesia and mild conscious sedation with

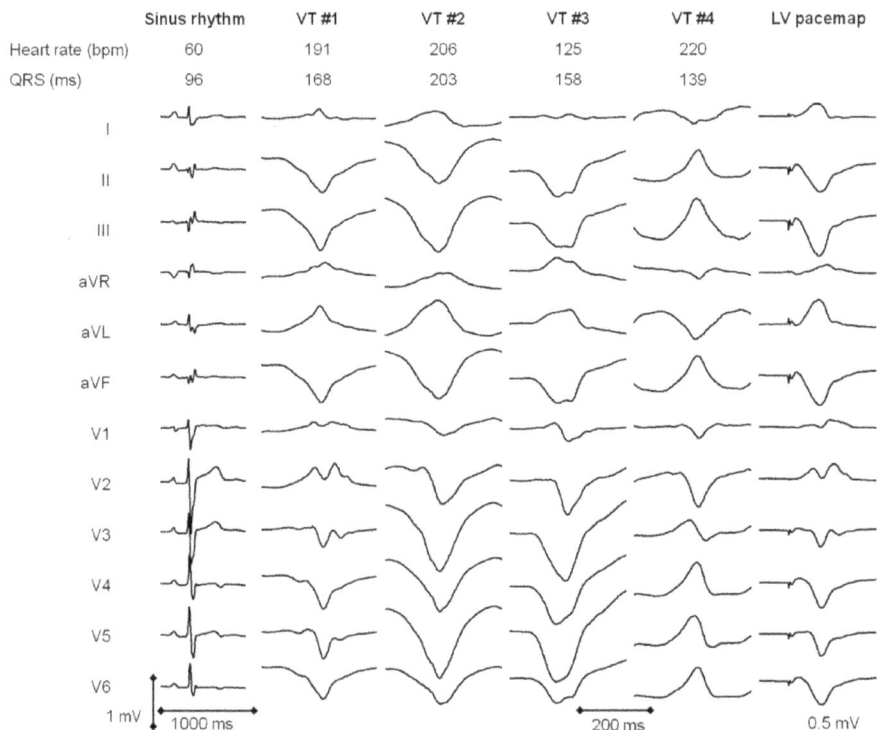

Figure 1 ECG in sinus rhythm, clinical ventricular tachycardia (VT #1) and three other induced VT morphologies during the electrophysiological procedure (VT #2 – #4). The pacemap for VT #1 is shown in the last column corresponding to the site marked by an asterisk in Figure 3.

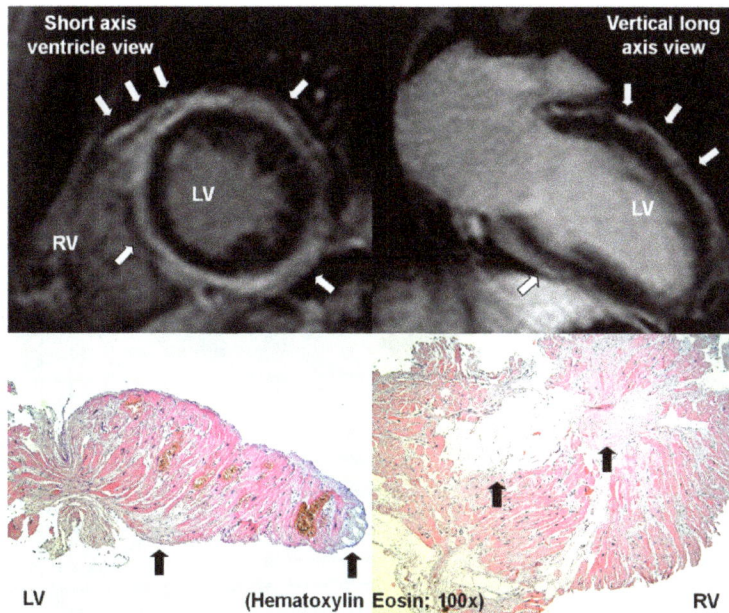

Figure 2 Distribution of late gadolinium enhancement (arrows) in short axis (left upper panel) and vertical long axis view (right upper panel) was distributed circumferentially in the subepicardial left ventricular free wall myocardium with discrete progression to the adjacent mid-anterior free wall of the right ventricle. Note the subendocardial involvement at the RV aspect of the interventricular septum. Histological assessment of endomyocardial samples: from the left ventricular site of abnormal electrograms indicated by the cross in Figure 3 (left bottom panel); from right ventricular aspect of the interventricular septum (right bottom panel). Arrows indicate abnormal fibrosis and adipose tissue. Staining: hematoxylin-eosin. Magnified 100 times.

midazolam and alfentanyl. At the beginning of the procedure, clinical VT of 191 bpm and RBBB morphology (Figure 1, VT #1) was induced by programmed LV stimulation. This was unexpectedly poorly tolerated, so the procedure was continued with substrate mapping in sinus rhythm (3.5 mm irrigated-tip catheter, NaviStar Thermocool, D-curve and CARTO 3, Biosense Webster Inc., Diamond Bar, CA, USA). The procedure was guided by intracardiac echocardiography (AcuNav Diagnostic Ultrasound Catheter, Acuson – Siemens, Mountain View, CA, USA). The LV was accessed by a transseptal approach using a steerable sheath (Agilis, St. Jude Medical Inc., St. Paul, MN, USA) in order to enable subsequent endomyocardial biopsy. As expected, endocardial LV bipolar mapping did not reveal low-voltage areas <1.5 mV. There were a limited number of sites with abnormal electrograms, which were located only at the apicoseptal LV region (Figure 3). Stimulus-to-QRS (S-QRS) delay did not exceed 20 ms in any of them. The best, but far from optimum, pacemap (Figure 1) for the clinical VT was achieved in the mid-inferior LV septum where the morphology of bipolar electrograms was fairly normal. Despite this finding, RF energy (Stockert EP Shuttle, Biosense Webster Inc., Diamond Bar, CA, USA; setting: 30 W, <40°C, 30 ml/min) was delivered at this site and its close vicinity. After the initial ablation, we were unable to re-induce the VT of clinical morphology. However, three other non-clinical VTs (of 206, 125 and

220 bpm), all of left bundle branch block (LBBB) pattern, were observed (Figure 1, VT #2 - #4). They were inducible by programmed stimulation from the RV/LV or by catheter manipulation and were either non-sustained or non-tolerated. The pacemapping for VT morphology #2 and #3 suggested an exit site at the mid-to-apical RV septum. VT morphology #4 had an inferior axis and its exit site was located at the anteroseptal portion of the right ventricular outflow tract (RVOT). Electroanatomical mapping of the RV identified dispersed regions of abnormal electrograms, predominantly at the septum and the anterior/septum portions of the RVOT, while the RV free wall including the inferolateral peritricuspid annulus region was generally not affected. Maximum scar involvement was found at the RV aspect of the IVS, where sites with discrete late potentials and slow conduction zones (maximum S-QRS of 50 ms) were identified (Figure 3). Substrate-based ablation was performed rather extensively at the RV aspect of the midseptum from the inferior to middle segments up to the proximity of right bundle branch (contralateral to the exit of clinical VT #1 and close to the suspected exits of VT #2 and #3) as well as at the anterior portion of the RVOT (site of origin of VT #4).

An endomyocardial biopsy was performed prior to ablation, with an attempt to guide the catheter bioptome (7-F/104 cm biopsy forceps, Cordis, Bridgewater, NJ, USA) into affected regions according to electroanatomical mapping.

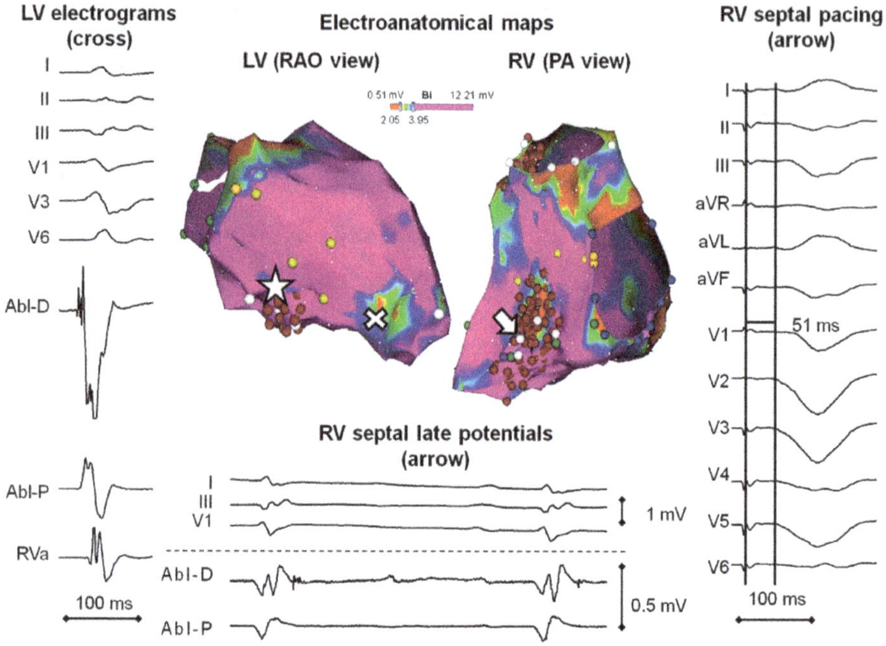

Figure 3 The bipolar voltage map of both ventricles in sinus rhythm. An atypical range (2–4 mV) for color-coding was used to highlight the areas of subtle reduction of bipolar voltages. The cross denotes the left ventricular apicoseptal region of abnormal electrograms where the endomyocardial biopsy was taken. The arrow indicates the site with a maximum stimulus-to-QRS interval at the right-sided interventricular septum. The asterisk shows the site of the pacemap for the clinical tachycardia at the left-sided interventricular septum site with normal electrograms.

Histological examination confirmed the presence of abnormal fibrous and adipose tissue with myocyte reduction in endomyocardial samples taken from both left and right aspects of the IVS (Figure 2). Mutation screening for desmosomal genes was not performed.

A cardioverter-defibrillator (ICD) was implanted and the patient was discharged on the same dosage of bisoprolol and trandolapril medication. No class I or III antiarrhythmic drugs were given. During the 18-month follow-up, the patient experienced only a single episode of monomorphic VT (243 bpm) when bisoprolol medication was discontinued by mistake. LV dilatation and mild dysfunction remained stable at regular check-ups.

Discussion

The phenotypic spectrum of arrhythmogenic cardiomyopathy includes either left dominant, right dominant or bi-ventricular variant. Isolated left and right ventricular abnormalities are at two extremes of the clinical manifestation of the disease [8]. There were no specific ECG abnormalities in the right precordial leads in our patient. The RV was not dilated and had normal kinetics. Typical regions involved in classic arrhythmogenic right ventricular cardiomyopathy (ARVC) (e.g. inferolateral peri-tricuspid area) were free of fibrofatty replacement according to both LGE CMR and electroanatomical mapping. The diagnosis of LDAC in this case was based on recently established clinical features of the disease [8]: ventricular arrhythmia of LV origin, repolarization abnormalities in inferolateral leads, mild LV dilatation with systolic dysfunction, and myocardial fibrofatty replacement assessed by LGE on CMR and confirmed by endomyocardial biopsy.

The designation as a purely LV entity might be questioned because a small region of fibrofatty replacement was present at the mid-anterior portion of the RV free wall, as assessed by LGE CMR. An additional region of abnormal electrograms was present at the anterior RVOT by electroanatomical mapping (not revealed by CMR), complemented by the observation that inducible VT #4 exited from this site. This is still compatible with LDAC because LV involvement including IVS clearly dominated and subtle RV regional abnormalities or the presence of additional arrhythmogenic substrate in RV has been observed in the majority of LDAC patients [8].

Although the presence of ventricular arrhythmias is an essential component of the clinical picture of LDAC, sustained monomorphic VT has been reported rarely. Besides the cases diagnosed post-mortem, the predominant arrhythmias were frequent ventricular premature beats or non-sustained VT of LV origin [8]. Sustained VT of RBBB morphology has been described only in a minority of patients: in 1 of 42 patients in Sen-Chowdry's cohort [8], in 3 of 7 carriers of a dominant desmoplakin mutation in single family [5] and in 3 more solitary case reports [3,10,11]. To the best of our knowledge, catheter ablation has never been performed for VT in an LDAC patient.

Similarly to classic ARVC, catheter ablation therapy in LDAC may be indicated in patients with recurrent VT despite therapy with antiarrhythmic drugs. In this case we preferred non-pharmacological treatment because of the considerable burden of arrhythmia, in order to prevent frequent ICD therapy and to avoid long-term medical therapy, which may be ineffective and/or associated with adverse effects.

Because of the non-transmural and rather homogeneous distribution of pathological tissue, electroanatomical mapping (both bipolar and unipolar) showed voltages almost invariably within the normal arbitrary range and thus was of little help. For this reason pre-procedural CMR was extremely valuable for tailoring the ablation strategy. It demonstrated from the very beginning that the clinical VT could only be effectively targeted by endocardial ablation from the RV aspect of IVS - the only site where the potential substrate was localized close to the endocardial surface. Any other LV targets would require an epicardial approach. Fortunately, VT #1 - #3 originated at the IVS. It is likely that the clinical VT (VT #1) originated from the RV subendocardium at the IVS with a preferential leftward exit, which could explain the RBBB morphology. Initial ablation at the LV aspect of the IVS probably modified the route of propagation. This explains why subsequent VT #2 and #3 had LBBB morphology. It is not known whether the initial LV ablation had any other impact besides changing the exit route.

Indeed, there was a preponderance of mappable arrhythmogenic substrate at the RV aspect of the IVS, although in sinus rhythm the abnormal electrograms were considerably masked by the fast activation of the septum from both sides via the intact His-Purkinje system conduction. Pacing from the LV would probably be helpful maneuver to reveal pathological electrograms or late potentials at the right side of the IVS, but this was not done in the present case. Ablation at the RV aspect of the IVS was performed rather extensively to target not only the critical zones of inducible VTs but also to homogenize the scar in order to prevent other VTs that did not manifest during the procedure.

Although the patient presented with VT of RBBB morphology, this case also suggests that, at least in theory, LDAC may manifest by ventricular arrhythmias of LBBB morphology alone. This might be taken into account when the clinical criteria of LDAC are refined in the future.

Endomyocardial biopsy guided by electroanatomical mapping confirmed the presence of fibrous and adipose tissue in samples obtained from both aspects of the IVS. Positive sampling from the right-sided IVS, fully affected by the pathological process, was expected in our case. The biopsy from the LV endomyocardium, without macroscopic signs of pathology by LGE CMR, was taken from the apicoseptal region of LV, which was the only

site with borderline abnormal electrograms. Such an approach could possibly increase the diagnostic yield, as already reported [12].

Because of structural heart disease that manifested by malignant ventricular arrhythmia and the existence of large-scale, potentially arrhythmogenic substrate, which could not be safely eliminated by catheter ablation, and because of the progressive nature of disease, the cardioverter-defibrillator was implanted for secondary prevention of sudden cardiac death. Despite the fact that single episode of VT was documented during the follow-up, it is likely that catheter ablation prevented frequent VT recurrences.

Conclusion
Left dominant arrhythmogenic cardiomyopathy is an infrequent structural heart disease, which rarely manifests with sustained monomorphic ventricular tachycardia. In this case, extensive circumferential LV involvement by fibrofatty replacement was distributed epicardially at the LV free wall and subendocardially at the RV aspect of the interventricular septum. Several VTs of both RBBB and LBBB morphology were amenable to endocardial radiofrequency catheter ablation.

Consent
Written informed consent was obtained from the patient to the publication of this case report and any accompanying images. A copy of the written consent is available for review by the Editor of this journal.

Abbreviations
LDAC: Left dominant arrhythmogenic cardiomyopathy; LV: Left ventricle; VT: Ventricular tachycardia; RBBB: Right bundle branch block; CMR: Cardiac magnetic resonance; LGE: Late gadolinium enhancement; IVS: Interventricular septum; RV: Right ventricle; S-QRS: Stimulus-to-QRS; LBBB: Left bundle branch block; RVOT: Right ventricular outflow tract; ARVC: Arrhythmogenic right ventricular cardiomyopathy; ICD: Implantable cardioverter-defibrillator.

Competing interests
The authors declare that they have no competing interests.

Authors' contributions
SH: attending physician, catheter ablation procedure, drafting of the manuscript; TP: referring physician, echocardiography and cardiac magnetic resonance imaging, follow-up of patient, drafting and revision of the manuscript; TK: endomyocardial biopsy; IV: histological examination, drafting the manuscript; MP: ICD implant and follow-up; AL: holder of the acknowledged grant, supervision of the study overall; DW: catheter ablation procedure, critical revision of the manuscript for important intellectual content. All authors read and approved the final manuscript.

Acknowledgements
Supported by PRVOUK-P35/LF1/5 and by project reg. no. CZ.2.16/3.1.00/24012 from OP Prague Competitiveness. We thank Barbara A. Danek for her help with language correction.

Author details
[1]2nd Department of Medicine – Department of Cardiovascular Medicine, First Faculty of Medicine, Charles University and General University Hospital in Prague, U Nemocnice 2, Prague 128 08, Czech Republic. [2]Institute of Pathology, First Faculty of Medicine, Charles University and General University Hospital in Prague, Studnickova 2, 128 00 Prague, Czech Republic.

[3]Department of Cardiology, Institute for Clinical and Experimental Medicine, Videnska 1958/9, Prague 140 21, Czech Republic.

References

1. Collett BA, Davis GJ, Rohr WB. Extensive fibrofatty infiltration of the left ventricle in two cases of sudden cardiac death. J Forensic Sci. 1994;39:1182–7.

2. Okabe M, Fukuda K, Nakashima Y, Arakawa K, Kikuchi M. An isolated left ventricular lesion associated with left ventricular tachycardia arrhythmogenic "left" ventricular dysplasia? Jpn Circ J. 1995;59:49–54.

3. Suzuki H, Sumiyoshi M, Kawai S, Takagi A, Wada A, Nakazato Y, et al. Arrhythmogenic right ventricular cardiomyopathy with an initial manifestation of severe left ventricular impairment and normal contraction of the right ventricle. Jpn Circ J. 2000;64:209–13.

4. De Pasquale CG, Heddle WF. Left sided arrhythmogenic ventricular dysplasia in siblings. Heart. 2001;86:128–30.

5. Norman M, Simpson M, Mogensen J, Shaw A, Hughes S, Syrris P, et al. Novel mutation in desmoplakin causes arrhythmogenic left ventricular cardiomyopathy. Circulation. 2005;112:636–42.

6. Bauce B, Rampazzo A, Basso C, Beffagna G, Daliento L, Frigo G, et al. Clinical profile of four families with arrhythmogenic right ventricular cardiomyopathy caused by dominant desmoplakin mutations. Eur Heart J. 2005;26:1666–75.

7. Sen-Chowdhry S, Syrris P, McKenna WJ. Desmoplakin disease in arrhythmogenic right ventricular cardiomyopathy: early phenotype studies. Eur Heart J. 2005;26:1582–4.

8. Sen-Chowdhry S, Syrris P, Prasad SK, Hughes SE, Merrifield R, Ward D, et al. Left-dominant arrhythmogenic cardiomyopathy: an under-recognized clinical entity. J Am Coll Cardiol. 2008;52:2175–87.

9. Coats CJ, Quarta G, Flett AS, Pantazis AA, McKenna WJ, Moon JC. Arrhythmogenic left ventricular cardiomyopathy. Circulation. 2009;120:2613–4.

10. Avella A, D'Amati G, Pappalardo A, Re F, Silenzi PF, Laurenzi F, et al. Diagnostic value of endomyocardial biopsy guided by electroanatomic voltage mapping in arrhythmogenic right ventricular cardiomyopathy/dysplasia. J Cardiovasc Electrophysiol. 2008;19:1127–34.

11. Szymański P, Klisiewicz A, Spiewak M, Szumowski L, Walczak F, Hoffman P. Left dominant arrhythmogenic cardiomyopathy- a newly defined clinical entity. Int J Cardiol. 2012;156:e60–1.

12. Hsiao CC, Kuo JY, Yun CH, Hung CL, Tsai CH, Yeh HI. Rare case of left-dominant arrhythmogenic right ventricular cardiomyopathy with dramatic reverse remodeling after cardiac resynchronization as an adjunct to pharmacological therapy. Heart Lung. 2012;41:e39–43.

17

Living with hypertrophic cardiomyopathy and an implantable defibrillator

Peter Magnusson[1,2]*, Jessica Jonsson[2], Stellan Mörner[3] and Lennart Fredriksson[2]

Abstract

Background: ICDs efficiently terminate life-threatening arrhythmias, but complications occur during long-term follow-up. Patients' own perspective is largely unknown. The aim of the study was to describe experiences of hypertrophic cardiomyopathy (HCM) patients with implantable defibrillators (ICDs).

Methods: We analyzed 26 Swedish patient interviews using hermeneutics and latent content analysis.

Results: Patients (aged 27–76 years) were limited by HCM especially if it deteriorates into heart failure. The ICD implies safety, gratitude, and is accepted as a part of the body even when inappropriate ICD shocks are encountered. Nobody regretted the implant. Both the disease and the ICD affected professional life and leisure time activities, especially at younger ages. Family support was usually strong, but sometimes resulted in overprotection, whereas health care focused on medical issues. Despite limitations, patients adapted, accepted, and managed challenges.

Conclusion: HCM patients with ICDs reported good spirit and hope even though they had to adapt and accept limitations over time.

Keywords: Content analysis, Hermeneutics, Hypertrophic Cardiomyopathy, Implantable cardioverter defibrillator, Interview, Qualitative

Background

The hypertrophic cardiomyopathy (HCM) phenotype is diagnosed when the left ventricular wall is thicker than 15 mm without any other explanation [1]. HCM prevalence is approximately 1:500 in the general population but 1:300 if genotypes are also included [2, 3]. A mutation is found in more than half of the cases and can be used for screening of family members [1]. Genetic screening is sometimes the way to diagnosis but an abnormal ECG or a murmur may lead to evaluation with echocardiography. Symptoms like shortness of breath, chest pain, tiredness, dizziness, or syncope are unspecific. Disease progression varies greatly, and atrial fibrillation and end-stage heart failure with low ejection fraction imply a worse prognosis [4, 5]. Sudden cardiac death (SCD) is difficult to predict but can be effectively prevented by inserting an implantable cardioverter defibrillator (ICD) [6–8] which terminates ventricular tachycardia or ventricular fibrillation by anti-tachycardia pacing or shock discharge. In survivors of cardiac arrest or ventricular tachycardia with hemodynamic compromise, implanting an ICD is standard practice defined as secondary prevention [1, 9]. For primary prevention patients, the decision to implant an ICD requires careful clinical judgement based on risk markers [1, 9]. Current guidelines also take into account the lifelong risk of complications and the impact of an ICD on lifestyle, socioeconomic status and psychological health [1]. However, knowledge gained from several studies on general ICD populations cannot be generalized, because HCM patients are generally younger, have an extended life expectancy, suffer from other symptoms, and have a genetic disease. Taken globally, these conditions may affect an individual's lifestyle, working life, family structure, leisure pursuits, and overall attitudes about life. Subasic concluded from 15 selected patients that living with HCM altered identity and generated fear and uncertainty [10]. Nevertheless, no previous study specifically addressed unselected HCM patients with

* Correspondence: peter.magnusson@regiongavleborg.se
[1]Cardiology Research Unit, Department of Medicine, Karolinska Institutet, Karolinska University Hospital/Solna, SE-171 76 Stockholm, Sweden
[2]Centre for Research and Development, Uppsala University/Region Gävleborg, SE-801 87 Gävle, Sweden
Full list of author information is available at the end of the article

ICDs. The aim of this study was to explore the individual experience of patients who had HCM and ICDs.

Methods

The methodology is inspired by hermeneutics and also by latent content analysis [11–13]. The most fundamental structure of understanding within hermeneutics is the hermeneutic circle. In this study it is visible 'both as a movement between tradition and the movement of the interpreter.' [14] This presupposes a consciousness of the fact that the researchers are situated within a tradition which imply structures of pre-understanding, but also are capable by reflection to alter this understanding. The circle can also be envisioned as a movement between the parts and the whole when interpreting a single interview and also as parts and a whole when several interviews are translated into each other.

Inclusion criteria, setting, procedures, and ethics

To cover essential aspects of the heterogeneous disease HCM we predefined the following maximum variation sampling variables: sex, age, time since diagnosis, primary/secondary indication of ICD, and a history of appropriate or inappropriate shock (Table 1). All patients, aged ≥18 years with at least 2 years history of a transvenous ICD due to HCM, were identified from the Swedish ICD Registry which has a complete coverage of all implants [15]. Patients with a postal address in the Region Gävleborg or Umeå University hospital and their affiliated hospitals were recruited.

Medical data were validated using medical records (PM, SM). The patients were contacted by phone by the investigators (PM or SM) and scheduled for an appointment with the interviewer (JJ). All patients came to the appointment, consented, and were subsequently interviewed (sample size, n = 26) between February and

Table 1 Characteristics of 26 interviewed HCM patients with history of ICD

Sex, age	Civic status	Child	Indication	ICD duration	ICD shock	Diagnosis	NYHA
M, 27	Cohabitate	0	primary	4.9	no	9	I
F, 32	Cohabitate	2	primary	2.4	no	17	II
F, 33	Cohabitate	2	secondary	6.3	no	14	I
M, 37	Divorced	1	primary	3.0	no	8	II
M, 42	Married	2	secondary	8.4	inappropriate	9	I
M, 48	Divorced	2	primary	4.8	no	30	I
M,49	Cohabitate	0	secondary	6.9	appropriate	7	II
F, 54	Cohabitate	1	primary	10.9	inappropriate	20	II
M,55	Single	0	secondary	8.0	appropriate	37	IIIB
M, 59	Married	2	primary	3.8	inappropriate	4	I
M, 59	Cohabitate	2	primary	1.0	no	32	IV/I[a]
F, 60	Married	3	secondary	10.9	inappropriate	20	I
M, 61	Married	2	primary	8.9	no	18	I
M, 61	Divorced	5	primary	11.3	inappropriate	45	IIIB
M, 63	Married	2	primary	16.6	appropriate	17	I
M, 64	Cohabitate	2	primary	3.0	no	4	I
F, 65	Single	1	primary	5.3	inappropriate	8	I
M, 65	Married	1	primary	5.1	no	42	I
M, 65	Married	2	primary	7.6	no	9	I
M, 67	Married	2	primary	3.2	no	4	II
F, 68	Married	4	primary	7.8	no	7	I
M, 69	Married	1	primary	4.5	no	5	I
M, 72	Divorced	7	secondary	3.5	no	20	II
F, 75	Divorced	0	primary	11.2	inappropriate	15	I
F, 75	Married	1	primary	9.8	inappropriate	14	IIIA
F, 76	Single	2	primary	5.2	no	7	I

M Male, *F* Female, *NYHA* New York Heart Association, *ICD* Implantable cardioverter defibrillator, *HCM* Hypertrophic cardiomyopathy
ICD duration refers to time (years) with an ICD and *Diagnosis* time (years) since first known diagnosis of HCM
[a]heart transplant due to NYHA IV, at the time of interview NYHA I

June 2015 either at the research department, outpatient clinic, or at home. The study was approved by the Regional Ethical committee in Uppsala (Dnr 2015/060). References to patients' identities have been omitted due to confidentiality.

The interviews

Following information about the study, written consent, questions about age and habitual status, an open-ended communication was initiated. An interview guide was constructed based on the aim of the study using a narrative, explorative approach. Based on the researcher's clinical experience and literature search in the field, the topics were developed. The topics covered wide areas of life experiences (see Appendix 1). The guide provided open-ended questions and also specific questions on each topic. This ensured that all relevant topics were addressed in each interview. The guide served as a narrative framework to achieve structure but encouraged the participants to speak freely and raise issues of concern to them. At the end of the interview, the guide was used to check for completeness. After each interview, a contact with their clinician was arranged or supported if the patient desired. Interviews were digitally audio-recorded and transcribed verbatim. The mean duration of interviews was 135 min (in total 58.6 h; range 81–210 min).

Analysis and interpretation of interviews

The analysis and interpretation of the interviews was guided both by an awareness of the movement in the hermeneutic circles, but also by latent content analysis as a means to condense and code the text (Table 2). All interviews were read as a holistic narrative and discussed among the researchers. Through repeated reading, the interviews were condensed into meaning units, according to the aim of the study. These condensed meaning units were shortened and labelled with a code. The text was decontextualized, meaning that codes were read

Table 2 Examples of content analysis and hermeneutic interpretation of narratives of hypertrophic cardiomyopathy and ICD

Condensed meaning unit	Code	Narrative themes	Theoretical themes
It is constantly in the back of my mind. And it has surely become more visible for me because I received this device. It is therefore something that reminds me every day. Earlier – before I received the device- it was a reminder when I was called in for a check-up. At that time it was longer between the occasions…but it is nothing…yeah…it is part of the person I am.	ICD is a reminder of disease. ICD is internalized and considered as part of the patient.	Implant decision, surgery, and wearing an ICD	Awareness Acceptance
Does the ICD affect your health? *Not at all. I used to let people touch it, feel what I have under my skin! I think it is kind of amusing.*	Appraisal focused strategy using humor but also denial.	ICD provides assurance	Adaptation
I am comfortable with it. It is such a security and I am so grateful for getting the opportunity to do it [ICD implant].	ICD implies safety and gratefulness.	ICD knowledge and worries	Gratitude
It [the ICD] is almost on the outside, it seems to me. One can feel the wires here…but that is the only thing. One has to be careful not the get a hit here when playing with the grandchildren.	Local problems superficial device system.	Implant decision, surgery, and wearing an ICD	Awareness Adaptation
After the cardiac arrest it was mostly like this: Have I done everything before I fall asleep? Have I said good-bye to everybody…But after the last shocks it was not like that, I woke up in the night and jumped out of the bed (laughter). *But now it is all right, now I don't wake up in the middle of the night.*	Anxiety after cardiac arrest and inappropriate shocks. Finally coping.	ICD knowledge and worries	Hope
Yes, it is after the shock it became worrisome…But I did not want to tell them (husband and son)…I think I keep a lot to myself. Sometimes it feels like I want to be alone…I don't want them to call me ten times a day: how are you? Is everything ok?	Anxious shortly after inappropriate shock. Does not share worries with close relatives.	Relationship and support	Adaptation
One can't just get too bogged down and worry. There are so many other things to be worried about. Damn, you have to live! That's how I feel.	Realistic view on risk of death. Accept risk.	Feeling healthy despite disease	Awareness Acceptance
About friends' concerns: I think they are ridiculous. But I say, oh God, what can I do about it? It's over when it's over…ha (laughter).	Fatalistic view on death. Dissociates from friends worries.		Hope
Brother of a sudden death victim: *My mom became very worried about that time…but that is nothing we talked about very much. That is the way my family works…The ostrich method…it just buries the head in the sand and pretends like there is nothing.*	Sudden death affects family but they do not talk about it.	Relationship and support	Awareness
I have such a bad background. They just dropped dead. On my mother's side they just died, it started in the 40s…one was just 13 and the other 17…and I have a cousin…she was only 25…	Aware of several cases of sudden cardiac death in the family.	Inheritance	Awareness

across interviews. Preliminary themes were interpreted and reflected upon, moving between parts and the whole. The process resulted in ten narrative themes and five theoretical themes, together 'unfolding a world in front of the text.' [16] Finally, all interviews were read again to verify the accuracy of interpretations and the reported themes (Table 2).

Results

Patient characteristics

Patient age ranged from 27 to 76 years (mean 57.7 years) and the majority (65.3%) was male. All New York Heart Association (NYHA) functional classes were represented. Time since the first known diagnosis of HCM varied (range 4–45 years, mean 16 years) Mean time with an ICD was 6.7 years and ranged from 2.4 to 16.6 years, with the exception of one patient who had an ICD for 1 year before explant due to heart transplant. Both primary (n = 20) and secondary ICD indications (n = 6) were represented. Experiences of at least one appropriate or inappropriate ICD shock were reported in 3 and 8 different patients, respectively. Characteristics of each participant are described in Table 1.

The findings of the study are presented as 10 narrative themes describing the experience of HCM patients living with an ICD. The order follows the narrative thread in the patients' interviews and serves to depict that some things often happen before other. In the discussion section these narrative themes are further interpreted and reflected upon at a more abstract level in the light of 5 theoretical themes.

HCM symptoms, diagnosis, and medication

Shortness of breath was the predominant HCM symptom, which was especially pronounced at exertion. Other symptoms were unspecific, such as tiredness, lack of stamina, syncope, and palpitations. Notably, no patient suffered from chest pain. ECG signs or a murmur sometimes lead to an echocardiography confirming HCM, but discovery also occurred during family screening or as a result of medical investigations for other reasons, including childbirth, general surgery, or when an infection, stroke, or cardiac arrest were managed.

The HCM diagnosis was often delayed and initially misdiagnosed as something else and the patients occasionally expressed worries about health providers' actual knowledge about the disease. This trust was particularly damaged when a relative experienced SCD. Patients with a family history of SCD were easily convinced of the value of an ICD, whereas patients with other risk markers, such as non-sustained ventricular tachycardia sometimes questioned the need of an ICD before implant. At the time of interview, the term hypertrophic cardiomyopathy and its abbreviation HCM were unknown to many and they called the disease *an enlarged heart, heart trouble,* or *heart thickness.* One young patient said, *Then* (at the time of implant) *they said hypertrophic cardiomyopathy...and I really understood it,* while others required their physicians to write the term down for them. The patients reported high compliance with the prescribed HCM related medications (beta-blocker or calcium-channel antagonist) despite lack of short-term symptom relief, but dosage was often lowered due to presumed side effects.

Inheritance

Although HCM is not always diagnosed early in life, women of childbearing age still reported that they wanted to have children despite the risks of passing on the condition to their children. One severely symptomatic older man said that he would have had fewer children if he had known what the disease progression would mean, but otherwise did not have much concern. Parents of young children pondered the consequences of genetic testing for their children. One couple talked openly to their child about HCM to avoid confusion. Even when patients received genetic counseling, they sometimes had only a vague understanding of how the disease can be passed on to their children. Cascade screening was challenging and sometimes impossible due to broken families, estrangements, and dysfunctional family dynamics, such as the young woman who could not be tested for HCM because her parents did not tell her that the disease ran in the family. No patient in the study blamed parents for their HCM.

Implant decision, surgery, and wearing an ICD

Few primary prevention patients had a clear idea about the risk markers that made them eligible for ICD implant and sometimes these patients were not initially motivated to get an ICD. The experience of the implant procedure varied and they often recalled considerable pain. Complications requiring surgery were tolerated but some patients thought that preoperative information was sometimes lacking. Others reported feelings of isolation: *When I was waiting for surgery, I felt like a chicken going into the slaughterhouse.*

All young patients disliked people staring at the scars from the implant procedure, especially when bathing, but after some years many joked about the scar and claimed the ICD was a part of their body. An elderly woman said she initially avoided certain clothes which exposed the device, but later on, this did not trouble her. Some male patients even let people touch the scar. When ICD patients were playing with children, the device served as a reminder of the disease and made it real. A mother of a 5-year old daughter called it *the life-saver* and her daughter said she wanted one as well. Descriptions like *my heart runs on batteries* were common and show awareness and acceptance of living with technology. Gratitude, trust, and security were expressed along with a feeling of privilege because it is such a costly device. However, the device sometimes caused local irritation and required padding when using a seat belt or carrying a backpack; patients sometimes said they needed a cushion when lying in certain positions in bed.

ICD knowledge and worries

A few patients knew that the ICD shock-function could temporarily be inhibited by magnet application; among patients who experienced inappropriate shocks this was common knowledge and some even had a magnet with them. Patients were worried about the lack of ICD-specific knowledge among health personnel. They had encountered this lack of knowledge in emergency care, primary care, and specialized care outside of cardiology units. The ICD card, which is provided to all patients, was considered helpful but there were suggestions for necklace or a bracelet with information, and one patient obtained one from a patient organization. Such easily visible identification could prove invaluable in an emergency situation, in which the patient was unable to communicate.

The difference between a pacemaker and an ICD was generally common knowledge among patients but they did not think this was known to the general public or among health care providers. The experience of the vibration alert function of some ICDs was sometimes confused with an ICD shock; some individuals realized this for the first time during their interview. The ICD device usually contraindicated medical investigations such as magnetic resonance imaging or transcutaneous electrical nerve stimulation which limited full access to health care. Some patients had reflected about deactivation in case of terminal illness and were concerned that health care providers would not recognize the ICD or distinguish it from a pacemaker at life's end.

ICD provides reassurance

All patients felt secure and grateful to receive an ICD. None regretted the decision to implant the ICD. They often had nicknames for the device, i.e. *my life-saver, the fire extinguisher, a friend of mine*, and *life insurance*. The word *secure* was announced numerous times by different patients. A young man whose father died suddenly at an early age felt overwhelmed and said, *Everybody should have one...I am protected but they are not....*

ICD shocks

Even patients who experienced several inappropriate shocks persevered and accepted the therapy as part of their new life. Some of them came to terms with the shocks within a couple of weeks and one woman said,

You know that it [the ICD] *actually works.* Other expressions were, *it was horrible, unpleasant, but I know I won't die from it and I know how it feels...it is just a dreadful feeling.* Another commented, *It is damn nasty, really nasty, but there is no pain afterwards and it feels like a strong electrical discharge.* Typically they described their first feelings as, *scary, nasty, unpleasant, horrible, terrible, dreadful,* and *ghastly.* Metaphors for the shock were *being hit by a stone*, and *being shot by a revolver*, and *I jumped a foot, and I was like a jumping jack.* The unpredictable nature of shock therapy was described as a *bolt from out of the blue*, but these victims of inappropriate shocks came to terms with the shock and actually felt reassured after a few weeks. One patient who got the opportunity to talk to her device physician the same day a shock occurred, felt immediate relief. Most of the time, repeated ICD shocks caused a witness to summon an ambulance. Close relatives who witnessed a shock might become overly protective or avoid situations like the one that preceded the last shock. Although patients typically coped with the situation at the time it happened, relatives were also influenced by the dramatic event. A 4-year-old daughter avoided physical contact with her father for a short time after he experienced several shocks. One exceptional case involved a disappointed patient who had experienced complications, including device system infection and several inappropriate shocks due to a fractured Sprint Fidelis lead. She had considered (but rejected) device explant in favor of an external defibrillator. She described her situation as, *I can never relax ... and be a human being again.* However, she appreciated the fact that her device had also delivered appropriate therapy. When experiencing an appropriate shock due to ventricular arrhythmia one patient typically fainted, but felt almost normal soon afterwards. It was a dramatic event for the people around him, but not for the patient who did not always seek medical attention after a shock. A survivor of a ventricular arrhythmia described his adrenergic response, *It was fantastic...I was sitting in a dark room and everything turned bright white.*

Feeling healthy despite disease

Individuals spontaneously described themselves as *healthy* and did not perceive themselves as victims of disease. Their identity did not change even though they had to undertake several changes in their life. They typically denied being sick because they had adapted to a new lifestyle and accepted their limitations: *My husband has energy but I have almost no energy*, and *I learned to live with it*, and *I listen more to my body...* Upon reflection, they occasionally did realize that they had experienced a life-altering event. These changes may have kept them away from certain activities and was most dramatic after surviving a cardiac arrest. As time passed, patients coped with these events, reoriented themselves, and achieved new goals. When asked about his heart problem, an older patient replied: *Maybe I do not need a device. I feel healthy.* In patients with systolic heart failure or atrial fibrillation, physical limitations such as shortness of breath and tiredness were pronounced and they considered that it was HCM, not the ICD, that was severely limiting life. HCM affected their professional opportunities and made them dependent on other people's help. Patients who had secondary prevention ICD felt safer and expressed gratitude that they had a new chance at life. For them, it was obvious that they had a severe disease but this did not make them give up their joy of living. Even though some secondary prevention patients admitted slight cognitive impairment, they still felt eager to continue their old activities. The family members of SCD survivors were often unable to continue ordinary life, expressed worries, and even suffered sleep disturbances according to the patients. In this group, it was common for partners to be overly protective of the ICD patient, especially when there were young children in the family. In general, young patients were more worried and felt more limited than older patients, who remembered the worries they had about their health during adolescence and early adulthood. A woman said, *My teenage years were difficult. I sometimes think: Why me? I am so nice, why couldn't she get it instead? Still, I think everything is crap but I have become wiser and gained more perspective.* Shortly after diagnosis, patients usually had a feeling of being different but later accepted and adapted to the lifestyle changes their condition demanded, and did not see themselves as stigmatized.

Leisure-time activities

In general, patients perceived their underlying HCM, rather than the ICD, as constituting the limit on their leisure-time activities. Athletic activities had to be avoided, modified, or restricted, and many patients were unsure about their recommended level of activity. Mountain trekking, badminton, ice hockey, soccer, dancing, swimming, and hunting sometimes had to be restricted, but patients adapted to these restrictions or switched to other activities. Young patients felt more limited by recommendations to restrict their activities than older patients did. In some cases, driving was restricted by the authorities but this restriction was not always communicated to the patient. In other instances, a concerned spouse might advise the patient against driving. Such advice was at times ignored. When the patient had to limit driving, this impacted both his leisure and professional activities. Physical intimacy was not affected by the device and patients did not express fear of shocks during sex. However presence of severe heart failure or comorbidity limited sexual performance. In fact, one patient who had intercourse the next day after ICD implant said, *We did it immediately when I came back from the hospital...just because I wanted to test it.*

Professional life

Inability to work was associated with symptoms of HCM or comorbidities, especially atrial fibrillation and progression to heart failure or cognitive impairment in cardiac arrest survivors. Younger patients were more worried about their work and sometimes struggled to reorient themselves professionally. These adaptations included less travelling, avoiding stressful situations, reducing their workload, and accepting being on sick leave now and then. Sometimes colleagues helped with certain tasks such as climbing a ladder or heavy lifting. With age, the concerns about working capacity diminished. Looking back, patients with an early onset of symptoms had military service exemptions but thought they were otherwise free to pursue their own career goals. A welder had to change his line of work specifically because of the ICD and other patients sometimes could not pursue work that involved driving or electromagnetic exposure. If this brought on economic constraints, patients adapted to their modified standard of living and did not report it as being problematic.

Relationship, support, and insurance

Following cardiac arrest, patients found their personal relationships were vastly changed. The survivor expressed gratitude, had a renewed appreciation for life, and modified goals and values. By contrast, the emotional response of family members was ambiguous...*The event has made us better connected but also creates problems...these worries can be really tiresome...on the other hand, we have a shared experience that somehow bonds us.* While patients were offered support, including referrals to psychology professionals from the health care system, family members were seldom involved. Generally, patients shared their feelings about their condition with the family, but occasionally the patients did not allow relatives to attend their clinical visits because they did not want them to worry, they expected it would result in overprotection and restrictions, or they wanted to make their own decisions independently but would introduce relatives later on. Occasionally (two patients) the disease was considered by the patient as a contributing factor in divorce. In younger patients, identification phenomena were observed, such as the man who became very anxious when he reached the age at which his father had died unexpectedly or when the child of an ICD patient said she wanted to get an ICD like her mother. In some cases when a patient and a family member went out for a walk, the family member would deliberately choose a less strenuous route to accommodate the patient. Having HCM caused emotional distress as well as physical symptoms in teenagers, who had an acute perception of themselves as being different from their peers.

No patient attended patient organization meetings, but a few had joined a Facebook group for ICD patients and one patient had found the American HCM patient association webpage. Older, highly symptomatic patients were less likely to use the internet as source of information than younger patients. Several patients expressed concern that they lacked information about their prognoses, which they considered the responsibility of their physicians to communicate to them. Not all of the information that patients found was considered beneficial. *The fact that athletes drop dead...it is not advantageous for me.* Furthermore, extensive talk and information about the disease sometimes conflicted with the patients' self-image of being normal. Another young patient said, *The less you know, the less ill you are.* Swedish citizens are covered by a national insurance that pays for medical expenses, including the ICD. In addition, private insurance compensated certain patients for disability. Patients reported unexpected problems when renewing coverage or trying to sign up for a new policy.

Discussion

Patients with ICDs due to HCM report various experiences and limitations throughout their lives, which is impacted by multiple external episodes in conjunction with their own personal traits. In the discussion, we want to introduce five theoretical themes, which we view as symbolic main threads in narratives presented in the result section. Despite the fact that these were individual perceptions, common theoretical themes emerged from them: awareness, adaptation, acceptance, gratitude, and hope (Fig. 1 and examples in Table 2). These themes were interpreted as influenced by the patients' level of knowledge, support, and perceived limitations.

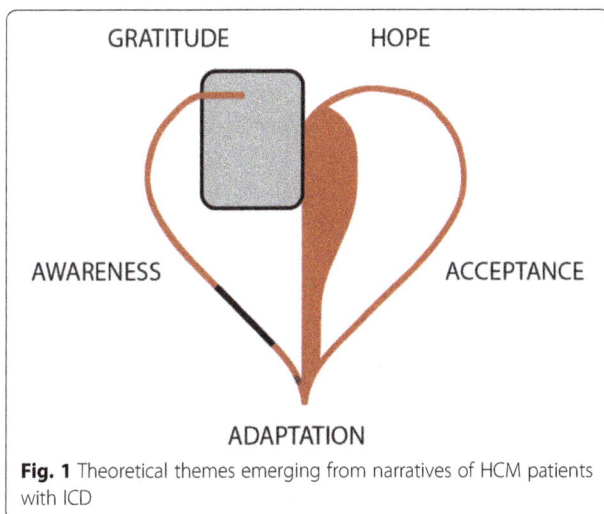

Fig. 1 Theoretical themes emerging from narratives of HCM patients with ICD

Even though HCM is the most common myocardial genetic disease, the awareness about HCM (even among health care providers) is often perceived as poor both among patients and their relatives [1, 10]. The lack of awareness about HCM and its terminology may be historical in nature, in that in the past, there have been >80 names to describe HCM [17] and its unspecific symptoms [1]. There is a lack of structured care for the HCM patient, who may ascribe this absence to ignorance of the disease. No patient had continued contact with any patient organization (there is currently no HCM specific support group in Sweden) and patients found social media irrelevant for communication about the disease. On the other hand, patients were grateful to the communications of their cardiologists, with whom they often had a long-term relationship. Patients acknowledged and appreciated the support they got from the cardiology clinic, although these clinics did not take a holistic approach and tended to limit themselves to device function and medical concerns. In particular, patients perceived that they did not get information about their prognoses, a finding supported by studies on general ICD patients [18–20]. Our patients did not expect emotional or existential support from health care systems, and turned to family instead. This could result in complicated situations. Patients sometimes reported that their family could be overprotective, imposing restrictions on them. On the other hand, family members could also be helpful, especially in doing physical tasks or coping with work situations, as previously described in general ICD populations [20, 21].

Many patients adapted, reduced their workload or even quit their jobs, which relieved stress and left time for them to enjoy family and friends but also limited social networking, leading to isolation and economic constraints [18]. This was more pronounced among younger patients in our study. This was described in a recent American study on HCM, in which investigators reported fear and identity changes among HCM patients [10]. In contrast, our patients adapted to their condition and accepted the limitations their disease put on them, but this did not change identity over their lifespan. Our patients were aware that their ICD offered protection from SCD and this resulted in gratitude and hope, which aligns with previous studies [22–25]. Before the ICD era, the health status of HCM patients assessed by questionnaires, was significantly lower than normal population [26]. While overall disease management has likely improved the situation, the authors feel that the ICD may also relieve some of the stress as it protects against potentially life-threatening SCD. Both primary and secondary indication patients appreciated their lives and considered the device a valuable life-saver contained within their body. It was accepted but constituted restriction and adaptation with regard to specific activities. The ICD was neither a reminder of death nor a cause for anxiety. This reassurance was also valid even after a history of ICD shocks (both appropriate and inappropriate). The time period after ICD shock for regaining calmness and acceptance was typically a few weeks, which is shorter than cross-sectional and longitudinal findings from other ICD populations but consistent with an actual time dependent improvement [19]. Patients with inappropriate shocks recalled an unpredictable, unpleasant episode that often led to urgent hospital visits, whereas appropriate shocks were not perceived as painful, probably because the patient received therapy while unconscious. Inappropriate shocks are often multiple, and are the major drawback of ICD therapy. Efforts are warranted to reduce this risk, especially in a HCM population with extended life expectancy [27]. However, even in the case of inappropriate shocks, our patients were reassured, accepted, and understood the benefits of the life-saving ICD. No patient in our study regretted having the ICD implanted. We believe that in addition to careful information about risk of shocks, patients should be given balanced, not exaggerated, information. Even though receiving an ICD shock is unpleasant and temporarily distressing, patients were surprised that it was not as bad as they expected it to be. Our results indicate that shock therapy affects the whole family and the spouse's response to therapy should not be ignored or trivialized [21, 24].

Patients thought that their everyday activities were restricted by HCM and comorbidity, rather than the ICD. This adaptation is supported by previous findings as in the general ICD populations [28, 29]. Overall, patients were able to adapt and accept obstacles over the course of their lives. Patients with HCM and ICDs encountered challenges, but still had a strong life spirit, great hope, and accepted the lifestyle adaptations they had to make, but were grateful to their device as a life-saver. HCM is a heterogeneous disease and only a subset of HCM patients are indicated for ICD therapy. Nevertheless, it is important to recognize in this diverse patient population that patients can still enjoy their lives, experience joy and hope, learn new things, and have meaningful communications and interactions with others.

Study strengths and weaknesses

This study focuses on ICD recipients specifically due to HCM, in a large cohort. We identified eligible patients from the validated Swedish ICD Registry which covers all implants [15]. The diagnosis of HCM was validated through reading of medical records to ensure

correctness of register data on ICD indication. All patients consented and participated in the interviews from the two regions which reduces selection and referral center bias. All patients were fluent in Swedish and were able to express themselves well. The interview guide fulfilled the purpose of covering different topics and was useful to catalyze elaborate and rich narratives. One of the study's strengths is the rich data, both in quantity and quality. The amount of data was also a challenge. Here the combination of latent content analysis to condense and bring order to the data combined with hermeneutics to analyze and interpret data was useful. The research team continuously reflected on the pre-understanding trough the discussions and repetitive readings of the texts to ensure that interpretations were grounded in data. Notably, self-reported experiences may differ from a relative's views and longitudinal experiences recalled by patients may be different than findings from studies using follow-up interviews. The explorative design is beneficial because it gives insight in a new field but findings need to be confirmed in further confirmative studies. However, the generalizability to other geographical areas and cultural contexts needs to be addressed in future studies.

Conclusions

HCM patients with ICDs perceive that their poor health is the result of the burden of HCM symptoms, especially shortness of breath at exertion. The slow progression of HCM allows patients to adapt to the disease and accept limitations it may impose. HCM patients feel hope and reassurance for the future despite their disease state. To some extent, patients reprioritize their lives from professional activities to value family from whom they seek support. Support is usually obtained from the family rather than health care professionals, whom they consider as mostly a technical service of disease management. They feel grateful to the life-saving ICD and they trust the device and consider it as an integral part of their body, which contributes to hope as they continue with their lives. Inappropriate as well as appropriate shocks may result in temporary concerns but patients usually cope with them (adapt and accept) and rationalize them within a short period of time. ICD treatment is well tolerated among HCM patients but knowledge about it varies substantially. This emphasizes the importance of raising awareness about HCM and increasing knowledge about the role of ICD therapy and tailored disease management in the care of HCM patients. Improvement of clinical care should facilitate awareness, adaptation, and acceptance during the patients' life course. This approach will give hope when encountering challenges.

Appendix 1

Table 3 The interview guide is a framework of the areas relevant to the exploration of the life experiences of HCM patients with ICDs. It should be considered a support tool for conducting the interview using an open question format

Background	How old are you?
	Do you live with anybody?
	Do you have children?
Early questions	What is it like to live with HCM and ICD?
	How and when did you get the HCM diagnosis?
	When did you get the ICD?
General health	What do think about your health?
	How do other people consider your health?
	In what way does the ICD affect your health?
	Has your health changed over time?
	What do think about your future health?
Professional life	Are you working/studying?
	Has your professional life been affected by HCM/ICD?
	Do you think your future career will be affected by HCM/ICD?
Leisure time	In what way has you leisure-time been affected?
	Do you exercise? How does that work?
	Did you get advice on activity levels? Do you follow this advice?
Family & Friends	Is family life affected by HCM/ICD?
	How did your relatives know about your HCM diagnosis and ICD?
	What do your family and close friends think about your having an ICD?
	What do your family and friends know about your HCM and ICD?
Driving	Do you have a driver's license? Which certificates?
	Is your driver's licenses affected by HCM/ICD?
	Did you drive for a living?
	What advice did you get about driving?
Insurance	Did your insurance company act differently based on your HCM/ICD?
Lifestyle	What kind of food do you eat? Alcohol? Smoking?
Medication	Which pharmaceutical drugs do you take?
	Do you take these prescribed drugs?
	Do think that these drugs relieve symptoms/cause side effects?
Diagnosis of HCM	What made them suspect HCM? How long did it take to be diagnosed?
ICD	When and why did they decide about the ICD?

Table 3 The interview guide is a framework of the areas relevant to the exploration of the life experiences of HCM patients with ICDs. It should be considered a support tool for conducting the interview using an open question format *(Continued)*

	What do you think about the information before ICD implant?
	Did you experience ICD shock (appropriate/inappropriate)?
	How was the implant procedure?
	Did you experience any surgical complications?
	Does the ICD give you a sense of security?
	Did you ever regret receiving an ICD?
	Do you know how to turn the ICD off?
	What is the difference between a pacemaker and an ICD?
Health care	What could be improved in health care in HCM and ICD?
	Did you ever contact a patient association?
	Do you use internet/social media? For HCM/ICD communication?
	What can the society do to improve care for HCM/ICD patients?
Sexuality	Is your sex life affected by HCM/ICD?
	Did you need medication to improve sexual performance?
Reproduction	What are your concerns about your child getting HCM?
Pregnancy	Did HCM/ICD affect your pregnancy?
Genetics	Have they found a mutation causing your HCM?
	Did the genetic counselling affect the family?
Sleep	How is your sleep quality?
	Has you sleep been affected by HCM/ICD?

Abbreviations
HCM: Hypertrophic cardiomyopathy; ICD: Implantable cardioverter defibrillator; NYHA: New York Heart Association; SCD: Sudden cardiac death

Acknowledgements
The authors acknowledge editing by Jo Ann LeQuang of LeQ Medical who reviewed the manuscript for American English use and Helena Wase who transcribed the interviews.

Funding
Region Gävleborg funded this research project.

Authors' contributions
PM: design, analysis, structuring and interpretation of data, writing the article, and coordination. JJ conducted the interviews and made critical revisions. SM interpreted the data, provided critical revision, and coordination. LF handled design, interpretation of data, critical revision, and coordination. All authors approved the manuscript for submission.

Competing interests
The authors declare that they have no competing interests.

Author details
[1]Cardiology Research Unit, Department of Medicine, Karolinska Institutet, Karolinska University Hospital/Solna, SE-171 76 Stockholm, Sweden. [2]Centre for Research and Development, Uppsala University/Region Gävleborg, SE-801 87 Gävle, Sweden. [3]Department of Public Health and Clinical Medicine, Umeå University, SE-90187 Umeå, Sweden.

References
1. Elliott PM, Anastasakis A, Borger MA, Borggrefe M, Cecchi F, Charron P, Hagege AA, et al. 2014 ESC guidelines on diagnosis and Management of Hypertrophic Cardiomyopathy: the task force for the diagnosis and management of hypertrophic Cardiomyopathy of the European Society of Cardiology (ESC). Eur Heart J. 2014;35:2733–79.
2. Maron BJ, Olivotto I, Spirito P, Casey SA, Bellone P, Gohman TE, et al. Epidemiology of hypertrophic cardiomyopathy-related death: revisited in a large non-referral-based patient population. Circulation. 2000;102:858–64.
3. Semsarian C, Ingles J, Maron MS, Maron BJ. New perspectives on the prevalence of hypertrophic cardiomyopathy. J Am Coll Cardiol. 2015;65:1249–54.
4. Vriesendorp PA, Schinkel AF, de Groot NM, van Domburg RT, Ten Cate FJ, Michels M. Impact of adverse left ventricular remodeling on sudden cardiac death in patients with hypertrophic cardiomyopathy. Clin Cardiol. 2014;37:493–8.
5. Pasqualucci D, Fornaro A, Castelli G, Rossi A, Arretini A, Chiriatti C, Targetti M, et al. Clinical Spectrum, therapeutic options, and outcome of advanced heart failure in hypertrophic Cardiomyopathy. Circ Heart Fail. 2015;8:1014–21.
6. Schinkel AF, Vriesendorp PA, Sijbrands EJ, Jordaens LJ, ten Cate FJ, Michels M. Outcome and complications after implantable cardioverter defibrillator therapy in hypertrophic cardiomyopathy: systematic review and meta-analysis. Circ Heart Fail. 2012;5:552–9.
7. Vriesendorp PA, Schinkel AF, Van Cleemput J, Willems R, Jordaens LJ, Theuns DA, van Slegtenhorst MA, et al. Implantable cardioverter-defibrillators in hypertrophic cardiomyopathy: patient outcomes, rate of appropriate and inappropriate interventions, and complications. Am Heart J. 2013;166:496–502.
8. O'Mahony C, Tome-Esteban M, Lambiase PD, Pantazis A, Dickie S, Mc Kenna WJ, Elliott PM, et al. A validation study of the 2003 American College of Cardiology/European Society of Cardiology and 2011 American College of Cardiology Foundation/American Heart Association risk stratification and treatment algorithms for sudden cardiac death in patients with hypertrophic cardiomyopathy. Heart. 2013;99:534–41.
9. Gersh BJ, Maron BJ, Bonow RO, Dearani JA, Fifer MA, Link MS, Naudu SS, et al. 2011 ACCF/AHA guideline for the diagnosis and treatment of hypertrophic cardiomyopathy: executive summary: a report of the American College of Cardiology Foundation/American Heart Association task force on practice guidelines. Circulation. 2011;124:2761–96.
10. Subasic K. Living with hypertrophic cardiomyopathy. J Nurs Scholarsh. 2013;45:371–9.
11. Gadamer H-G. Truth and method. New York: Continuum; 1993.
12. Krippendorff KH. Content analysis: an introduction to its methodology. 3rd ed. Thousand Oaks: Sage Publications; 2012. p. 355–70.
13. Ricoeur P. Hermeneutics and the human sciences. Cambridge: Cambridge University Press; 1995.
14. Gadamer H-G. Truth and method. New York: Continuum; 1993. p. 293.
15. Gadler F, Valzania C, Linde C. Current use of implantable electrical devices in Sweden: data from the Swedish pacemaker and implantable cardioverter-defibrillator registry. Europace. 2015;17:69–77.
16. Ricoeur P. Hermeneutics and the human sciences. Cambridge: Cambridge University Press; 1995. p. 93.
17. Maron BJ, Epstein SE. Hypertrophic cardiomyopathy: a discussion of nomenclature. Am J Cardiol. 1979;43:1242–4.
18. Flemme I, Hallberg U, Johansson I, Strömberg A. Uncertainty is a major concern for patients with implantable cardioverter defibrillators. Heart Lung. 2011;40:420–8.
19. Williams AM, Young J, Nikoletti S, McRae S. Getting on with life: accepting the permanency of an implantable cardioverter defibrillator. Int J Nurs Pract. 2007;13:166–72.
20. Kamphuis HC, Verhoeven NW, Leeuw R, Derksen R, Hauer RN, Winnubst JA. ICD: a qualitative study of patient experience the first year after implantation. J Clin Nurs. 2004;13:1008–16.
21. Fluur C, Bolse K, Strömberg A, Thylén I. Spouses' reflections on implantable cardioverter defibrillator treatment with focus on the future and the end-of-life: a qualitative content analysis. J Adv Nurs. 2014;70:1758–69.
22. McDonough A. The experiences and concerns of young adults (18-40 years) living with an implanted cardioverter defibrillator (ICD). Eur J Cardiovasc Nurs. 2009;8:274–80.
23. Flemme I, Johansson I, Strömberg A. Living with life-saving technology - coping strategies in implantable cardioverter defibrillators recipients. J Clin Nurs. 2012;21:311–21.
24. Rahman B, Macciocca I, Sahhar M, Kamberi S, Connell V, Duncan RE. Adolescents with implantable cardioverter defibrillators: a patient and parent perspective. Pacing Clin Electrophysiol. 2012;35:62–72.
25. Lang S, Becker R, Wilke S, Hartmann M, Herzog W, Löwe B. Anxiety disorders in patients with implantable cardioverter defibrillators: frequency, course, predictors, and patients' requests for treatment. Pacing Clin Electrophysiol. 2014;37:35–47.
26. Cox S, O'Donoghue AC, McKenna WJ, Steptoe A. Health related quality of life and psychological wellbeing in patients with hypertrophic cardiomyopathy. Heart. 1997;78:182–7.
27. Magnusson P, Gadler F, Liv P, Mörner S. Hypertrophic Cardiomyopathy and implantable defibrillators in Sweden: inappropriate shocks and complications requiring surgery. J Cardiovasc Electrophysiol. 2015;26:1088–94.
28. Hoogwegt MT, Kupper N, Jordaens L, Pedersen SS, Theuns DA. Comorbidity burden is associated with poor psychological well-being and physical health status in patients with an implantable cardioverter-defibrillator. Europace. 2013;15:1468–74.
29. Johansen JB, Pedersen SS, Spindler H, Andersen K, Nielsen JC, Mortensen PT. Symptomatic heart failure is the most important clinical correlate of impaired quality of life, anxiety, and depression in implantable cardioverter-defibrillator patients: a single-centre, cross-sectional study in 610 patients. Europace. 2008;10:545–51.

18

Maternal and fetal prognosis of subsequent pregnancy in black African women with peripartum cardiomyopathy

Nobila Valentin Yaméogo[1], André Koudnoaga Samadoulougou[1], Larissa Justine Kagambèga[2], Koudougou Jonas Kologo[1], Georges Rosario Christian Millogo[1], Anna Thiam[1], Charles Guenancia[3,4*] (iD) and Patrice Zansonré[1]

Abstract

Background: The aim of this study was to describe maternal and fetal outcomes after pregnancy complicated by peripartum cardiomyopathy (PPCM).

Methods: We included women that had subsequent pregnancy (SSP) after PPCM and assessed maternal prognosis and pregnancy outcomes, in-hospital up to one week after discharge. Clinical and echocardiographic data were collected comparing alive and deceased women. Factors associated with pregnancy outcomes were assessed.

Results: Twenty-nine patients were included, with a mean age of 26.7 ± 4.6 years and a mean gravidity number of 2.3 ± 0.5 of. At the last medical control before subsequent pregnancy, there was no congestive heart failure, the mean left ventricular diastolic diameter (LVDD) was 53 ± 4 mm and the left ventricular ejection fraction (LVEF) was $\geq 50\%$ in 13 cases (44.8%).
Maternal outcomes were marked by 14 deaths (48.3%). Among the factors tested in univariate analysis, LVEF at admission had an excellent receiver-operating characteristic (ROC) curve to predict maternal mortality (AUC = 0.95; 95% CI 0.87–1, $p < 0.001$), with a cut off value of < 40% (sensitivity = 93% and specificity = 87%). Concerning fetal outcomes, baseline LVEF had the best area under the curve (AUC) to predict abortion or prematurity among all variables (AUC = 0.75; 95% CI 0.58–092, $p = 0.003$), with a cut-off value of < 50% (sensitivity = 79%, specificity = 67%).

Conclusions: SSP outcomes are still severe in our practice. Maternal mortality remains high and is linked to ventricular systolic function at admission (due to pregnancy), while fetal outcomes are linked to baseline LVEF before pregnancy.

Keywords: Peripartum cardiomyopathy, Subsequent pregnancy, Prognosis, Burkina Faso

Background

Peripartum cardiomyopathy (PPCM) is a rare form of heart failure of unknown etiology that occurs between the last month of pregnancy up to 6 months postpartum [1–3]. Although previous studies suggested that approximately 50% of patients with PPCM recover a normal cardiac function, with 25% having persistently reduced heart function stable on medications and 25%

progressing to severe heart failure, more recent research [4, 5] suggests that severe outcomes have been reduced, with survival rates as high as 90 to 95% thanks to contemporary medical and device therapy. The Burkina Faso PPCM registry has been prospectively collecting data from women suffering from PPCM since 2010, and estimates the incidence of PPCM around 1/3800 births. According to this registry, even though contraception is prescribed to PPCM women, we noted that some of them get pregnant again.. However, there is a concern that such pregnancy may be associated with an increased risk of recurrence of cardiomyopathy [1–3, 6].

* Correspondence: charles.guenancia@gmail.com
[3]Department of Cardiology, University Hospital, 14 rue Paul Gaffarel, 21079 Dijon CEDEX, France
[4]PEC2, UFR Sciences de Santé, University Bourgogne Franche-Comté, Dijon, France
Full list of author information is available at the end of the article

The objective of this study was to determine the incidences and the associated factors of maternal and fetal outcomes of first subsequent pregnancy (SSP) among women with a history of peripartum cardiomyopathy.

Methods

Study population

The Burkina-Faso registry of PPCM prospectively includes women diagnosed with PPCM in the university hospital of Ouagadougou and Saint Camille hospital of Ouagadougou. The criteria for the diagnosis of the initial peripartum cardiomyopathy include the development of congestive heart failure within 1 month before delivery to 5 months after delivery in the absence of any another identifiable cause of heart failure; and evidence of depressed left ventricular function, defined as a left ventricular ejection fraction (LVEF) of less than 45% (Simpson method), as measured by echocardiography [7]. Women from the PPCM registry who were hospitalized during a subsequent pregnancy (despite medical advice not to become pregnant after PPCM) were prospectively included from 2012 to 2016. In-hospital to one week post discharge data were collected. We assessed clinical condition, left ventricular diameters and LVEF, tricuspid annular plan systolic excursion (TAPSE) and systolic pulmonary arterial pressure. Delta (%) values of these parameters were assessed as follows: (value at admission – baseline value) / baseline value. Maternal and fetal mortality, pregnancy issues, way of delivery and newborn weight were also appreciated. We compared alive and deceased women to identify the factors associated with maternal death. We also conducted a second analysis focused on fetal prognosis to identify factors associated with miscarriage or prematurity in these women.

Echocardiographic data collection

- Baseline echocardiographic data are the data from the last cardiac echography before subsequent pregnancy (SSP). This echography was performed on average 2.6 months before pregnancy.
- Admission echocardiographic data come from echography performed on admission during or after SSP.
- During hospitalization, echocardiography was performed weekly until one week post discharge.

Statistical methods

Continuous variables are presented as means ± standard deviations (SD) when normally distributed or medians and ranges otherwise. Categorical variables are presented as numbers (percentages). For continuous data, normality was checked by the Kolmogorov–test. The characteristics of the deceased and alive groups were compared using the exact Mann-Whitney test for continuous variables and the Chi-square or Fisher's exact test for categorical variables as appropriate. All of the tests were two-sided, and a p value less than 0.05 was considered significant.

To examine determinants of death events, we examined the area under the receiver-operating characteristic (ROC) curve (plot of sensitivity versus 1 – specificity for all possible cut-off values for classifying predictions) for LVEF, systolic Pulmonary arterial pressure (sPAP) and TAPSE with the best sensitivity and specificity according to the Youden index [8]. The cut-off value is given in the results section. Areas under the ROC curves were compared using the method of DeLong et al. [9] for paired data.

All analyses were performed using SPSS 20.0 0 (SPSS, Inc., Chicago, IL, USA) and MedCalc 13.3.1 (MedCalc Softaware, Mariakerke, Belgium).

Results

Patient characteristics

During the inclusion period, 29 women followed in the PPCM registry were hospitalized while pursuing a subsequent pregnancy. The mean age was 26.7 ± 4.6 years, with predominance of low socio-economic status. The diagnosis of cardiomyopathy had been made before delivery in 4 women (all of them in the seventh months of pregnancy), during the first month after delivery in 20 women, and between two and six months after delivery in 5 women (3 women in the second month after delivery, 1 in the third month, and 1 in the fifth month). No case of preeclampsia, chronic hypertension, severe anemia or history of hyperthyroidism was identified. Clinical and echocardiographic characteristics of patients during subsequent pregnancy in both groups alive vs deceased (*according to the occurrence of maternal death during subsequent pregnancy*) are summarized in Table 1.

Maternal outcomes

The mean LVEF in the total cohort of 29 women at the last follow-up before pregnancy was 49.9 ± 5.1% and decreased significantly to 37.6 ± 4.7% after the first subsequent pregnancy with a mean delta LVEF of – 19.3 ± 9%.

Fourteen (14) women died (48.3%). There was no statistically significant difference between alive and deceased women concerning socioeconomic status, left ventricular and right ventricular systolic function before subsequent pregnancy (baseline). At the time of hospitalization (during the subsequent pregnancy) (Table 1), congestive heart failure ($p < 0.001$), with lower left and right ventricular function was more frequently observed in women who died after pregnancy than in the group of surviving patients.

Table 1 Clinical and echocardiographic characteristics according to the occurrence of death during subsequent pregnancy after PPCM

n (%), median (interquartile range), mean ± SD	Total population	Alive patients ($n = 15$)	Deceased patients ($n = 14$)	p
Baseline data				
Age	26.7 ± 4.6	26 ± 5	28 ± 6	0.44
Low socio-economic status	22 (75.8)	12 (80)	9 (64)	0.43
Gravidity	2.3 ± 0.5	2.2 ± 0.6	2.4 ± 0.5	0.26
Baseline LVEF after the first PPCM (%)	49.9 ± 5.2	50 ± 6	50 ± 7	0.99
Baseline LVEF after the PPCM < 50%	16 (55.2)	7 (47)	9 (64)	0.46
Baseline LVEF after the first PPCM < 45%	5 (17.2)	2 (13)	4 (29)	0.39
Baseline LVEDD after the PPCM (mm)	53.3 ± 3.6	54 ± 4	53 ± 5	0.88
Baseline sPAP after the PPCM (mmHg)	29.2 ± 4.2	28 ± 5	30 ± 5	0.26
Baseline TAPSE after the PPCM (mm)	18.2 ± 2.4	19 ± 3	17 ± 3	0.10
Follow-up data (at the time of hospitalization)				
Delay between last follow-up and hospitalization (month)	17 ± 6	15 ± 6	18 ± 6	0.27
Congestive heart failure	19 (65.5)	6 (40)	14 (100)	< 0.001
LVEF (%)	37.6 ± 4.7	44 ± 6	33 ± 6	< 0.001
LVEF < 40%	14 (48.3)	2 (13)	13 (93)	0.001
Delta LVEF (%)	−19.3 ± 9	- 11 ± 10	−32 ± 15	< 0.001
LVEDD (mm)	57.5 ± 3.9	59 ± 4	56 ± 5	0.05
Delta LVEDD (%)	8 ± 6	11 ± 11	5 ± 7	0.09
sPAP (mmHg)	37.9 ± 5.4	34 ± 5	42 ± 5	< 0.001
Delta sPAP (%)	19 ± 8	17 ± 10	27 ± 15	0.07
TAPSE (mm)	16.8 ± 3.2	19 ± 3	14 ± 4	< 0.001
TAPSE < 17 mm	11 (37.9)	1 (7)	10 (71)	< 0.001
TAPSE < 18 mm	13 (44.8)	2 (13)	11 (79)	< 0.001
Delta TAPSE (%)	- 7.5 ± 5	3 ± 17	−15 ± 27	0.03
Pregnancy data				
Abortion	6 (20.6)	2 (13)	4 (29)	0.39
Prematurity	8 (27.6)	4 (27)	4 (29)	1
Full-term pregnancy	51.7	9 (60)	6 (43)	0.47
Newborn weight (g)	2385 ± 286	2350 ± 500	2380 ± 300	0.90

PPCM peripartum cardiomyopathy, *LVEF* left ventricular ejection fraction, *LVEDD* left ventricular end diastolic diameter, *sPAP* systolic pulmonary arterial pressure, *TAPSE* tricuspid annular plan systolic excursion

To find out if echocardiographic data (at the last follow-up and at admission) could predict mortality after pregnancy, we built ROC curves using variables with a strong statistical association to death in univariate analysis: LVEF (at last follow-up (=baseline), at admission and delta LVEF), sPAP (at last follow-up, at admission and delta sPAP), and TAPSE (at last follow-up, at admission and delta TAPSE). The AUC were compared to determine the best variable, and the best cut-off value. Among these variables, LVEF at admission (AUC = 0.95; 95% CI 0.87–1, $p < 0.001$), TAPSE at admission (AUC = 0.879; 95% CI 0.74–1, $p = 0.001$) and sPAP at admission (AUC = 0.85; 95% CI 0.71–0.99, p = 0.001) were strongly and significantly associated to death (Figs. 1, 2, 3). Comparing the AUC of these 3 variables at the time of admission (data not shown), there was no statistically significant difference. The best cut-offs for these variables are detailed within the figures.

Pregnancies outcomes

Miscarriage occurred in six cases. Among the 23 women with a living child after subsequent pregnancy, 13 had a normal vaginal delivery, and 10 were delivered by cesarean. The mean newborn weight was 2385 ± 286 g. Miscarriage and prematurity were associated with baseline LVEF and baseline TAPSE as shown in Table 1. Baseline LVEF had the best AUC to predict SSP outcomes among all variables (AUC = 0.75; 95% CI

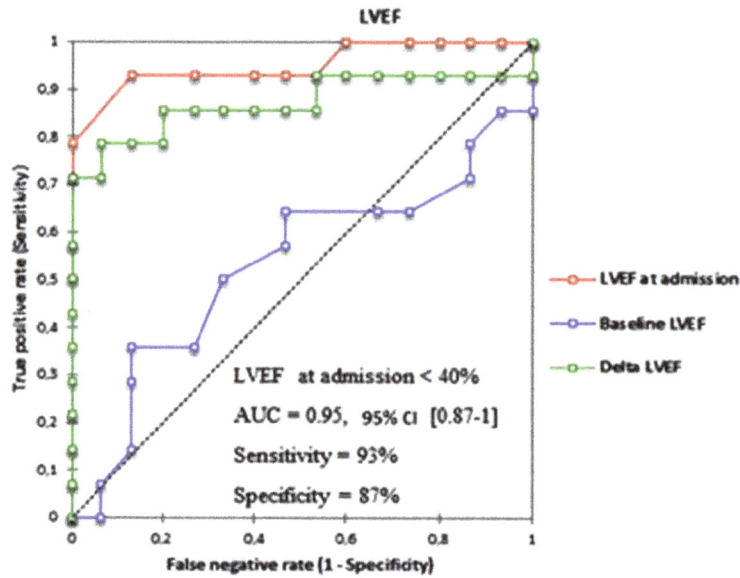

Fig. 1 ROC curves with optimal cut-off values of LVEF (admission, baseline and delta) to predict mortality

0.58–092, $p = 0.003$), with a cut-off value of < 50% (sensitivity = 79%, specificity = 67%).Four newborn (that 3 preterm) died, all from neonatal infection.

Discussion

Maternal outcomes

Our study demonstrated that when women with SSP did not benefit from cardiac follow-up, the issue can be fatal.

Mortality was remarkably high in our study, probably because the women were lost from clinical follow-up during the pregnancy period.

In several studies [10–12], SSP was responsible for maternal death in about 0.5 to 1%. This contrasts with

our results. This can be explained by the fact that our patients were lost from follow-up and the lack of therapeutic means. Indeed follow-up enables an effective management of heart failure, pregnancy and delivery. During this follow-up, normalization of left ventricular function does not guarantee an uncomplicated SSP as demonstrated by some authors in America and Europe. In their study, approximately 20% of such patients are also at risk of moderate to severe deterioration of left ventricular function, which persists after delivery in 20 to 50% of cases [10–12].

We demonstrated that left ventricular ejection fraction decreased during SSP.

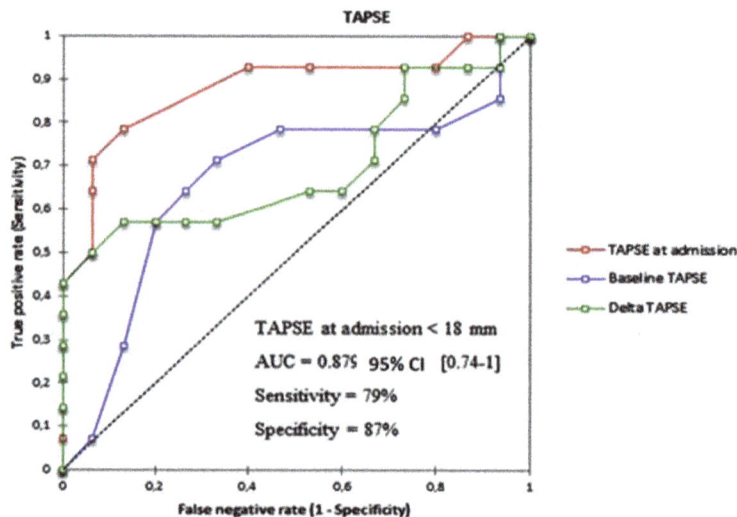

Fig. 2 ROC curves of TAPSE (admission, baseline and delta) to predict mortality

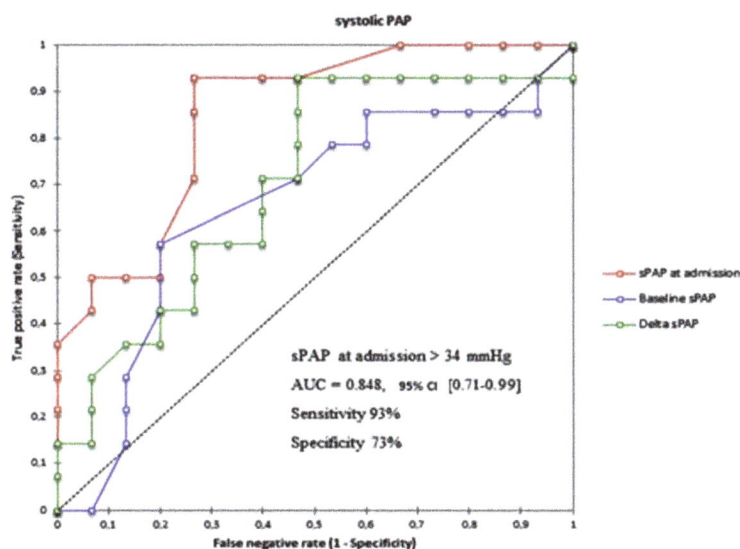

Fig. 3 ROC curves of sPAP (admission, baseline and delta) to predict mortality

Factors associated with maternal death

The best determinant of maternal death in our study was the left ventricular ejection fraction at admission and the percentage of loss of left ventricular ejection fraction. The best cut-off value of left ventricular ejection fraction to predict mortality during first SSP in our study was a LVEF at admission < 40% [Sensitivity = 93%, Specificity = 87%].

All previous studies were based on left ventricular function, but right ventricular function was not studied. We demonstrate that right ventricle systolic function also has an important role in the prediction of maternal mortality during SSP. We appreciated right ventricular systolic function by TAPSE, but we also measured systolic pulmonary arterial pressure to determine if sPAP could predict mortality during SSP.

We found that all these parameters were associated to maternal death. These results underline that right ventricular function must be taken into account to estimate maternal outcomes of SSP. In a study by Elkayam et al. [10], medical pregnancy interruption was used in some cases to prevent maternal outcomes. In their study, maternal mortality was very low compared to our result, but medical pregnancy interruption was more frequent.

All our results demonstrate that PPCM women with SSP are very fragile. They must benefit from a rigorous follow-up including echocardiographic assessment.

Pregnancy outcomes and infant morbi-mortality

Pregnancy outcomes were also poor. We noted that miscarriage and prematurity were associated with baseline left ventricular ejection fraction and baseline TAPSE.

This can be explained by the fact that low baseline left ventricular ejection fraction compromises fetal development. The same reason can explain why our new borns had all small birth weight.

Elkayam et al. [10] demonstrated that abortion rate is very high (20.4%), and prematurity is two times more frequent in women with persistent baseline left ventricular dysfunction. In our study, not only baseline left ventricular ejection, but also baseline TAPSE was responsible for pregnancy outcomes.

Infant mortality

Death occurred predominately in premature new borns (3/4). There was no maternal nor fetal factor linked to these deaths. However, as we know, prematurity is a factor of mortality in new born babies.

Limitations

Our study included only a small number of PPCM women but it is to the best of our knowledge the biggest African study on SSP outcomes.

A recruitment bias has to be acknowledged: only hospitalized women were included, due to loss of follow-Up. Indeed, from the 166 women included in the registry, 38 were lost to follow-up. From these lost to follow-up women, 29 were hospitalized during a SSP and 9 were missing. None of the 128 patients followed in the registry had so far a SSP. Among the 9 patients missing, uncomplicated pregnancies could have occurred. Thus, the mortality rate of SSP described in our study could be slightly overestimated.

Conclusions

Some women with a history of PPCM hope to get pregnant again. They are therefore at risk because pregnancy outcomes are unknown.

This study demonstrated that subsequent pregnancy after peripartum cardiomyopathy has poor maternal and fetal prognosis.

Maternal mortality is very high and associated with LVEF at admission, TAPSE at admission and sPAP at admission. On the other hand, pregnancy outcomes were linked to baseline LVEF and baseline TAPSE.

In these conditions, we advise physicians, to systematically explain to PPCM patients the severity of their pathology, the possibility of evolution and to give them a drafted document that contains recommendations in this situation (subsequent pregnancy risk, medical conditions to get pregnant, necessity to continue follow-up).

Abbreviations

AUC: Area under the curve; LVDD: Left ventricular diastolic diameter; LVEF: Left Ventricular Ejection Fraction; PPCM: Peripartum cardiomyopathy; ROC: Receiver-Operating Characteristic; SD: Standard deviations; sPAP: Systolic pulmonary arterial pressure; SSP: Subsequent pregnancy; TAPSE: Tricuspid annular plan systolic excursion

Acknowledgements

We wish to thank Joëlle Hamblin for English assistance.

Authors' contributions

YNV initiated the study in the cardiology department. The protocol was read and corrected by ZP, KLJ, HJ and SAK. Data collection was done by YNV, ZP, KLJ, SAK, KKJ, MGRC and TA. Data analysis was done by GC. The manuscript was edited by YNV, KLJ and GC. Then all the authors read and corrected the manuscript and gave their approval for publication.

Competing interests

The authors declares that they have no competing interest.

Author details

[1]Department of Cardiology, Yalgado Ouedraogo University Hospital, Ouagadougou, Burkina Faso. [2]Medical Sciences Department, University of Ouagadougou, Ouagadougou, Burkina Faso. [3]Department of Cardiology, University Hospital, 14 rue Paul Gaffarel, 21079 Dijon CEDEX, France. [4]PEC2, UFR Sciences de Santé, University Bourgogne Franche-Comté, Dijon, France.

References

1. Sliwa K, Hilfiker-Kleiner D, Petrie MC, Mebazaa A, Pieske B, Buchmann E, Regitz-Zagrosek V, Schaufelberger M, Tavazzi L, van Veldhuisen DJ, Watkins H, Shah AJ, Seferovic PM, Elkayam U, Pankuweit S, Papp Z, Mouquet F, McMurray JJ. Current state of knowledge on aetiology, diagnosis, management, and therapy of peripartum cardiomyopathy: a position statement from the Heart Failure Association of the European Society of Cardiology Working Group on peripartum cardiomyopathy. Eur J Heart Fail. 2010 Aug;12(8):767–78.
2. Heider AL, Kuller JA, Strauss RA, Wells SR. Peripartum cardiomyopathy: review of the literature. Obstet Gynecol Surv. 1999;54:526–31.
3. Pearson GD, Veille JC, Rahimtoola S, Hsia J, Oakley CM, Hosenpud JD, Ansari A, Baughman KL. Peripartum cardiomyopathy: National Heart, Lung, and Blood Institute and Office of Rare Diseases (National Institutes of Health) workshop recommendations and review. JAMA. 2000;283:1183–8.
4. Felker GM, Thompson RE, Hare JM, Hruban RH, Clemetson DE, Howard DL, Baughman KL, Kasper EK. Underlying causes and long-term survival in patients with initially unexplained cardiomyopathy. N Engl J Med. 2000;342:1077–84.
5. Cooper LT, Mather PJ, Alexis JD, Pauly DF, Torre-Amione G, Wittstein IS, Dec GW, Zucker M, Narula J, Kip K, McNamara DM; IMAC2 Investigators. Myocardial recovery in peripartum cardiomyopathy: prospective comparison with recent onset cardiomyopathy in men and nonperipartum women. J Card Fail 2012; 18:28–33.
6. Witlin AG, Mabie WC, Sibai BM. Peripartum cardiomyopathy: an ominous diagnosis. Am J Obstet Gynecol. 1997;176:182–8.
7. Howlett JG1, McKelvie RS, Costigan J, Ducharme A, Estrella-Holder E, Ezekowitz JA, Giannetti N, Haddad H, Heckman GA, Herd AM, Isaac D, Kouz S, Leblanc K, Liu P, Mann E, Moe GW, O'Meara E, Rajda M, Siu S, Stolee P, Swiggum E, Zieroth S; Canadian cardiovascular society.. The 2010 Canadian cardiovascular society guidelines for the diagnosis and management of heart failure update: heart failure in ethnic minority populations, heart failure and pregnancy, disease management, and quality improvement/assurance programs. Can J Cardiol 2010; 26: 185–202.
8. Youden WJ. Index for rating diagnostic tests. Cancer. 1950;3(1):32–5.
9. DeLong ER, DeLong DM, Clarke-Pearson DL. Comparing the areas under two or more correlated receiver operating characteristic curves: a nonparametric approach. Biometrics. 1988;44(3):837–45.
10. U E, Tummala PP, Rao K, Akhter MW, Karaalp IS, Wani OR, Hameed A, Gviazda I, Shotan A. Maternal and fetal outcomes of subsequent pregnancies in women with peripartum cardiomyopathy. N Engl J Med. 2001;344:1567–71.
11. Sliwa K, Forster O, Zhanje F, Candy G, Kachope J, Essop R. Outcome of subsequent pregnancy in patients with documented peripartum cardiomyopathy. Am J Cardiol. 2004;93(11):1441–3.
12. Elkayam U. Pregnant again after peripartum cardiomyopathy: to be or not to be? Eur Heart J. 2002;23:753–6.

19

Left ventricular non-compaction cardiomyopathy with coronary artery anomaly complicated by ventricular tachycardia

Gustav Mattsson[1]* [iD], Abdullah Baroudi[2], Hoshmand Tawfiq[1] and Peter Magnusson[1,3]

Abstract

Background: Non-compaction cardiomyopathy (NCCM) is characterized by prominent trabeculations, deep intertrabecular recesses, and a thick non-compacted endocardial myocardium. Prevalence in the general population remains unclear, but echocardiography series report 0.05%. During fetal development muscle fibers and trabeculae should compact into a solid myocardium and when this fails, NCCM occurs. The condition is genetic, even though acquired forms have been described. Worsening myocardial dysfunction may lead to heart failure and/or arrhythmias.

Case presentation: A 52-year-old man presented with heart failure. The diagnosis of NCCM was confirmed after echocardiography and cardiac magnetic resonance tomography. Interestingly, the angiogram revealed a coronary anomaly, in which the circumflex artery rose aberrantly from the right coronary artery. Due to left ventricular ejection fraction being less than 35% despite optimal pharmacological therapy, an implantable cardioverter defibrillator (ICD) was implanted and four years later a ventricular tachycardia was terminated by antitachycardia pacing.

Conclusion: We describe a case of NCCM with a concomitant coronary anomaly, in which systolic myocardial dysfunction developed. The ICD subsequently terminated a life-threatening ventricular arrhythmia, which supports risk stratification based on low ejection fraction and possibly coronary anomaly.

Keywords: Cardiac imaging, Cardiac magnetic resonance, Cardiomyopathy, Coronary artery anomaly, Echocardiography, Heart failure, implantable cardioverter defibrillator, Non-compaction cardiomyopathy, Sudden cardiac death, Ventricular tachycardia

Background

Non-compaction cardiomyopathy (NCCM) was first described in 1984 as a clinical entity and is a heterogeneous cardiomyopathy that can occur at any age [1, 2]. Congenital NCCM is caused by a defect in compaction of muscle fibers during fetal development, resulting in a spongiform myocardium. It appears that NCCM can also be acquired, for example due to athlete's heart [3]. In a large hospital cohort the prevalence was 0.05%, and there seems to be an increased awareness among clinicians about NCCM [4]. Echocardiographic diagnosis is based on four criteria (Jenni criteria): absence of other cardiac abnormalities, end-systolic ratio between non-compacted endocardial myocardium and compacted epicardial myocardium of >2, localization of hyper-trabeculation to the apex/mid-inferior/mid-lateral areas, and color doppler showing blood flow from the ventricle into deep intertrabecular recesses without communication with coronary vessels [5]. Some patients with NCCM are asymptomatic, others develop heart failure with reduced systolic ejection fracture (EF). NCCM may increase the risk of ventricular tachycardia, and the risk of thromboembolism, likely due to reduced

* Correspondence: gustav.mattsson@regiongavleborg.se
[1]Centre for Research and Development, Uppsala University/Region Gävleborg, SE-801 87 Gävle, Sweden
Full list of author information is available at the end of the article

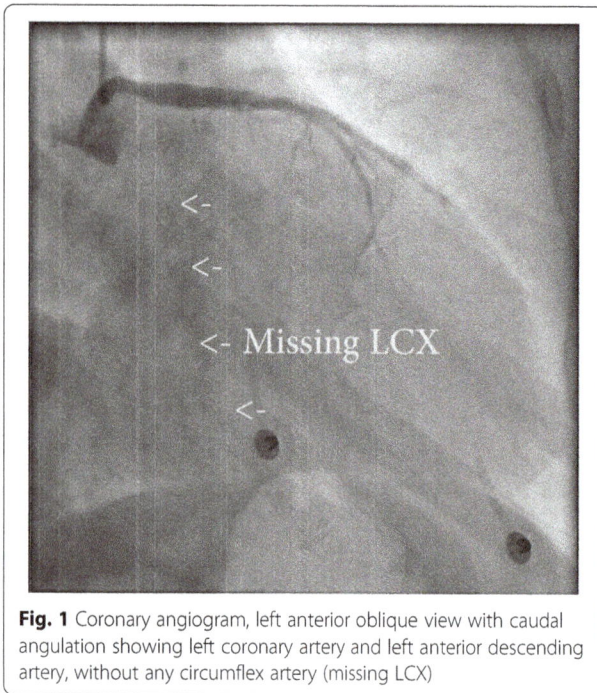

Fig. 1 Coronary angiogram, left anterior oblique view with caudal angulation showing left coronary artery and left anterior descending artery, without any circumflex artery (missing LCX)

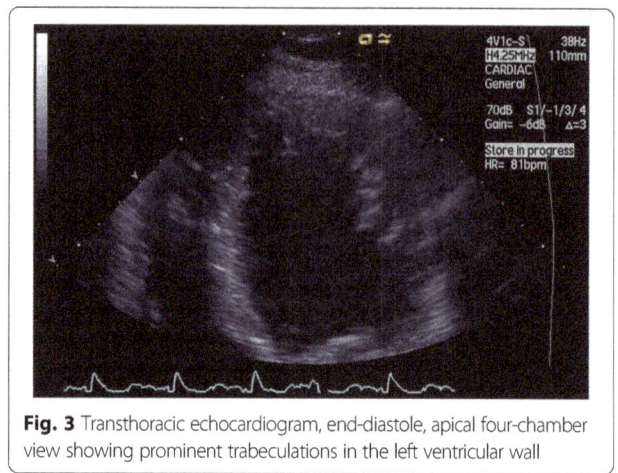

Fig. 3 Transthoracic echocardiogram, end-diastole, apical four-chamber view showing prominent trabeculations in the left ventricular wall

blood flow in the intertrabecular recesses [6]. NCCM exhibits familial clustering, with point prevalence of phenotype being 30% in first-degree relatives [7]. Genes encoding sarcomeric and cytoskeletal proteins have been implicated in NCCM, as well as genes previously linked to such disorders as hypertrophic cardiomyopathy, mitochondrial diseases, Barth syndrome, and myotonic dystrophy [8].

Case presentation

A 52-year-old man presented with dyspnea, chest discomfort, and palpitations upon exertion. His parents had confirmed ischemic heart disease. ECG at rest showed sinus rhythm, premature ventricular complexes and poor R-wave progression in precordial leads V_1 to V_4. The first echocardiography revealed general hypokinesia, predominantly in the anterior wall, thin walls without dilatation, EF around 35%, and high and pointy E-waves, indicative of a restrictive pattern. He reached 200 W on cycle ergometer exercise testing, but with frequent premature ventricular complexes. Angiography (Figs. 1 and 2.) showed no signs of coronary artery disease. Surprisingly, a coronary anomaly was revealed, in that the circumflex coronary artery (LCX) originated from the right coronary artery (RCA). At this point, cardiac magnetic resonance (CMR) imaging did not provide any further diagnostic clues. The situation was complicated by atrial fibrillation that was electrically converted but recurred at two-year follow-up. Another echocardiogram (Figs. 3, 4 and 5) was performed that for the first time raised suspicion of NCCM with

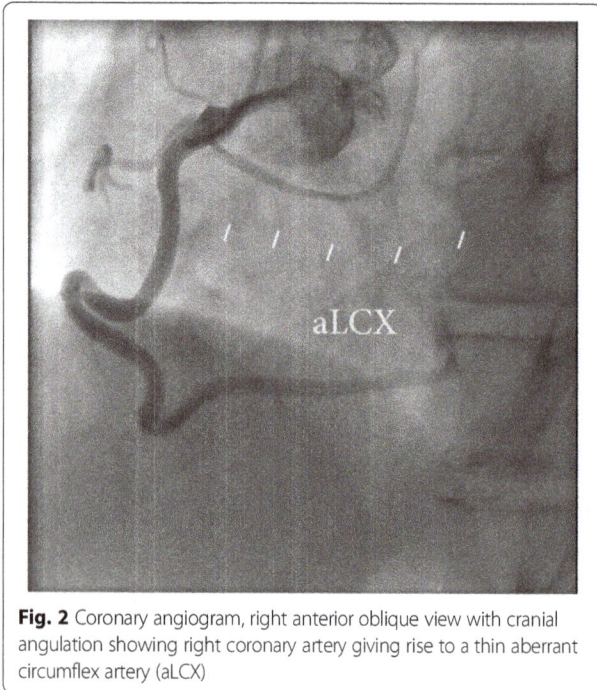

Fig. 2 Coronary angiogram, right anterior oblique view with cranial angulation showing right coronary artery giving rise to a thin aberrant circumflex artery (aLCX)

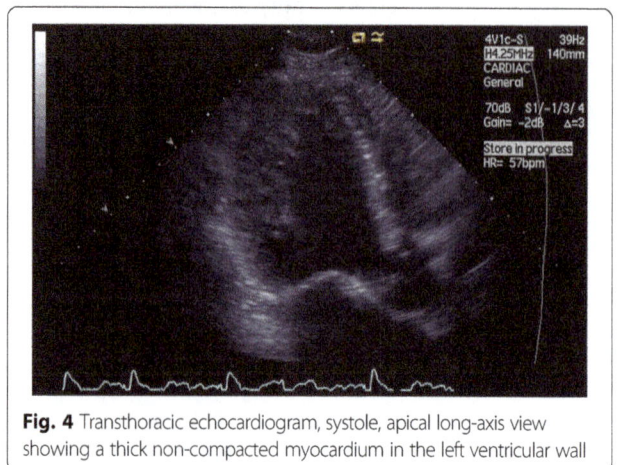

Fig. 4 Transthoracic echocardiogram, systole, apical long-axis view showing a thick non-compacted myocardium in the left ventricular wall

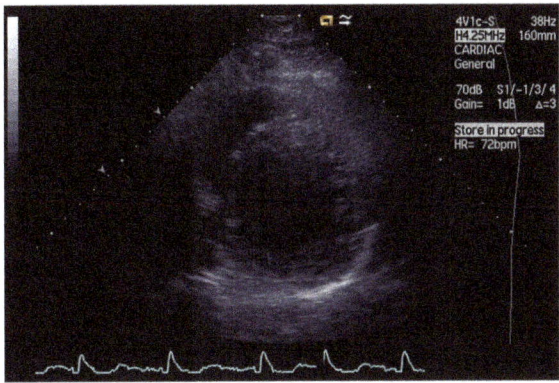

Fig. 5 Transthoracic echocardiogram, end-diastole, parasternal short axis view showing hypertrabeculation of the inferolateral left ventricular wall

EF around 30%. There were hypokinesia and deep intramyocardial recesses in the left ventricular wall. The ratio of non-compacted to compacted myocardium was 2.4 measured in the apical long-axis view, mid-inferior, at end-systole.

The patient was referred to a tertiary center for evaluation including right ventricular catheterization and endomyocardial biopsy that did not suggest any alternative diagnoses. Repeated echocardiograms confirmed the diagnosis of NCCM. An implantable cardioverter defibrillator (ICD) with a single lead (QRS < 120 ms)

was offered to the patient for primary prevention of sudden cardiac death (SCD). Four years later, antitachycardia pacing terminated a life-threatening monomorphic ventricular tachycardia of 200 beats per minute (Fig. 6.). The patient has been followed for another three years and is on beta-blocker, angiotensin receptor blocker, and eplerenone therapy. In that time, he has had no further arrhythmias requiring ICD therapy and is New York Heart Association (NYHA) functional class II. The CARE guidelines were followed in the writing of this report.

Discussion and conclusions

Clinical presentations of NCCM are heterogeneous and 35% have no hypertrophy or dilation of the ventricle. NCCM in the absence of arrhythmia seem to have similar survival rates as the general population [6]. Patients with NCCM with arrhythmia, are believed to have worse prognosis than patients with similar arrhythmias alone. Other forms of NCCM include dilated, hypertrophic, and restrictive pattern. NCCM typically affects the left ventricle, but biventricular and isolated right ventricular manifestations do occur [6]. There is no specific therapy for NCCM, but if heart failure is present this should be treated according to guidelines [9]. In our patient, metoprolol, enalapril, and eplerenone were titrated. The classic triad of NCCM consists of thromboembolism together with arrhythmia and heart failure. Anticoagulation is advocated

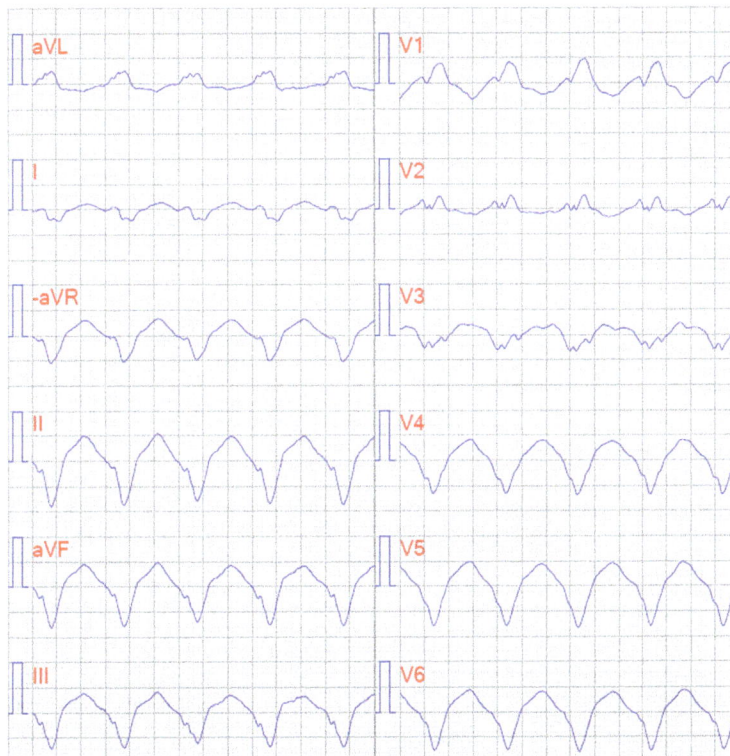

Fig. 6 Electrocardiogram of monomorphic ventricular tachycardia, 200 beats per minute (paper speed 50 mm/s)

if NCCM is associated with either atrial fibrillation, severe heart failure, confirmed thrombus, or previous thromboembolism [10]. In our patient, anticoagulation with warfarin was initiated due to atrial fibrillation and heart failure.

The Jenni echocardiography criteria are widely used but they can be difficult to validate and there is a lack of consensus about them [5]. CMR can provide additional value with borderline cases or in patients in whom differential diagnoses like hypertrophic cardiomyopathy are difficult to rule out. An end-diastolic ratio between non-compacted and compacted layers of >2.3 is considered diagnostic [11]. Late gadolinium enhancement in trabeculae is indicative of fibrosis and correlates with clinical severity [12].

This case report describes concomitant NCCM and aberrant LCX arising from the RCA, which occurs in 0.37% of angiograms [13]. Other coronary anomalies have previously been described together with NCCM, a single coronary artery of anomalous origin [14], as well as an anomaly including four arteries arising from the RCA with an LCX arising directly from the aorta [15]. How common coronary anomalies are in patients with NCCM is unknown, because the rarity of both conditions makes this difficult to study. Given the common pathogenesis of abnormalities in embryogenesis, an overrepresentation is plausible. The presence of coronary anomalies provides a challenge in risk stratification for SCD. The anomaly present in this case, aberrant LCX from the RCA, is generally not linked to an increased risk of SCD. In cases where the aberrant LCX travels between the aorta and the pulmonary artery, increased SCD has been reported, likely caused by compression or angulation of the artery [13].

The efficacy of ICD treatment in preventing death from arrhythmia is well established [16]. The European Society of Cardiology guidelines regarding SCD state that NCCM without further risk factors is not an indication for ICD. It is suggested to use the same criteria for risk stratification in NCCM as in non-ischemic, dilated cardiomyopathy [17]. ICDs should be offered to survivors of ventricular arrhythmias regardless of the underlying cardiac etiology. ICD should be offered as primary prophylaxis to NCCM patients with EF ≤35% and NYHA functional class II-III despite at least three months of optimal pharmacological therapy, and an otherwise reasonable life expectancy. Despite the limitations of EF estimation in individual patients, it still provides the best discriminator for risk stratification in most cardiomyopathy types [17, 18]. We believe that the current approach of risk stratification is advisable until more specific data of NCCM are available. The ICD in our patient terminated a life-threatening arrhythmia.

This should encourage careful risk stratification in NCCM based on generalized knowledge from other cardiomyopathies.

Abbreviations
CMR: Cardiac magnetic resonance; EF: Ejection fraction; ICD: Implantable cardioverter defibrillator; LCX: Circumflex coronary artery; NCCM: Non-compaction cardiomyopathy; NYHA: New York Heart Association; RCA: Right coronary artery; SCD: Sudden cardiac death

Acknowledgements
Images of the coronary angiogram were provided by Lasse Hellsten, and echocardiography exams by Ann-Charlotte Larsson. Jo Ann LeQuang of LeQ Medical reviewed the manuscript for American English use.

Funding
There is no funding pertaining to the manuscript.

Authors' contributions
GM: design, data collection, major writing AB: design, writing HT: patient management, critical revision PM: idea, design, writing, patient and project management. All authors read and approved the final manuscript.

Competing interests
The authors declare that they have no competing interests.

Author details
¹Centre for Research and Development, Uppsala University/Region Gävleborg, SE-801 87 Gävle, Sweden. ²Department of Medicine, Kiruna sjukhus, Region Norrbotten, SE-981 28 Kiruna, Sweden. ³Cardiology Research Unit, Department of Medicine, Karolinska Institutet, SE-171 76 Stockholm, Sweden.

References
1. Engberding R, Bender F. Identification of a rare congenital anomaly of the myocardium by two-dimensional echocardiography: persistence of isolated myocardial sinusoids. Am J Cardiol. 1984;53:1733–4.
2. Elliott P, Andersson B, Arbustini E, Bilinska Z, Cecchi F, Charron P, et al. Classification of the cardiomyopathies: a position statement from the European Society of Cardiology working group on myocardial and pericardial diseases. Eur Heart J. 2008;29:270–6.
3. Gati S, Chandra N, Bennett RL, Reed M, Kervio G, Panoulas VF, et al. Increased left ventricular trabeculation in highly trained athletes: do we need more stringent criteria for the diagnosis of left ventricular non-compaction in athletes? Heart. 2013;99:401–8.
4. Ritter M, Oechslin E, Sütsch G, Attenhofer C, Schneider J, Jenni R. Isolated noncompaction of the myocardium in adults. Mayo Clin Proc. 1997;72:26–31.
5. Jenni R, Oechslin E, Schneider J, Attenhofer Jost C, Kaufmann PA. Echocardiographic and pathoanatomical characteristics of isolated left ventricular non-compaction: a step towards classification as a distinct cardiomyopathy. Heart. 2001;86:666–71.
6. Towbin JA, Lorts A, Jefferies JL. Left ventricular non-compaction cardiomyopathy. Lancet. 2015;386:813–25.
7. Bhatia NL, Tajik AJ, Wilansky S, Steidley DE, Mookadam F. Isolated noncompaction of the left ventricular myocardium in adults: a systematic overview. J Card Fail. 2011;17:771–8.
8. Finsterer J. Cardiogenetics, neurogenetics, and pathogenetics of left ventricular hypertrabeculation/noncompaction. Pediatr Cardiol. 2009;30:659–81.
9. Ponikowski P, Voors AA, Anker SD, Bueno H, Cleland JG, Coats AJ, et al. 2016 ESC guidelines for the diagnosis and treatment of acute and chronic heart failure: the task force for the diagnosis and treatment of acute and chronic heart failure of the European Society of Cardiology (ESC) developed with

the special contribution of the heart failure association (HFA) of the ESC. Eur Heart J. 2016;37:2129–200.

10. Finsterer J, Stöllberger C, Towbin JA. Left ventricular noncompaction cardiomyopathy: cardiac, neuromuscular, and genetic factors. Nature reviews. Cardiology. 2017;14:224–37.

11. Petersen SE, Selvanayagam JB, Wiesmann F, Robson MD, Francis JM, Anderson RH, et al. Left ventricular non-compaction: insights from cardiovascular magnetic resonance imaging. J Am Coll Cardiol. 2005;5(46):101–5.

12. Dodd JD, Holmvang G, Hoffmann U, Ferencik M, Abbara S, Brady TJ, et al. Quantification of left ventricular noncompaction and trabecular delayed hyperenhancement with cardiac MRI: correlation with clinical severity. Am J Roentgenol. 2007;189:974–80.

13. Villa AD, Sammut E, Nair A, Rajani R, Bonamini R, Chiribiri A. Coronary artery anomalies overview: the normal and the abnormal. World J Radiol. 2016;8:537–55.

14. Park JS, Shin DG, Kim YJ, Hong GR, Kim W, Lee SH, et al. Left ventricular noncompaction with a single coronary artery of anomalous origin. Int J Cardiol. 2007;119:35–7.

15. Iacovelli F, Pepe P, Contegiacomo G, Alberotanza V, Masi F, Bortone AS, et al. A striking coronary artery pattern in a grown-up congenital heart disease patient. Case Rep Cardiol. 2016;2016:5482578.

16. Goldenberg I, Gillespie J, Moss AJ, Hall WJ, Klein H, McNitt S, et al. Long-term benefit of primary prevention with an implantable cardioverter-defibrillator: an extended 8-year follow-up study of the multicenter automatic defibrillator implantation trial II. Circulation. 2010;122:1265–71.

17. Priori SG, Blomström-Lundqvist C, Mazzanti A, Blom N, Borggrefe M, Camm J, et al. 2015 ESC guidelines for the Management of Patients with ventricular arrhythmias and the prevention of sudden cardiac death: the task force for the management of patients with ventricular arrhythmias and the prevention of sudden cardiac death of the European Society of Cardiology (ESC). Endorsed by: Association for European Paediatric and Congenital Cardiology (AEPC). Eur Heart J. 2015;36:2793–867.

18. Bardy GH, Lee KL, Mark DB, Poole JE, Packer DL, Boineau R, et al. Amiodarone or an implantable cardioverter-defibrillator for congestive heart failure. N Engl J Med. 2005;352:225–37.

20

Left ventricular short-axis systolic function changes in patients with hypertrophic cardiomyopathy detected by two-dimensional speckle tracking imaging

Jun Huang*⬥, Zi-Ning Yan, Yi-Fei Rui, Li Fan, Chang Liu and Jie Li

Abstract

Background: Hypertrophic cardiomyopathy (HCM) is a genetic disease was characterised by left ventricular hypertrophy (LVH), myocardial fibrosis, fiber disarray. The short-axis systolic function is important in left ventricle function.

Methods: Forty one healthy subjects and 37 HCM patients were enrolled for this research. Parasternal short-axis at the basal, middle, and apical levels were acquired by Echocardiography. The peak systolic circumferential strain of the endocardial, the middle and the epicardial layers, the peak systolic radial strain, and the peak systolic rotational degrees at different short-axis levels were measured by 2-dimensional speckle tracking imaging (2D–STI).

Results: The peak systolic circumferential strain of the septum and anterior walls in HCM patients was significantly lower than normal subjects. All of the peak systolic radial strain in HCM patients was significantly lower than normal subjects. The rotational degrees at the base and middle short-axis levels in HCM patients were larger than normal subjects. The interventricular septal thickness in end-diastolic period correlated to the peak systolic circumferential strain of the septum wall.

Conclusions: The short-axis systolic function was impaired in HCM patients. The peak circumferential systolic strain of the different layers, peak systolic radial strain and rotation degrees of the different short-axis levels detected by 2D–STI are very feasible for assessing the short-axis function in HCM patients.

Keywords: Two-dimensional speckle tracking imaging, Hypertrophic cardiomyopathy, Circumferential, Radial, Strain

Background

Hypertrophic cardiomyopathy (HCM) is a common cardiac disease [1, 2]. As the universal use of the echocardiography, computer tomography, and magnetic resonance imaging, the discovery of HCM have increased annually [3–6]. The disease is characterized by thickening the ventricular myocardium walls [7]. It is a genetic disorder of the myocardium caused by mutations in cardiac sarcomeric proteins. The pathology of HCM is the gross of the cardiac myocardial hypertrophy and fiber disarray.

HCM patients often asymptomatic throughout life, but someone may have severe symptoms like sudden cardiac death at a young age [8, 9].

Two-dimensional speckle tracking imaging (2D–STI) can assess myocardial function accurately [10]. Currently, researches mainly focussed on myocardial function by detected the global myocardial strain, strain rate and torsion [11–16]. As we know, a normal myocardium is contained three layers: endocardial, middle myocardial and epicardial layers [17, 18]. Endocardial and epicardial layers are longitudinal oriented, and the middle myocardial is circumferential oriented. When the longitudinal and circumferential

* Correspondence: 305669112@qq.com
Department of Echocardiography, the Affiliated Changzhou No.2 People's Hospital of Nanjing Medical University, Changzhou, China

myocardium contract and relax, the cardiac myocardium deformation occurs in three directions: longitudinally, circumferentially, and radially. Our previous study showed that in HCM patients, the longitudinal function was damaged, even with normal LV ejection fraction [19], however, short-axis cardiac function as circumferentially and radially is also essential like longitudinally function. So, in this study, we mainly analysed the short-axis function in HCM patients.

Of data, detect the peak circumferential systolic strain of endocardial, middle myocardial, and epicardial layers in HCM patients is rare. The innovations of this study were ① Measure the peak systolic circumferential strain of endocardial, middle myocardial, and epicardial layers in patients with HCM. ② Measure the peak systolic radial strain in HCM patients. ③ Measure the peak systolic rotation degrees at the different short-axis levels in HCM patients, then to assess the changes in the left ventricular systolic function at the short-axis levels in HCM patients.

Methods

Ethical approvals
Recruitment to the study followed a full explanation of our methods including the fact that there was no risk of harm. Written informed consent was accepted. The Human Subjects Committee of Changzhou No. 2 People's Hospital approved this study.

Study sample
Thirty seven HCM patients and 41 age- and gender-matched healthy subjects were enrolled for the research. The diagnosis of HCM was based on the transthoracic echocardiography findings, and the inclusion criteria were as follows [20]: M-mode and/or 2D echocardiographic evidence of wall thickness ≥ 15 mm in one or more LV myocardial segments and non-dilated left ventricle (LV). All enrolled HCM patients were had septal wall hypertrophy and with/without other LV walls hypertrophy, in the absence of another cardiac disease causing LVM hypertrophy, such as hypertensive heart diseases, aortic valve stenosis. The normal subjects had no evidence of family histories of HCM, hypertension, and any other diseases. All of the physical examination tests, the electrocardiogram and the echocardiography were normal.

Conventional 2D Doppler echocardiography
Thirty seven HCM patients and 41 normal subjects all had conventional 2D Doppler echocardiography (Vivid E9, GE Healthcare, Horten, Norway), Left atrial diameter (LAD), interventricular septal thickness in end-diastolic period (IVSD) and LV posterior wall thickness in end-diastolic period (LVPWD) were

measured in the parasternal long axis view of the left ventricular by M-mode. Biplane Simpson's method was used to measure the LV ejection fractions (LVEF). The peak velocities during early diastole (Ve) and late diastole (Va) of the anterior mitral valve were measured by pulsed-wave Doppler, and the ratio of Ve/Va was calculated. ECG leads were connected to each individual in all groups. Hold on the breath, standard high frame rate (60–90/s) of the parasternal short-axis views at the base, middle and apex of three consecutive were acquired for offline analysis.

Data analysis for LV systolic function
We analysis the short-axis views at the base, middle and apex using 2D–STI software (2D–Strain, EchoPac PC version 113, GE Healthcare, Horten, Norway). Used the button SAX-MV, SAX-PM and SAX-AP to sketched the endocardial, respectively, then the software would create a region of interest (ROI) automatically which contained endocardial, middle myocardial and epicardial layers, then adjusted the ROI to make the myocardium included well. Approved the ROI, the software would divide the LV into six segments, and then the peak systolic circumferential strain of endocardial, middle myocardial and epicardial layers, the peak radial systolic strain and the different short-axis rotation degrees could be calculated and recorded.

Statistical analysis
All of the analysis was performed using a commercially available package (SPSS 17.0. SPSS Inc., Chicago, IL, USA). Whether the distribution of the data in all subjects was normal were assessed by Kolmogorov-Smirnov's test. If the data distribution was normal, differences between HCM patients and normal subjects were compared with an independent student t-test, for variables with a non-normal distribution, the nonparametric Mann-Whitney test was used. The correlation between the IVSD and the peak circumferential systolic strain of endocardial, middle myocardial, and epicardial layers, the radial systolic strain used the correlations test. Pearson correlation was used if the data distribution was normal, however, Spearman correlation was chosen if the data distribution was non-normal distribution. Data were presented as the mean ± s.d.. Difference was considered statistically significant in all tests when the P-value was less than 0.05.

Results

Basic information in HCM patients and the normal subjects
The values of LAD, IVSD and LVPWD in HCM patients were larger than normal subjects ($p < 0.001$). There were no significant difference in LVEDV, LVESV, LVEF, Ve, Va and Ve/Va ($p > 0.05$) (Table 1).

Table 1 The basic Information in HCM patients and control subjects from conventional Two-Dimensional Doppler Echocardiography (mean ± s.d)

	HR (bpm)	LAD (mm)	IVSD (mm)	LVPWD (mm)	LVEDV (ml)	LVESV (ml)	LVEF (%)	Ve (m/s)	Va (m/s)	Ve/Va
HCM (37)	72 ± 13	42 ± 5	19 ± 4	10 ± 1	80 ± 17	27 ± 9	67 ± 6	0.75 ± 0.16	0.62 ± 0.23	1.39 ± 0.57
Normal (41)	72 ± 12	35 ± 3	9 ± 1	9 ± 1	80 ± 12	29 ± 7	65 ± 6	0.84 ± 0.15	0.69 ± 0.18	1.29 ± 0.39
P-Value	0.900	**< 0.001**	**< 0.001**	**< 0.001**	0.845	0.354	0.137	0. 207	0.143	0.367

LAD left atrial diameter, HR heart rate, IVSD interventricular septal thickness in end-diastolic period, LVPWD left ventricular posterior wall thickness in end-diastolic period, LVEDV left ventricular end-diastolic volume, LVESV left ventricular end-systolic volume, LVEF left ventricular ejection fraction, Ve the peak velocity during early diastole of anterior mitral leftlet, Va the peak velocity during late diastole of anterior mitral leftlet bold number is specify the significance of the comparision

Table 2 Comparision of the peak systolic circumferential strain of endocardial, the middle myocardial and epicardial layers and peak systolic radial strain in HCM patients and control subjects (mean ± s.d.)

| LV Walls | PSCS (%) | | | | | | | | | | | | PSRS (%) | | |
| | Endocardial | | | Middle myocardial | | | Epicardial | | | | | | | | |
	HCM (37)	Normal (41)	P-value	HCM (37)	Normal (41)	P-value	HCM (37)	Normal (41)	P-value	HCM (37)	Normal (41)	P-value
Ant-Septum	**−29.16 ± 6.26**	**−34.16 ± 5.42**	**< 0.001**	**−16.79 ± 4.58**	**−23.62 ± 4.62**	**< 0.001**	**−9.36 ± 3.83**	**−15.95 ± 4.29**	**< 0.001**	**23.89 ± 9.82**	**40.22 ± 12.50**	**< 0.001**
Anterior	**−24.73 ± 6.43**	**−28.23 ± 7.01**	**0.025**	**−13.92 ± 4.61**	**−18.83 ± 5.53**	**< 0.001**	**−7.24 ± 3.73**	**−11.91 ± 4.70**	**< 0.001**	**27.12 ± 9.75**	**41.06 ± 11.92**	**< 0.001**
Lateral	−22.33 ± 5.32	−20.95 ± 6.45	0.310	−12.45 ± 3.25	−12.58 ± 4.56	0.884	−6.18 ± 2.58	−6.61 ± 3.82	0.568	33.65 ± 11.52	**42.27 ± 11.73**	**0.002**
Posterior	**−22.62 ± 8.15**	**−17.66 ± 7.45**	**0.006**	**−13.20 ± 4.95**	**−10.58 ± 4.89**	**0.021**	−7.11 ± 3.22	−5.60 ± 3.60	0.055	**37.25 ± 13.33**	**43.26 ± 11.59**	**0.036**
Inferior	−26.47 ± 7.79	−23.87 ± 7.64	0.141	−15.89 ± 5.37	−14.93 ± 5.46	0.437	−8.94 ± 4.12	−8.50 ± 4.16	0.639	35.66 ± 14.20	**43.59 ± 11.83**	**0.009**
Septum	−31.73 ± 7.12	−34.08 ± 6.58	0.134	**−19.68 ± 5.00**	**−23.53 ± 5.28**	**0.002**	**−12.08 ± 4.14**	**−15.75 ± 4.89**	**< 0.001**	**27.88 ± 11.55**	**42.39 ± 12.63**	**< 0.001**

PSCS peak systolic circumferential strain, PSRS peak systolic radial strain
bold number is specify the significance of the comparision

The peak systolic circumferential strain in different myocardium layers

The trend of the peak systolic circumferential strain of endocardial, middle myocardial, and epicardial layers of all the subjects was: endocardial > middle myocardial > epicardial. The strain absolute values of the anterseptum and anterior walls (in all layers) in HCM patients had significant lower than normal subjects. The strain absolute values of the septum wall (middle and epicardial layers) in HCM patients had significant lower than normal subjects. The strain absolute values of the posterior wall (endocardial and middle layers) in HCM patients had significant larger than normal subjects. Although the other walls had no significant difference, the absolute values of HCM patients were larger than normal subjects. (Table 2, Fig. 1).

The peak systolic radial strain

All of the peak systolic radial strain in HCM patients was significantly lower than normal subjects. (Table 2, Fig. 2).

Rotation degrees at different short-axis levels

In the systolic period, the LV apex wall rotated counterclockwise, whereas the LV basal wall rotated clockwise in all subjects. Middle LV rotation was clockwise in HCM patients. The absolute values of peak systolic rotational degrees in the basal and middle short-axis levels in HCM patients had significant larger than normal subjects. (Table 3).

The correlation between IVSD and the peak systolic circumferential strain in different myocardium layers, the peak systolic radial strain

The IVSD correlated well to the peak systolic circumferential strain of endocardial, middle myocardial, and epicardial layers of the septum wall (Endocardial: $r = 0.445$, $p = 0.006$, Middle myocardial: $r = 0.458$, $p = 0.004$, Epicardial: $r = 0.373$, $p = 0.023$). There was no correlation between IVSD and the peak systolic radial strain ($r = -0.230$, $p = 0.170$) (Table 4, Fig. 3).

Discussion

HCM is a genetic disease, and mainly was characterized by left ventricular hypertrophy [21]. The systolic function detects by conventional echocardiography like LVEF is often normal, so the subclinical LV dysfunction cannot be identified by 2D conventional echocardiography. Peak short-axis systolic myocardial strain detect by 2D–STI can reflect the systolic function accurately. As we know, the peak circumferential strain of endocardial, middle myocardial, and epicardial layers in HCM patients is little reported.

Tigen K et al. [22] detected the LV systolic function by measuring the circumferential strain of the HCM patients, and found that the circumferential strain was significantly lower in patients with HCM compared with those of normal subjects. From the results, we found that, in the hypertrophied LVM, the LV peak systolic circumferential strain was decreased, and in nonhypertrophied myocardium, the strain value was increased. In HCM patients, LV hypertrophy, myocardial

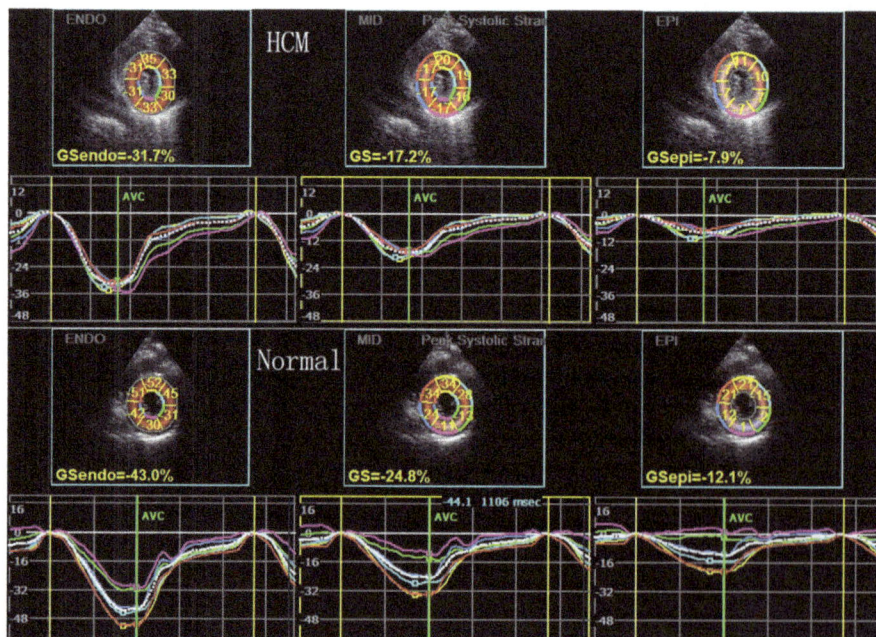

Fig. 1 The peak systolic circumferential strain of the endocardial, the middle and the epicardial layers of left ventricular in HCM patients and normal subjects

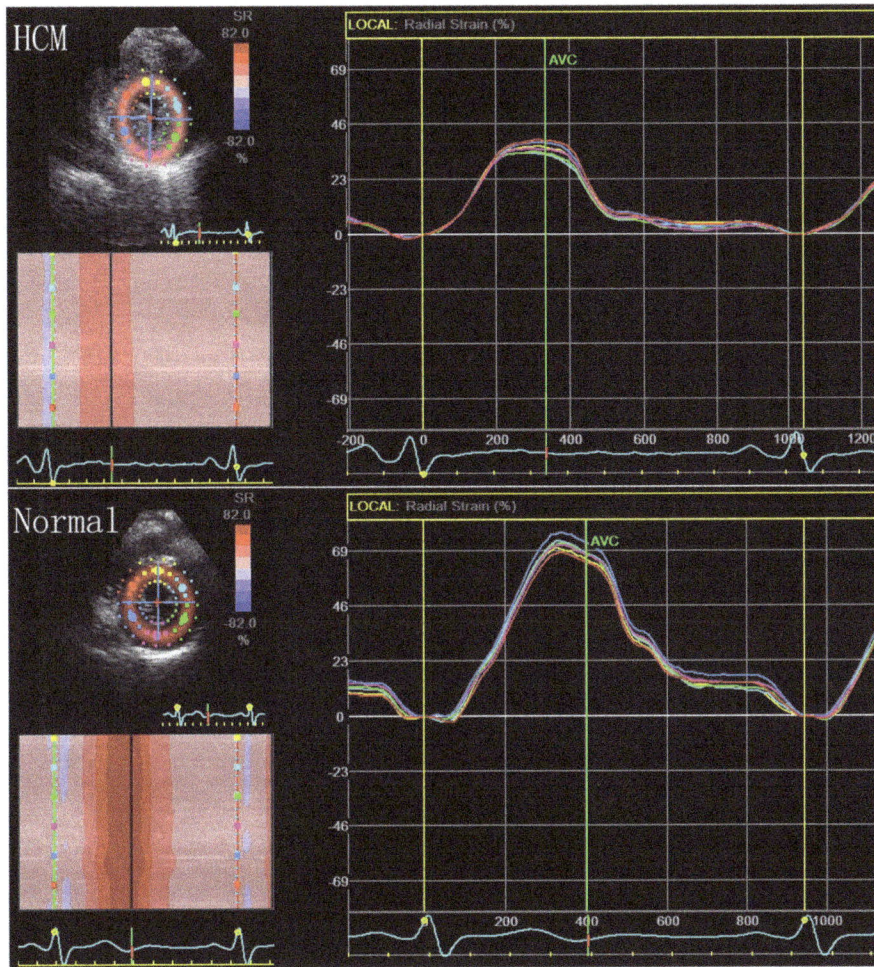

Fig. 2 The peak systolic radial strain of left ventricular in HCM patients and normal subjects

fibrosis, fiber disarray in the LV myocardium maybe a reason for the results. Once the LV was hypertrophy, the sequence of endocardial, middle myocardial, and epicardial layers had changed. The segmental systolic function was impaired. In order to maintain the normal LV systolic function, the non- hypertrophied myocardium enhanced their peak systolic circumferential strain. HCM patients with non- hypertrophied myocardium appeared to compensate for the early systolic changes via increased circumferential strain in order to keep the normal LV systolic function.

Yajima R et al. [8] found regional peak radial strain in basal, middle and apical levels were all significantly lower in HCM subjects than those in normal subjects. Our results were according to their results. Peak systolic radial strain in HCM patients was significantly lower than in the normal subjects. In HCM patients, decreased LV peak systolic radial strain appears not only in hypertrophied LVM, but also in non-hypertrophied myocardium. Peak systolic radial strain can reflect the systolic function very conveniently and accurately.

Table 3 The rotational degrees at different short-axis levels in HCM patients and normal subjects (mean ± s.d.)

	Rotational degrees in different short-axis levels		
	Basal (°)	Middle (°)	Apex (°)
HCM (37)	−11.27 ± 5.14	−3.90 ± 4.86	4.84 ± 7.34
Normal (41)	−4.65 ± 6.65	−0.87 ± 5.98	6.42 ± 7.35
P-Value	**< 0.001**	**0.017**	0.346

bold number is specify the significance of the comparision

Table 4 The correlation between IVSD and the peak systolic circumferential strain of endocardial, the middle myocardial and epicardial layers and peak radial strain in HCM patients

	PSCS			PSRS
	Endocardial	Middle	Epicardial	
r-value	0.445	0.458	0.373	−0.230
p-value	**0.006**	**0.004**	**0.023**	0.170

PSCS peak systolic circumferential strain, *PSRS* peak systolic radial strain
bold number is specify the significance of the comparision

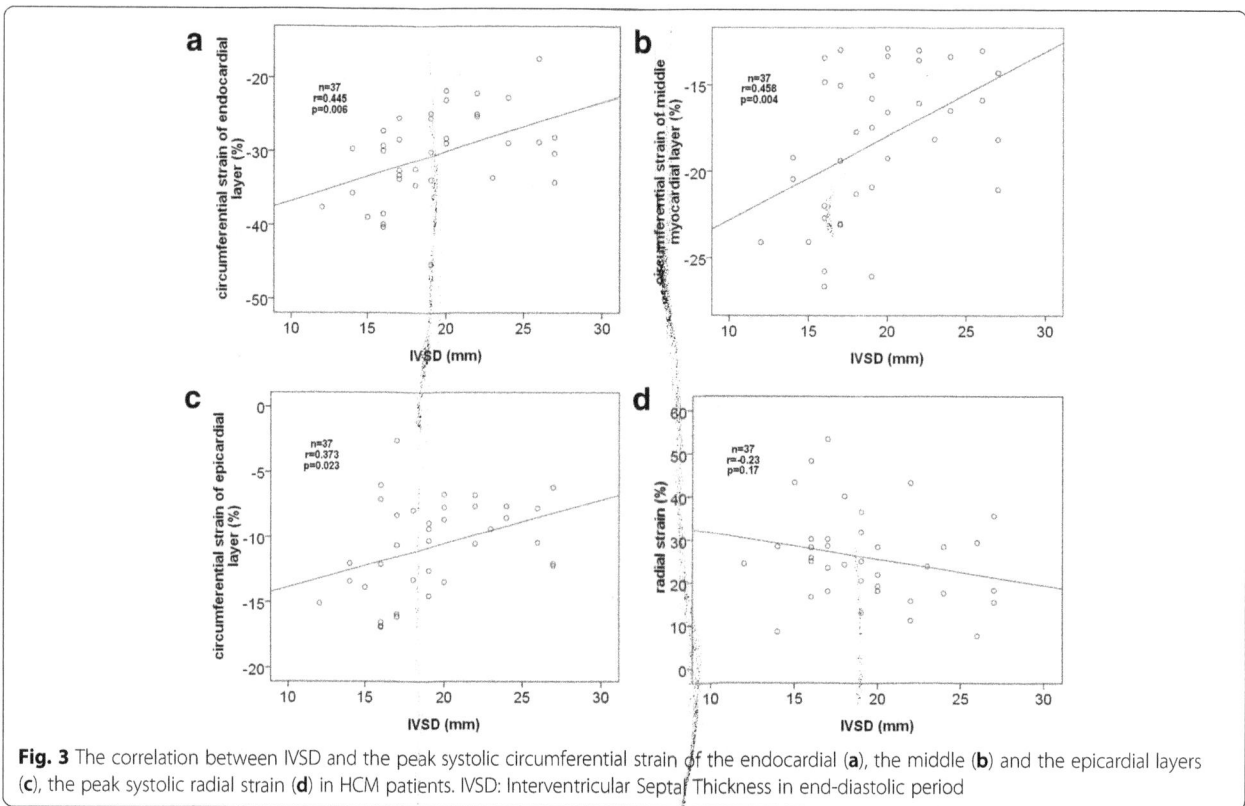

Fig. 3 The correlation between IVSD and the peak systolic circumferential strain of the endocardial (**a**), the middle (**b**) and the epicardial layers (**c**), the peak systolic radial strain (**d**) in HCM patients. IVSD: Interventricular Septal Thickness in end-diastolic period

Zhang HJ et al. [23] investigated whether left ventricular twist analysis can detect the extent of myocardial fibrosis in patients with HCM, and found that, left ventricular twist mechanics are associated with the extent of myocardial fibrosis, and LV-twist assessment by STI may be clinically useful. Carasso S et al. [24] found middle LV rotation was clockwise (opposite to normal), they found that, in both HCM and normal subjects, LV rotation, viewed from the apex, was clockwise at the base, and count-clockwise at the apex, the difference was in the middle level. Ni XD et al. [25] found that in normal subject the transition from basal clockwise rotation to apical counterclockwise rotation is located at the papillary muscle level. Our research was according with the previous studies. The base-to-apex twist plane in HCM patients was changed. The peak rotational degrees at the base and middle short-axis levels in HCM patients were larger than normal subjects. Sengupta PP et al. [26] told us in the LV myocardial wall, the myofibers geometry changes smoothly from a right-handed helix in the endocardium to a left-handed helix in the epicardium such that the helix angle varies continuously from positive at the endocardium to negative at the epicardium. When the myofibres contract and relax, the cardiac have three motions: longitudinal, circumferential and radial, also produced the rotational motion. The pathogenesis of abnormal rotation at the middle level and the different rotation degrees are not clear. When the LV fibrosis,

hypertrophied and stiffening, the LV myofibres were remodeling, the original balance of endocardial, middle myocardial, and epicardial myofibres was changed. Because the longitudinal and radial function were decreased in HCM patients, so for another possible reason was, in order to keep normal LV systolic function. HCM patients enhanced the peak rotational degrees at the base and middle short-axis levels.

The IVSD correlated well to the peak circumferential systolic strain of endocardial, middle myocardial, and epicardial layers of the septum wall, we concluded that, the more thickening of IVSD, the more circumferential systolic function was impaired. Through the correlation analysis, we found that the thickening of IVSD in HCM patients was consistent with its systolic function. There was not any correlation between IVSD and the peak systolic radial strain of the septum wall ($r = -0.230$, $p = 0.170$), we concluded that, the thickening of IVSD had no internal relationship with peak systolic radial strain.

Conclusions

According to this research, we know the short-axis systolic function is impaired despite the presence of preserved LVEF in patients with HCM. The peak circumferential systolic strain of the different layers, peak systolic radial strain and rotation degrees of the different short-axis levels detected by 2D–STI are very sensitive for assessing the systolic function in HCM patients. In the clinical implication, the study can help us to know the early cardiac dysfunction of HCM patients, then to give them early treatment and assess the effect after the treatment.

Limitations

The greatest limitation of this study is that the relationship of decreasing short axis functions to a clinical outcome or event is not investigated. Another important limitation is the small number of patients. The third limitation is that we don't evaluate the relationship with other image techniques, such as cardiac MR, SPECT.

Abbreviations

2D–STI: 2-dimensional speckle tracking imaging; HCM: Hypertrophic cardiomyopathy; IVSD: Interventricular septal thickness in end-diastolic period; LAD: Left atrial diameter; LVEDV: Left ventricular end-diastolic volume; LVEF: Left ventricular ejection fraction; LVESV: Left ventricular end-systolic volume; LVH: Left ventricular hypertrophy; LVPWD: LV posterior wall thickness in end-diastolic period; Va: The peak velocities during late diastole of the anterior mitral valve; Ve: The peak velocities during early diastole of the anterior mitral valve

Acknowledgements
The authors would like to thank the department of Echocardiography, the Affiliated Changzhou No.2 People's Hospital of Nanjing Medical University.

Funding
none

Authors' contributions
HJ, YZN and RYF designed the study and carried out the study, data collection and analysis, HJ wrote and revised the manuscript, RYF and FL revised the manuscript, LC, LJ and FL designed part of the experiments, and collected the HCM patients and normal subjects. HJ and LJ performed the statistical analysis. All authors read and approved the final manuscript.

Competing interests
The authors declare that they have no competing interests.

References
1. Hensley N, Dietrich J, Nyhan D, Mitter N, Yee MS, Brady M. Hypertrophic cardiomyopathy: a review. Anesth Analg. 2015;120:554–69.
2. He XW, Song ZZ. Evaluation Of left ventricular function, rotation, twist and untwist in patients with hypertrophic cardiomyopathy. Exp Clin Cardiol 2013;18: e47–e49.
3. Shah PM, Gramiak R, Kramer DH. Ultrasound localization of left ventricular outflow obstruction in hypertrophic obstructive cardiomyopathy. Circulation. 1969;40:3–11.
4. Baccouche H, Maunz M, Beck T, Gaa E, Banzhaf M, Knayer U, et al. Differentiating cardiac amyloidosis and hypertrophic cardiomyopathy by use of three-dimensional speckle tracking echocardiography. Echocardiography. 2012;29:668–77.
5. Nagueh SF, Bierig SM, Budoff MJ, Desai M, Dilsizian V, Eidem B, Goldstein SA, et al. American Society of Echocardiography; American Society of Nuclear Cardiology; Society for Cardiovascular Magnetic Resonance; Society of Cardiovascular Computed Tomography. American Society of Echocardiography clinical recommendations for multimodality cardiovascular imaging of patients with hypertrophic cardiomyopathy: endorsed by the American Society of Nuclear Cardiology, Society for Cardiovascular Magnetic Resonance, and Society of Cardiovascular Computed Tomography. J Am Soc Echocardiogr. 2011;24:473–98.
6. Olivotto I, Maron MS, Autore C, Lesser JR, Rega L, Casolo G, et al. Assessment and significance of left ventricular mass by cardiovascular magnetic resonance in hypertrophic cardiomyopathy. J Am Coll Cardiol. 2008;52:559–66.
7. Bing W, Knott A, Redwood C, Esposito G, Purcell I, Watkins H, et al. Effect of hypertrophic cardiomyopathy mutations in human cardiac muscle alpha-tropomyosin (Asp175Asn and Glu180Gly) on the regulatory properties of human cardiac troponin determined by in vitro motility assay. J Mol Cell Cardiol. 2000;32:1489–98.
8. Yajima R, Kataoka A, Takahashi A, Uehara M, Saito M, Yamaguchi C, et al. Distinguishing focal fibrotic lesions and non-fibrotic lesions in hypertrophic cardiomyopathy by assessment of regional myocardial strain using two-dimensional speckle tracking echocardiography: comparison with multislice CT. Int J Cardiol. 2012;158:423–32.
9. Kauer F, van Dalen BM, Michels M, Soliman OI, Vletter WB, van Slegtenhorst M, et al. Diastolic abnormalities in normal phenotype hypertrophic cardiomyopathy gene carriers: a study using speckle tracking echocardiography. Echocardiography. 2013;30:558–63.
10. Notomi Y, Lysyansky P, Setser RM, Shiota T, Popović ZB, Martin-Miklovic MG, et al. Measurement of ventricular torsion by two-dimensional ultrasound speckle tracking imaging. J Am Coll Cardiol. 2005;45:2034–41.
11. Hurlburt HM, Aurigemma GP, Hill JC, Narayanan A, Gaasch WH, Vinch CS, et al. Direct ultrasound measurement of longitudinal, circumferential, and radial strain using 2-dimensional strain imaging in normal adults. Echocardiography. 2007;24:723–31.
12. Sengupta PP, Tajik AJ, Chandrasekaran K, Khandheria BK. Twist mechanics of the left ventricle: principles and application. JACC Cardiovasc Imaging. 2008;1:366–76.
13. Hartlage GR, Kim JH, Strickland PT, Cheng AC, Ghasemzadeh N, Pernetz MA, et al. The prognostic value of standardized reference values for speckle-tracking global longitudinal strain in hypertrophic cardiomyopathy. Int J Cardiovasc Imaging. 2015;31:557–65.
14. Takano H, Isogai T, Aoki T, Wakao Y, Fujii Y. Feasibility of radial and circumferential strain analysis using 2D speckle tracking echocardiography in cats. J Vet Med Sci. 2015;77:193–201.
15. Urbano Moral JA, Arias Godinez JA, Maron MS, Malik R, Eagan JE, Patel AR, et al. Left ventricular twist mechanics in hypertrophic cardiomyopathy assessed by three-dimensional speckle tracking echocardiography. Am J Cardiol. 2011;108:1788–95.
16. Orta Kilickesmez K, Baydar O, Bostan C, Coskun U, Kucukoglu S. Four-dimensional speckle tracking echocardiography in patients with hypertrophic cardiomyopathy. Echocardiography. 2015;32:1547–453.
17. Greenbaum RA, Ho SY, Gibson DG, Becker AE, Anderson RH. Left ventricular fibre architecture in man. Br Heart J. 1981;45:248–63.
18. Henein MY, Gibson DG. Editorial normal long axis function. Heart. 1999;81:111–3.
19. Huang J, Yan ZN, Fan L, Rui YF, Song XT. Left ventricular systolic function changes in hypertrophic cardiomyopathy patients detected by the strain of different myocardium layers and longitudinal rotation. BMC Cardiovasc Disord. 2017;17:214.
20. Gersh BJ, Maron BJ, Bonow RO, Dearani JA, Fifer MA, Link MS, et al. American College of Cardiology Foundation/American Heart Association task force on practice guidelines; American Association for Thoracic Surgery; American Society of Echocardiography; American Society of Nuclear Cardiology; Heart Failure Society of America; Heart Rhythm Society; Society for Cardiovascular Angiography and Interventions; Society of Thoracic Surgeons. 2011 ACCF/AHA guideline for the diagnosis and treatment of hypertrophic cardiomyopathy: a report of the American College of Cardiology Foundation/American Heart Association task force on practice guidelines. Circulation. 2011;124:e783–831.
21. Urbano-Moral JA, Rowin EJ, Maron MS, Crean A, Pandian NG. Investigation of global and regional myocardial mechanics with 3-dimensional speckle tracking echocardiography and relations to hypertrophy and fibrosis in hypertrophic cardiomyopathy. Circ Cardiovasc Imaging. 2014;7:11–9.

22. Tigen K, Sunbul M, Karaahmet T, Dundar C, Ozben B, Guler A, et al. Left ventricular and atrial functions in hypertrophic cardiomyopathy patients with very high LVOT gradient: a speckle tracking echocardiographic study. Echocardiography. 2014;31:833–41.

23. Zhang HJ, Wang H, Sun T, Lu MJ, Xu N, Wu WC, et al. Assessment of left ventricular twist mechanics by speckle tracking echocardiography reveals association between LV twist and myocardial fibrosis in patients with hypertrophic cardiomyopathy. Int J Cardiovasc Imaging. 2014;30:1539–48.

24. Carasso S, Yang H, Woo A, Vannan MA, Jamorski M, Wigle ED, et al. Systolic myocardial mechanics in hypertrophic cardiomyopathy: novel concepts and implications for clinical status. J Am Soc Echocardiography: official Publ Am Soc Echocardiography. 2008;21:675–83.

25. Ni XD, Huang J, Hu YP, Xu R, Yang WY, Zhou LM. Assessment of the rotation motion at the papillary muscle short-axis plane with normal subjects by two-dimensional speckle tracking imaging: a basic clinical study. PLoS One. 2013;8:e83071.

26. Sengupta PP, Tajik AJ, Chandrasekaran K, Khandheria BK. Twist mechanics of the left ventricle. principles and application JACC Cardiovascular imaging. 2008;1:366–76.

21

Temporarily increased stroke rate after Takotsubo syndrome: need for an anticoagulation?

Nadine Abanador-Kamper[1]* ⓘ, Lars Kamper[2], Judith Wolfertz[1], Marc Vorpahl[1], Patrick Haage[2] and Melchior Seyfarth[1]

Abstract

Background: Previous studies have reported slightly higher stroke rates in Takotsubo Syndrome compared to acute myocardial infarction. Our goal was to evaluate the temporal course of stroke rates and left ventricular recovery in patients with Takotsubo Syndrome.

Methods: We retrospectively examined the clinical and imaging data of 72 patients with Takotsubo Syndrome. The data collected came from January 2005 to March 2017. Left ventricular performance was evaluated by cardiovascular magnetic resonance imaging (MRI) in all patients during the acute phase of Takotsubo Syndrome and in a follow-up scan 2 months later. Acute stroke and major adverse clinical events, such as myocardial infarction or recurrence of Takotsubo Syndrome and death, were also determined for each patient at 30 days and 12 months after initial presentation.

Results: The MRI scans performed during the acute phase of Takotsubo Syndrome demonstrated apical ballooning with anterior wall motion dysfunction in 65 (90%) patients. Imaging performed 2 months later demonstrated resolution of this in 97% of those patients. Median left ventricular ejection fraction also significantly increased between both scans (49.5% vs. 64.0%, $P < 0.001$). We observed 9 (12%) events in the study population within 12 months of the initial diagnosis of Takotsubo Syndrome. Stroke had an event rate of 2.8% after 30 days and 4.2% after 12 months.

Conclusions: Apical ballooning was found in the majority of our Takotsubo Syndrome patients on the MRI scans performed at presentation. This finding was subsequently associated with higher than expected stroke rates within 30 days of diagnosis and with rapid recovery of left ventricular function within 2 months of diagnosis. This suggests that rapid improvement in left ventricular morphology and function may facilitate the formation of cardiac emboli and consequently increase stroke rates in Takotsubo Syndrome. Although no guidelines currently exist for the treatment of Takotsubo Syndrome, these results may point to a potential role for temporary oral anticoagulation in high-risk patients. Future studies should examine if stroke rates after Takotsubo Syndrome have been underestimated.

Keywords: Takotsubo syndrome, Stroke event, Cardiovascular magnetic resonance imaging

* Correspondence: nabanador@gmail.com
[1]Department of Cardiology, Helios University Hospital Wuppertal, University Witten/Herdecke, Germany; Center for Clinical Medicine Witten/Herdecke University Faculty of Health, Wuppertal, Germany
Full list of author information is available at the end of the article

Background

Large anterior wall myocardial infarction is associated with an increased risk of stroke. [1]. Apical ballooning and temporal anterior wall dysfunction in Takotsubo syndrome (TTS) may also lead to a higher risk for acute cardioembolic complications. Registries reporting long-term outcome data for TTS have found stroke rates of 1–1.7% [2, 3]. The aim of this study was to evaluate the temporal course for the risk of stroke in TTS patients.

Methods

We evaluated 72 patients with TTS in our tertiary care center from January 2005 until March 2017. The diagnosis was established according to the Mayo Clinic diagnostic criteria [4]. The criteria included reversible left ventricular wall motion abnormalities extending beyond a single coronary territory, absence of significant (> 50%) coronary artery stenosis or plaque rupture, new electrocardiogram abnormalities or elevation of cardiac biomarkers, and absence of myocarditis or late gadolinium enhancement on cardiovascular magnetic resonance imaging (MRI). Patients who were diagnosed with TTS and who had a cardiac MRI performed during the hospital stay (MRI scan < 30 days after admission) were included. Exclusion criteria were history of myocardial infarction, coronary bypass surgery, and congenital heart disease. Acute stroke and major adverse clinical events (MACE), which were defined as a composite of myocardial infarction, recurrence of TTS, or death, were evaluated for each patient after 30 days and after 12 months. All patients with acute coronary syndrome were initially treated according to the current guidelines, which include antiplatelet medication. After confirming the diagnosis of TTS medication was individually adapted. The patients who later had a stroke were not previously treated with anticoagulation due to absence of classical indications.

We performed the contrast-enhanced cardiac MRI using a 1.5 T MRI scanner (Philips; Intera Achieva; Best, Netherlands) in all patients during the acute phase of TTS in order to analyze global and regional left ventricular function and to assess myocardial injury.

The MRI protocol included two-dimensional turbo gradient echo sequences in state of the art steady-state free precession technique. These sequences were performed in short axis, four-chamber, two-chamber and three-chamber views of the left ventricle. For the assessment of myocardial oedema, T2-weighted black blood turbo-spin-echo sequences with fat saturation pre-pulse in short axis and in four-chamber views with slice thickness of 8 mm and gap 0 mm covering the complete left ventricle were performed (echo time 90 ms, flip angle 90°, reconstruction matrix 512). These sequences were previously validated [5–9].

For Late Gadolinium Enhancement (LGE) image acquisition, a three-dimensional inversion-recovery turbo gradient echo sequence of the left and right ventricle was performed in the long and short axis views. LGE images were scanned after an interval of 10–15 min post-injection of 0.2 mmol/kg of gadoteridol (Prohance®, Bracco-Imaging, Konstanz, Germany).

Follow-up MRI scans were performed 2 months after initial presentation to reassess global and regional left ventricular function and myocardial injury.

A commercially available software-tool (CMR/CVI 42, Version 4.0, Circle Cardiovascular Imaging Inc., Calgary, Canada) was used for the cardiac MRI image analysis. Assessment of left ventricular functional parameters included determination of global left ventricular ejection fraction (LVEF), left ventricular end-diastolic volumes and wall motion abnormalities (WMA). The WMA were classified as apical, midventricular, or basal ballooning of the left ventricle. Apical ballooning was specifically defined as WMA of the left ventricular apex, all four apical segments, and a minimum of four affected midventricular segments, which was based on the AHA 17-segment model for the analysis of regional left ventricular function [10]. Midventricular ballooning was defined as WMA of all midventricular segments. Basal ballooning was defined as only WMA of all basal segments.

A region was quantitatively described as having myocardial oedema when the signal intensity threshold was > 2 standard deviations (SD) above that of remote normal myocardium in T2-weighted sequences [9].Myocardial oedema volumes (T2-size) were expressed as percentage of the total left ventricular mass.

LGE was defined as hyperenhancement of myocardium that was ≥5 SD above that of the signal intensity threshold of remote normal myocardium, as previously described [11]. A semi-automated quantification in each short axis slice of the entire left ventricle and right ventricle was used for LGE image analysis. Myocardial

Table 1 Description of study population

Demographic findings	Study population ($n = 72$)
Age (y)	68.8 ± 17.5
Female (n)	67 (93.1%)
Cardiovascular risk factors	
Arterial hypertension	49 (68.1%)
Diabetes mellitus	7 (9.7%)
Current smoking	9 (12.5%)
Hyperlipidemia	20 (27.8%)
Obesity (BMI)	24 (15–39)
Family history for MI	16 (22.2%)

Data is presented as number of patients and percentage. Age, is presented as mean and standard deviation. Body Mass Index is presented as median with minimum and maximum range. *BMI* Body mass index, *MI* myocardial infarction

Table 2 Data of MACE

MACE			
	Total	After 30 days	After 12 months
Total events	9 (12%)	4 (5.6%)	9 (12%)
Stroke	3 (4.2%)	2 (2.8%)	3 (4.2%)
Death	4 (5.6%)	1 (1.4%)	4 (5.6%)
MI/TTS	2 (2.8%)	1 (1.4%)	2 (2.8%)

Data is presented as number of patients and percentage. Death events are counted of all causes. *MACE* major adverse clinical events, *MI* myocardial infarction, *TTS* Takotsubo syndrome

scarring volumes (LGE size) were expressed as percentage of the total left or right ventricular mass.

The local ethics committee (University Witten/Herdecke) approved this study and patients gave written informed consent. Patients or their treating physicians were contacted by telephone for the standardized interview used for MACE assessment.

Statistical analysis was performed using STATA/IC 14.2 software (Stat Corp, LP, Texas, USA). Categorical variables are described by frequencies; continuous data are expressed as median with maximum – minimum or interquartile range or with mean and standard deviation. To test if distribution of parameters of the two MRI scans were different Wilcoxon matched-pairs signed-ranks test was used. A two-sided P value of less than 0.05 was considered to indicate statistical significance.

Results

Patients had a mean age of 68.8 ± 17.5 years. The majority were female patients (93%). Patient characteristics are presented in Table 1. We observed 9 (12%) MACE in the study population within 12 months (Table 2). Stroke had an event rate of 2.8% after 30 days and 4.2% after 12 months. Left ventricular thrombus formation (Fig. 1, Additional file 1: Video S1) was found in a patient with acute stroke (Fig. 2). There was no prior anticoagulation in any of the patients who suffered a stroke. The mortality rate was 1.4% after 30 days. After 12 months, three patients had died from non-cardiac events. Two patients had a myocardial infarction or recurrence of TTS (1.4% after 30 days; 2.8% after 12 months).

Initial MRI was performed in all patients shortly after presentation with TTS (median: 2d; IQR 1–4), and a follow-up scan was conducted 2 months later (IQR 1.3–2.9) in 63 (88%) patients. Apical ballooning was initially observed in 65 (90%) patients and resolved in 97% of those patients within 2 months (Table 3). Apical ballooning was initially detected in

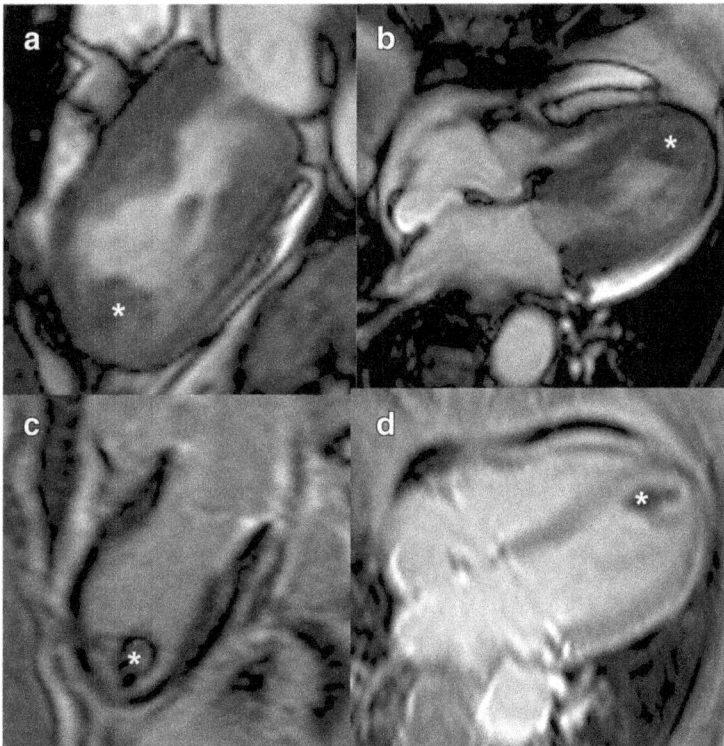

Fig. 1 Cardiovascular magnetic resonance imaging of a patient with apical ballooning due to Takotsubo Syndrome. Apical left ventricular thrombus formation (asterisks) in the end-systolic two-chamber view (**a**) and four-chamber view (**b**). Inversion recovery sequence shows a lack of Late Gadolinium Enhancement in the myocardial tissue (**c**) and confirms thrombus in the sequence with long inversion time (**d**)

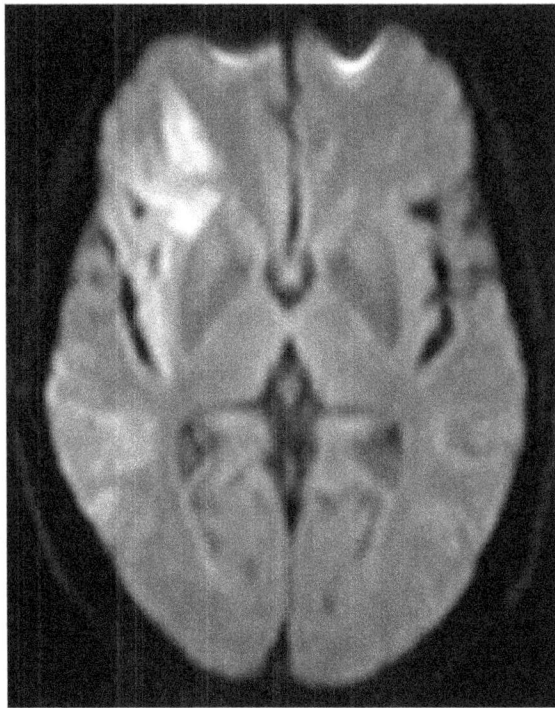

Fig. 2 Diffusion-weighted brain MRI of patient who had left ventricular thrombus formation. The scan demonstrates an ischemic stroke in the territory of the right middle cerebral artery

all patients who later suffered a stroke. In all of these cases, stroke events occurred before apical ballooning resolved in the follow-up MRI scan.

Median LVEF significantly increased between both scans (49.5% vs. 64.0%, $P < 0.001$). Myocardial oedema

Table 3 Description of differences between MRI parameters of initial MRI ($n = 72$) and follow-up scan ($n = 63$)

MRI parameters	MRI I	MRI II	p-value
LV function			
LVEF (%)	49.5 (25–73)	64 (49–84)	< 0.001
LVEDVI (ml/m^2)	76.5 (47.0–112.0)	73 (46.0–101.0)	0.198
LV ballooning n (%)			
anterior	65 (90)	2 (3)	< 0.001
midventricular	7 (10)	0	0.493
basal	0	0	
Myocardial injury (%)			
T2 Volume	13.5 ± 11.3	0.6 ± 2.4	< 0.001
LGE Volume	0.0 ± 0.0	0.0 ± 0.0	

LV ballooning is presented as number of patients and percentage. LVEF, LVEDVI are presented as median with minimum and maximum range. LGE (myocardial scarring) and T2 volumes (myocardial oedema) are presented as mean with standard deviation. *MRI* Cardiovascular magnetic resonance imaging, *AW* anterior wall, *LVEF* left ventricular ejection fraction, *LVEDVI* left ventricular end diastolic volume index, *LV* left ventricular, *LGE* late gadolinium enhancement
P-values in italic indicates statistical significance

decreased significantly between the two MRI scans. LGE was not detected in these TTS patients (Table 3).

Discussion

Prior studies have reported stroke rates of 0.5–0.9% [1, 12] in acute myocardial infarction and slightly higher stroke rates of 1–1.7% in TTS [2, 3]. A small prospective registry of TTS patients found that 1% of the 209 registry patients suffered a stroke and that all of those with a stroke had progressive LV thrombus formation despite therapeutic doses of heparin or treatment with clopidogrel or aspirin within the acute event [2]. There was a trend towards a lower LVEF in patients with LV thrombus formation and a significantly higher rate of right ventricular involvement. However, quantitative analysis of the regional WMA found in these patients were not precisely performed. Interestingly, the incidence of LV thrombi detection within the first 5 days was relatively high at 3% and might even be an underestimate in this registry due to the fact that not every patient underwent imaging by cardiac MRI. Contrast enhanced MRI is known to be highly sensitive for the detection of LV thrombi in acute myocardial infarction [13].

A larger, prospective registry reported a stroke / transient ischemic attack rate of 1.7% per patient-year. Apical ballooning was found in 81.7% of the enrolled patients; however, precise descriptions of the WMA in the stroke patients were again not supplied. In our study, we found a higher stroke rate (2.8%) in TTS patients within the first 30 days. One explanation for this might be that we also found more apical ballooning with severe anterior WMA. The most common WMA in our study were associated with apical ballooning, which was found in 90% of patients and resolved in 97% of them. Previous studies support this finding; although, the percentage of TTS patients with apical ballooning in these studies was found to be approximately 82% [3, 14]. The higher stroke rate seen in our study may, in part, be secondary to the fact that we also observed more apical ballooning in the TTS patients and that these patients then experienced significant recovery of left ventricular function within 2 months of presentation. Indeed, all of the patients who suffered a stroke had apical ballooning, which resolved completely upon subsequent imaging. Thus, we suggest that rapid changes in left ventricular morphology may facilitate the formation of cardiac emboli and that the risk of stroke after TTS may currently be underestimated.

At this time, there are no standard therapeutic recommendations for TTS available. We propose that oral anticoagulation for 2 months or until recovery of ventricular function might decrease the risk of stroke in TTS.

Study limitations

A limitation of the study is its retrospective design and the relatively small, single-center cohort. A larger, prospective, multicenter study would be better powered to confirm our hypothesis.

Conclusions

In conclusion, our findings suggest that apical ballooning with severe anterior WMA followed by a rapid improvement in left ventricular morphology and function may facilitate the formation of cardiac emboli and consequently increase stroke rates in TTS. No guidelines currently exist for the treatment of TTS, but our results point to a potential role for oral anticoagulation in high-risk patients until recovery of left ventricular function.

Abbreviations

AW: Anterior Wall; IQR: Interquartile range; LGE: Late Gadolinium Enhancement; LV: Left ventricular; LVEF: Left ventricular ejection fraction; MACE: Major adverse clinical events; MRI: Magnetic Resonance Imaging; SD: Standard Deviations; TTS: Takotsubo-Syndrome; WMA: Wall Motion Abnormalities

Acknowledgements

We especially thank Lisa C. Costello-Boerrigter, MD, PhD, HELIOS Klinikum Erfurt for support and critical revision of the manuscript. We thank the staff of the cardiovascular magnetic imaging department of the Helios University Hospital Wuppertal.

Funding

This study was supported by HELIOS Kliniken GmbH, [Grant ID 058848]. Funding was used for data analysis and statistical assistance by a certified biometrician.

Authors' contributions

NAK and LK have contributed equally in developing the design of the study, data acquisition, and editing of the manuscript. JW, MV, PH and MS have contributed in design of the study and to critical revision of the manuscript. All authors have read and approved of the manuscript and ensure that this is the case.

Competing interests

The authors declare that they have no competing interests.

Author details

[1]Department of Cardiology, Helios University Hospital Wuppertal, University Witten/Herdecke, Germany; Center for Clinical Medicine Witten/Herdecke University Faculty of Health, Wuppertal, Germany. [2]Department of Diagnostic and Interventional Radiology, Helios University Hospital Wuppertal, University Witten/Herdecke, Germany; Center for Clinical Medicine Witten/Herdecke University Faculty of Health, Wuppertal, Germany.

References

1. Loh E, Sutton MS, Wun CC, Rouleau JL, Flaker GC, Gottlieb SS, et al. Ventricular dysfunction and the risk of stroke after myocardial infarction. N Engl J Med. 1997;336:251–7.
2. Schneider B, Athanasiadis A, Schwab J, Pistner W, Gottwald U, Schoeller R, et al. Complications in the clinical course of tako-tsubo cardiomyopathy. Int J Cardiol. 2014;176:199 205.
3. Templin C, Ghadri JR, Diekmann J, Napp LC, Bataiosu DR, Jaguszewski M, et al. Clinical features and outcomes of Takotsubo (stress) cardiomyopathy. N Engl J Med. 2015;373:929–38.
4. Prasad A, Lerman A, Rihal CS. Apical ballooning syndrome (Tako-Tsubo or stress cardiomyopathy): a mimic of acute myocardial infarction. Am Heart J. 2008;155:408–17.
5. Aletras AH, Tilak GS, Natanzon A, Hsu L-Y, Gonzalez FM, Hoyt RF, et al. Retrospective determination of the area at risk for reperfused acute myocardial infarction with T2-weighted cardiac magnetic resonance imaging: histopathological and displacement encoding with stimulated echoes (DENSE) functional validations. Circulation. 2006;113:1865–70.
6. Friedrich MG, Abdel-Aty H, Taylor A, Schulz-Menger J, Messroghli D, Dietz R. The salvaged area at risk in reperfused acute myocardial infarction as visualized by cardiovascular magnetic resonance. J Am Coll Cardiol. 2008;51:1581–7.
7. Fuernau G, Eitel I, Franke V, Hildebrandt L, Meissner J, de Waha S, et al. Myocardium at risk in ST-segment elevation myocardial infarction comparison of T2-weighted edema imaging with the MR-assessed endocardial surface area and validation against angiographic scoring. JACC Cardiovasc Imaging. 2011;4:967–76.
8. Phrommintikul A, Abdel-Aty H, Schulz-Menger J, Friedrich MG, Taylor AJ. Acute oedema in the evaluation of microvascular reperfusion and myocardial salvage in reperfused myocardial infarction with cardiac magnetic resonance imaging. Eur J Radiol. 2010;74:e12–7.
9. Wright J, Adriaenssens T, Dymarkowski S, Desmet W, Bogaert J. Quantification of myocardial area at risk with T2-weighted CMR: comparison with contrast-enhanced CMR and coronary angiography. JACC Cardiovasc Imaging. 2009;2:825–31.
10. Cerqueira MD, Weissman NJ, Dilsizian V, Jacobs AK, Kaul S, Laskey WK, et al. Standardized myocardial segmentation and nomenclature for tomographic imaging of the heart. A statement for healthcare professionals from the cardiac imaging Committee of the Council on clinical cardiology of the American Heart Association. Int J Cardiovasc Imaging. 2002;18:539–42.
11. Schulz-Menger J, Bluemke DA, Bremerich J, Flamm SD, Fogel MA, Friedrich MG, et al. Standardized image interpretation and post processing in cardiovascular magnetic resonance: Society for Cardiovascular Magnetic Resonance (SCMR) board of trustees task force on standardized post processing. J Cardiovasc Magn Reson Off J Soc Cardiovasc Magn Reson. 2013;15:35.
12. Buss NI, Friedman SE, Andrus BW, DeVries JT. Warfarin for stroke prevention following anterior ST-elevation myocardial infarction. Coron Artery Dis 2013; 24:636–41.
13. Mollet NR, Dymarkowski S, Volders W, Wathiong J, Herbots L, Rademakers FE, et al. Visualization of ventricular thrombi with contrast-enhanced magnetic resonance imaging in patients with ischemic heart disease. Circulation. 2002;106:2873–6.
14. Eitel I, von Knobelsdorff-Brenkenhoff F, Bernhardt P, Carbone I, Muellerleile K, Aldrovandi A, et al. Clinical characteristics and cardiovascular magnetic resonance findings in stress (takotsubo) cardiomyopathy. JAMA. 2011;306: 277–86.

22

Left ventricular systolic function changes in hypertrophic cardiomyopathy patients detected by the strain of different myocardium layers and longitudinal rotation

Jun Huang*[iD], Zi-Ning Yan, Li Fan, Yi-Fei Rui and Xiang-Ting Song

Abstract

Background: Impairment of left ventricular (LV) longitudinal function has an important role in hypertrophic cardiomyopathy (HCM). This research investigated an association between the longitudinal strain of different myocardial layers, longitudinal rotation and the LV systolic function of HCM patients.

Methods: The research was performed on 36 HCM patients and 36 healthy subjects. The peak systolic longitudinal strain of the subendocardial, midmyocardial, and subepicardial layers was measured using 2-dimensional speckle tracking echocardiography (2D–STE). The apical long-axis and 4- and 2- chamber views were acquired via 2D Doppler echocardiography. The curve of the longitudinal rotation was traced at 17 timepoints in the analysis of 2 cardiac cycles.

Results: Compared with healthy subjects, in HCM patients regional LV peak systolic longitudinal strain was less, not only in hypertrophied LV myocardium, but also in non-hypertrophied myocardium. The rotational degrees of the midmyocardial-septal, apex, and lateral wall of HCM patients were significantly different from that of normal subjects, as follows. In HCM patients, clockwise longitudinal rotation was found. The interventricular septum thickness at end-diastole positively correlated with the peak longitudinal systolic strain of the subendocardial, the midmyocardial, and the subepicardial layers. The area under ROC curve values for subendocardial, midmyocardial and subepicardial layers in HCM patients were 0.923, 0.938, 0.948.

Conclusion: In HCM patients, the longitudinal function was damaged, even with normal LV ejection fraction. The peak longitudinal systolic strain of the subendocardial, midmyocardial, and subepicardial layers, and the longitudinal rotation detected by 2D–STE, are very sensitive predictors of systolic function in patients with HCM.

Keywords: Left ventricular, Hypertrophic cardiomyopathy, Strain, Longitudinal rotation

* Correspondence: 305669112@qq.com
Department of Echocardiography, ChangZhou No.2 People's Hospital
Affiliated to NanJing Medical University, ChangZhou 213003, China

Background

Hypertrophic cardiomyopathy (HCM) is a common clinical heart disease. It is a genetic disorder of the myocardium caused by mutations in cardiac sarcomeric proteins, with asymmetric hypertrophy of the left ventricle, right ventricle, or both [1–3]. The interventricular septum is always involved. Based on the degree of left ventricular (LV) outflow tract obstruction, HCM can be categorized at rest as non-obstructive (no obstruction or provocation), labile, or obstructive, with peak gradients <30 mmHg, >30 mmHg only during provocation, and >30 mmHg, respectively [4]. Most patients with HCM present with no clinical symptoms, but signs are often found during echocardiography, computed tomography scan, or magnetic resonance imaging [5–7]. Some patients may suffer sudden cardiac death due to ventricular tachycardia or fibrillation [8].

With the development of various imaging techniques, especially echocardiography, the discovery and diagnosis of HCM by conventional 2-dimensional ultrasound is becoming more easy and convenient. While the LV ejection fraction (LVEF) can sometimes reflect the systolic function of the left ventricle, it is not reliable, as the LVEF of most HCM patients is normal. Tissue Doppler imaging detects velocity and strain and is one of the most used echocardiography methods [9, 10], but angle dependency is not reproducible [11]. Two-dimensional (2D) speckle tracking echocardiography (STE) is a new technique that tracks frame-to-frame movement of natural acoustic markers. This enables the measurement of velocity, strain, strain rate, and torsion so that the ventricular or atrium function can be assessed [12–16]. While 2D–STE is angle-independent, out-of-plane motion often makes the results not particularly accurate [17]. Three-dimensional (3D)-STE can be used to assess LV function [18, 19], but the frame rate prevents accuracy, and therefore 3D–STE depends on the quality of 2D images for acquisition and suffers in lower temporal and spatial resolution [20].

To evaluate the changes in LV longitudinal systolic function in HCM patients, the following are innovations of the present study: The anatomy of normal myocardium consists of subendocardial, middle wall and subepicardial myocardial fibers, Using multilayer strain to analysis the LV function is a new method, so the first aim is to measure the peak systolic longitudinal strain of the subendocardial, midmyocardial, and subepicardial layers in patients with HCM; Longitudinal rotation as a new marker has received little attention. The LR means the rotational motion in the long axis of heart, but the origin of LR is still unclear, so the second aim is to Phase a hypothesis that there was longitudinal rotation of the cardiac in HCM patients, measure the longitudinal rotation in HCM patients; and tracing the curve of the LV longitudinal rotation motion in HCM patients by 2D–STE, and then to verify the hypothesis. Last to assess the changes in LV longitudinal systolic function in HCM patients.

Methods

Ethical approval

The Human Subjects Committee of Changzhou No. 2 People's Hospital approved this study. Written informed consent was obtained from the each couple enrolled in the study.

Study sample

Thirty-six HCM patients and 36 age-and gender-matched healthy (normal control) subjects were enrolled. The diagnosis of HCM was based on the following M-mode and 2D echocardiographic evidence of wall thickness ≥ 15 mm in one or more LV myocardial segments and non-dilated left ventricle (LV). In addition to the absence of another cardiac or systemic disease capable of producing the magnitude of hypertrophy evident in patients with HCM, such as the valve diseases valve stenosis, hypertensive heart diseases, and coronary heart disease. Apical HCM patients were excluded for the study. If the ECG showed LBBB, HCM patients were excluded for the study. All enrolled HCM patients were non-obstructive, based on the degree of LV outflow tract obstruction, there was no obstruction at rest or provocation (peak gradient <30 mmHg). All enrolled HCM patients were had septal wall hypertrophy and with/without other LV walls hypertrophy.

The normal control subjects had no evidence or family history of HCM, hypertension, diabetes mellitus, or any other disease; all of the physical examination tests, the electrocardiogram, and the echocardiograph were normal. Recruitment to the study followed a full explanation of our methods, including that there was no risk of harm.

Conventional 2D Doppler echocardiography

All 36 HCM patients and 36 normal subjects underwent conventional 2D Doppler echocardiography (Vivid E9, GE). Left atrial diameter, interventricular septum thickness at end-diastole (IVSD), and LV posterior wall thickness in end-diastole (LVPWD) were measured in the parasternal long axis view of the LV by M-mode. Simpson's biplane method was used to measure the LVEF. The peak early and late diastolic mitral annular velocities (Ve and Va, respectively) were measured by pulsed-wave Doppler, and the ratio of early diastolic inflow-to-late diastolic flow at the mitral valve (Ve/Va) was calculated.

In each group, ECG leads were connected to each individual. For offline analysis, the following were acquired: hold on the breath, standard high frame rate (60–90/s) of the apical long-axis, and 4 and 2-chamber views of 3 consecutive cycles.

Data analysis for LV systolic function

We analyzed the apical long-axis and 4- and 2- chamber views using 2D–STE software (2D–Strain, EchoPac PC v.7.x.x, GE Healthcare, Horten, Norway). Each of the LAX, A4C, and A2C options were used to sketch the LV subendocardial layer. The aortic valve closure time in the apical long-axis view was confirmed. The software then automatically created a region of interest (ROI) which contained the subendocardial, midmyocardial, and subepicardial layers. The ROI was adjusted to include the myocardial as well. In the ROI, the software divided the LV into 6 segments. The peak systolic longitudinal strain of the subendocardial, midmyocardial, and subepicardial layers were calculated.

We defined longitudinal rotation as the global rotation of the LV cross section. The subendocardium layer was displayed by using the SAX-MV of the Echopac in the apical 4-chamber view. The software automatically created a ROI that included the subendocardial, midmyocardial, and subepicardial layers. The ROI was adjusted to include the subendocardial and subepicardial layers. The LV region was divided into five segments: base-septal, midmyocardial-septal, apex, midmyocardial-lateral and base-lateral. The segmental longitudinal rotation of the LV was assessed in the same view via 2D–STE.

The longitudinal rotational degrees in the apical 4-chamber views were measured at 17 timepoints in the analysis of 2 cardiac cycles (each measured from onset-to-onset of the QRS wave): onset of QRS wave; mitral valve closure; mid-isovolumic contraction; aortic valve opening; 25%, 50%, and 75% of ejection phase; aortic valve closure; mid-isovolumic relaxation; mitral valve opening; peak early diastole and end of early diastole; onset, peak, and end of atrial filling; onset of the second QRS wave; and aortic valve opening of the second heart cycle [21–23].

The time between mitral valve closure and aortic valve opening was considered the isovolumic contraction. The time from aortic valve opening to aortic valve closure was considered the ejection period. The time between aortic valve closure and mitral valve opening was defined as isovolumic relaxation. The time from mitral valve opening to mitral valve closure was the diastole period.

Statistical analysis

All of the analysis was performed using SPSS 17.0 software (SPSS, Chicago, IL, USA). Data are presented as the mean ± standard deviation. Any difference was considered statistically significant in all tests when the P-value was less than 0.05. To determine normality, the distribution of the peak longitudinal systolic strain of the subendocardial, midmyocardial, and subepicardial layers in all subjects was assessed using the Kolmogorov-Smirnov's test. If the data distribution was normal,

differences between the HCM patients and normal subjects were compared with an independent Student's t-test. For variables with a non-normal distribution, the nonparametric Mann-Whitney test was used. The correlation between the IVSD and the peak longitudinal systolic strain of the subendocardial, midmyocardial, and subepicardial layers was determined by Pearson's correlation if the data distribution was normal. For variables with a non-normal distribution, Spearman's correlation was chosen. We defined the peak longitudinal systolic strain values of different layers in control subjects as the normal state, and considered the values of HCM patients as abnormal. The values for measuring the peak longitudinal systolic strain of subendocardial, midmyocardial and subepicardial in HCM patients were determined from receiver operating characteristic (ROC) curve analysis. Yoden's index was selected for the cut-off point which can give the best composite of specificity and sensitivity.

Results

Basic information in HCM patients and the normal subjects

There were significant differences in left atrial diameter, IVSD, LVPWD ($P < 0.01$; Table 1). In HCM patients, the left atrial diameter, IVSD, and LVPWD were significantly larger than in the control subjects. Between the HCM and control subjects the following were statistically similar: LVEDV, LVESV, LVEF, Ve and Va and Ve / Va, ($P > 0.05$).

Table 1 Basic Information in HCM patients and normal subjects from conventional Two-Dimensional Doppler Echocardiography (mean ± s.d.)

	HCM (36)	Normal (36)	P-Value
Age(yrs)	47 ± 14	46 ± 12	0.703
Male gender(%)	64	61	
HR(bpm)	72 ± 12	73 ± 12	0.343
LAD(mm)	42 ± 5	35 ± 4	<0.001
IVSD(mm)	19 ± 4	9 ± 1	<0.001
LVPWD(mm)	10 ± 1	9 ± 1	<0.001
LVEDV(ml)	80 ± 18	84 ± 11	0.099
LVESV(ml)	27 ± 9	30 ± 8	0.333
LVEF(%)	67 ± 6	65 ± 6	0.087
Ve(m/s)	0.79 ± 0.26	0.85 ± 0.15	0.205
Va(m/s)	0.62 ± 0.23	0.69 ± 0.18	0.167
Ve/Va	1.45 ± 0.67	1.31 ± 0.36	0.259

LAD left atrial diameter, *HR* heart rate, *IVSD* interventricular septal thickness in end-diastolic period, *LVPWD* left ventricular posterior wall thickness in end-diastolic period, *LVEDV* left ventricular end-diastolic volume, *LVESV* left ventricular end-systolic volume, *LVEF* left ventricular ejection fraction, *Ve* the peak velocity during early diastole of anterior mitral leftlet, *Va* the peak velocity during late diastole of anterior mitral leftlet

Peak systolic longitudinal strain in different myocardium layers

The trend of the peak systolic longitudinal strain of the subendocardial, midmyocardial, and subepicardial layers in all the subjects was: subendocardial > midmyocardial > subepicardial (Table 2, Fig. 1). All systolic peak longitudinal strains were different between the HCM and normal subjects. In HCM patients, the LV peak systolic longitudinal strain was lower than in the normal subjects, not only in hypertrophied LV myocardium, but also in non-hypertrophied myocardium.

Segmental longitudinal rotation

The lateral wall rotated counter-clockwise, whereas the septum wall rotated clockwise in the normal subjects, the rotational degree was similar, whereas the direction was opposite (Table 3, Fig. 2). When the segmental longitudinal rotation of HCM patients and normal subjects were compared, the rotational degree of the midmyocardial-septal, apex, and the lateral wall of HCM patients was significantly different relative to that of the normal subjects. The rotational motion of the LV septal, apex, and lateral walls in HCM patients were impaired.

Globe longitudinal rotation of LV curves in the cardiac

The longitudinal rotation degrees in normal subjects was <3°, around the zero baseline for a small angle movement. In HCM patients, the clockwise longitudinal rotation was found (Table 4, Fig. 3).

Correlation between IVSD and the peak longitudinal systolic strain in myocardial layers

The IVSD positively correlated with the peak longitudinal systolic strain of the subendocardial, midmyocardial, and subepicardial layers in the HCM patients (subendocardial, $r = 0.353$, $P = 0.035$; midmyocardial, $r = 0.407$, $P = 0.014$; subepicardial, $r = 0.444$, $P = 0.007$; (Table 5, Fig. 4). Therefore, patients with higher IVSD

had higher peak longitudinal systolic strain in the different myocardial layers.

ROC analysis for detecting the accuracy of the different layers of the peak longitudinal systolic strain in HCM patients

Area under ROC curves allowing determination of optimal cut-off values for sensitivity, specificity, and accuracy for the peak longitudinal systolic strain of different layers in assessing the LV function. The area under ROC curve values for subendocardial, midmyocardial and subepicardial layers in HCM patients were 0.923, 0.938, 0.948. The sensitivity was higher for peak longitudinal systolic strain of midmyocardial layer (97.2%) than for the subendocardial and subepicardial layers (94.4% and 91.7%). Specificity was higher for peak longitudinal systolic strain of subepicardial layer (88.9%) than for the subendocardial and midmyocardial layers (80.6% and 83.3%). The cut-off values of the subendocardial, midmyocaidial and subepicardial were −19.43%, −16.33% and −15.33%. (Fig. 5).

Reproducibility and repeatability

Interobserver measurement of the global strain and LR were determined by having a second investigator measure all chosen subjects. For intraobserver variability, all subjects were analyzed twice by one investigator, and the second intraobserver measurements were "blinded" to results from the initial measurements. The results for the intraobserver and interobserver variabilities for the peak systolic global strain of subendocardial, midmyocardial and subepicardial layers and longitudinal rotation degrees upon repeated measurements in all study patients were shown in Table 6.

Discussion

This study investigated the differences in LV longitudinal systolic function of HCM patients relative to healthy

Table 2 Comparison of the peak systolic longitudinal strain of the subendocardial, midmyocardial and subepicardial layers in HCM patients and normal subjects (mean ± s.d.)

		Subendocardial			Midmocardial			Subepicardial		
		HCM(36) (%)	Normal(36) (%)	P-Value	HCM(36) (%)	Normal(36) (%)	P-Value	HCM(36) (%)	Normal(36) (%)	P-Value
3-CH	AnterSeptal	−15.95 ± 5.19	−25.80 ± 4.59	< 0.001	−11.32 ± 4.23	−21.05 ± 3.45	< 0.001	−8.50 ± 3.70	−17.55 ± 2.77	< 0.001
	Posterior	−16.96 ± 5.13	−24.18 ± 3.97	< 0.001	−13.43 ± 4.35	−20.40 ± 3.67	< 0.001	−10.94 ± 3.77	−17.50 ± 3.61	< 0.001
4-CH	Lateral	−17.19 ± 7.11	−24.33 ± 3.77	< 0.001	−13.08 ± 6.11	−20.32 ± 3.39	< 0.001	−10.20 ± 5.37	−17.32 ± 3.24	< 0.001
	Septal	−16.70 ± 5.41	−24.11 ± 3.61	< 0.001	−13.73 ± 4.71	−20.75 ± 3.15	< 0.001	−11.91 ± 4.24	−18.30 ± 2.85	< 0.001
2-CH	Anterior	−15.30 ± 6.69	−23.77 ± 3.46	< 0.001	−11.10 ± 5.89	−20.31 ± 2.89	< 0.001	−8.36 ± 5.20	−17.80 ± 2.55	< 0.001
	Inferior	−17.74 ± 5.21	−25.40 ± 4.24	< 0.001	−14.50 ± 4.30	−21.96 ± 3.61	< 0.001	−12.58 ± 3.88	−19.41 ± 3.11	< 0.001
Global		−16.75 ± 4.13	−23.99 ± 3.05	< 0.001	−13.44 ± 3.68	−20.64 ± 2.59	< 0.001	−10.85 ± 3.28	−17.82 ± 2.28	< 0.001

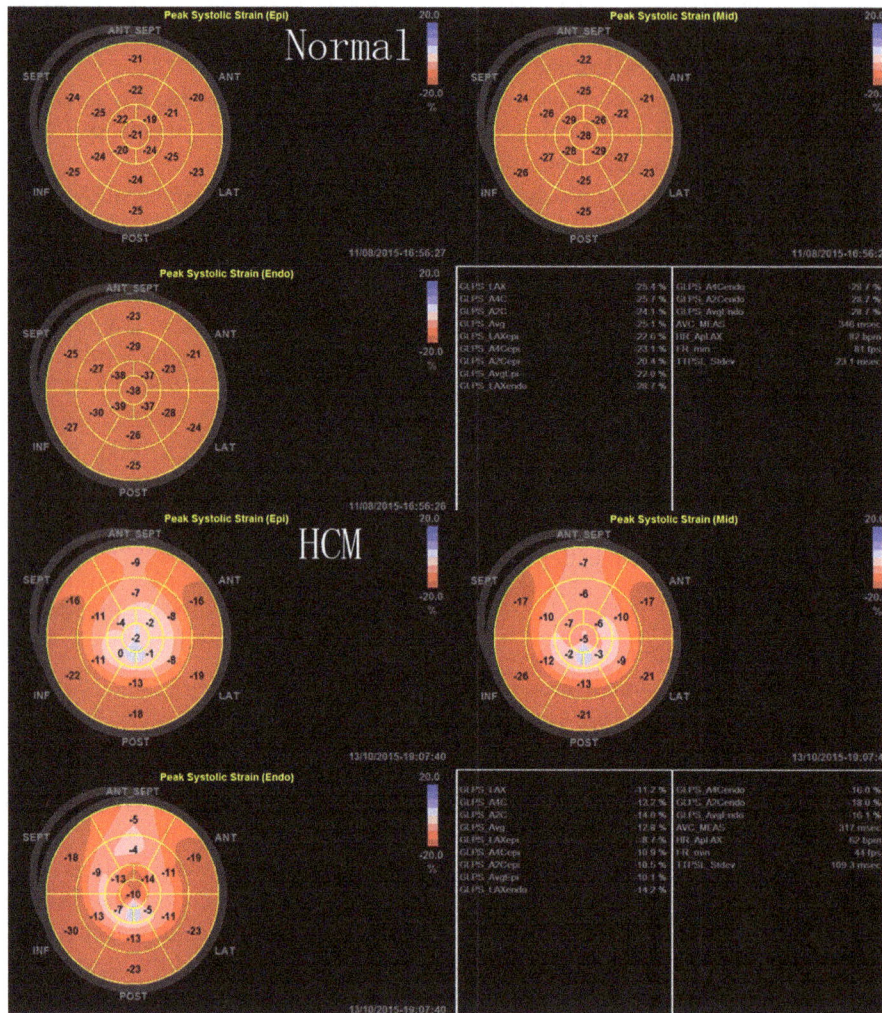

Fig. 1 The bull's eyes of the peak systolic longitudinal strain of the subendocardial, midmyocardial and subepicardial layers between normal subjects and HCM patients

subjects, with 4 main findings. First, in HCM patients decreased regional LV peak systolic longitudinal strain appeared not only in hypertrophied LV myocardium, but also in non-hypertrophied myocardium. Clockwise longitudinal rotation was found in the HCM patients, and the interventricular septum thickness at end-diastole positively correlated with the peak longitudinal systolic strain of the different layers. Finally, the area under the ROC curve values for the subendocardial, midmyocardial and subepicardial layers were 0.923, 0.938, 0.948, respectively. The sensitivity was higher for peak longitudinal systolic strain of the midmyocardial layer (97.2%) than for the subendocardial and subepicardial layers (94.4% and 91.7%). Specificity was higher for the peak longitudinal

Table 3 Comparison of the peak segmental and global longitudinal rotational degrees in the systolic period between HCM patients and normal subjects (mean ± s.d.)

	Base-Septal(°)	Mid-Septal(°)	Apex(°)	Mid-lateral(°)	Base-lateral(°)	Global
HCM (36)	−9.45 ± 2.65	−7.90 ± 3.08	−5.07 ± 3.61	−2.49 ± 4.85	0.15 ± 6.14	−4.92 ± 2.65
Normal (36)	−9.21 ± 3.11	−4.52 ± 4.01	1.28 ± 3.42	6.38 ± 3.63	9.66 ± 3.63	0.02 ± 2.42
P-Value	0.687	< 0.001	< 0.001	< 0.001	< 0.001	< 0.001

Base-Septal the base of the septal wall, *Mid-Septal* the middle of the septal wall, *Apex* the apex of the left ventricular, *Mid-lateral* the middle of the lateral wall, Base-lateral: the base of the lateral wall

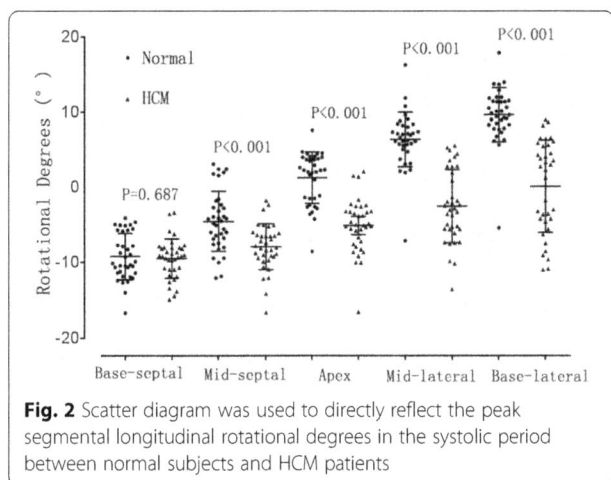

Fig. 2 Scatter diagram was used to directly reflect the peak segmental longitudinal rotational degrees in the systolic period between normal subjects and HCM patients

systolic strain of the subepicardial layer (88.9%) than for the subendocardial and midmyocardial layers (80.6% and 83.3%). Cut-off values for the subendocardial, midmyocardial and subepicardial layers were −19.43%, −16.33% and −15.33%.

HCM is a very common and important cardiac disease. LV hypertrophy, myocardial fibrosis, and fiber disarray in the LV myocardium has been reported as the major

Table 4 Longitudinal rotational degrees in HCM patients and normal subjects at 17 different points in two cardiac cycles (mean ± s.d.)

Points	HCM (36)		Normal (36)	
	Time(ms)	Rotation Degree(°)	Time(ms)	Rotation Degree(°)
Q	0	0	0	0
MVC	25 ± 7	−0.19 ± 0.36	25 ± 6	−0.12 ± 0.32
IVS	48 ± 8	−0.70 ± 0.79	45 ± 7	−0.13 ± 0.62
AVO	73 ± 13	−1.47 ± 1.55	65 ± 13	−0.17 ± 0.98
25%	147 ± 15	−3.29 ± 2.40	142 ± 15	−0.22 ± 2.24
50%	220 ± 21	−4.57 ± 2.63	219 ± 18	−0.02 ± 2.44
75%	293 ± 29	−4.92 ± 2.65	296 ± 23	0.02 ± 2.42
AVC	367 ± 37	−4.38 ± 2.53	373 ± 28	−0.41 ± 2.35
IVR	409 ± 35	−3.63 ± 2.30	402 ± 30	0.61 ± 2.17
MVO	451 ± 43	−2.86 ± 2.17	431 ± 37	−0.71 ± 1.97
E-Peak	534 ± 53	−2.12 ± 1.86	507 ± 41	0.36 ± 1.39
E-End	716 ± 95	−1.38 ± 1.29	658 ± 70	0.68 ± 1.09
A-Onset	808 ± 190	−1.26 ± 1.21	749 ± 104	−0.52 ± 0.90
A-Peak	848 ± 128	−0.74 ± 0.92	809 ± 104	0.34 ± 0.80
A-End	890 ± 141	−0.28 ± 0.53	854 ± 105	−0.11 ± 0.41
Q-2	904 ± 147	0	875 ± 98	0
AVO-2	971 ± 152	−1.16 ± 0.89	940 ± 103	−0.18 ± 1.05

When viewed from the above values, positive values of the rotation degree were considered as count-clockwise rotation, while negative values were considered as clockwise rotation
MVC mitral valve closure, *IVS* isovolumic contraction, *AVO* aortic valve opening, *AVC* aortic valve closure, *IVR* isovolumic relaxation, *MVO* mitral valve opening

structural myocardial abnormalities in HCM patients [4], and systolic function is damaged thereby. LV hypertrophy is the result of compensatory myocardial function.

Systolic function by conventional measurements, such as LVEF, cannot detect cardiac myocardium impairment; microscopic abnormalities result in intrinsic functional abnormalities [24]. Cardiac function has been determined based on velocity, strain, strain rate, degrees of rotation, and torsion using 2D–STE in many heart diseases, including cardiomyopathy, coronary heart disease, and hypertension [8, 25–28]. However, to measure the peak systolic strain of the subendocardial, midmyocardial, and subepicardial layers is a novel method for adjudging myocardium function. One of the innovations of the present study was to use 2D–STE to measure the peak systolic longitudinal strain of the subendocardial, midmyocardial, and subepicardial layers in HCM patients, and then evaluate longitudinal systolic function in HCM patients relative to that of healthy individuals.

In the present study, the peak systolic longitudinal strain of the subendocardial, midmyocardial, and subepicardial layers in both HCM and healthy individuals was: subendocardial > middle myocardial > subepicardial. A normal myocardium consists of the subendocardium, middle, and subepicardium fibers. Longitudinally oriented fibers of the subendocardium and subepicardium lead to longitudinal contraction, and middle wall fibers that are circumferentially oriented lead to circumferential shortening. Differences in contraction of the subepicardial and subendocardial layers lead to high subendocardial strain. The subendocardial region is responsible for most of the longitudinal deformation.

The present result was consistent with previous studies [4, 21]. By detecting the peak systolic longitudinal strain of the subendocardial, midmyocardial, and subepicardial layers, our data showed attenuation of longitudinal systolic function of the LV myocardium in HCM patients. Popovic et al. [29] also demonstrated that myocardial fibrotic lesions in the LV myocardium were associated with reduced longitudinal strain in HCM patients, and fibrotic lesions and wall thickening were predictors of lower longitudinal strain. Kofflard et al. [30] considered that the decrease in coronary flow reserve in HCM patients predisposed to myocardial ischemia. According to the research, they found that in HCM patients, hemodynamic (LV end-diastolic pressure, LV outflow tract gradient), echocardiographic (indexed LV mass) and histological (% luminal area of the arterioles) changes are responsible for a decrease in coronary flow reserve. Because of these changes, the systolic function in HCM patients was impaired. From our present results, we conclude that longitudinal function was damaged in HCM patients, and longitudinal

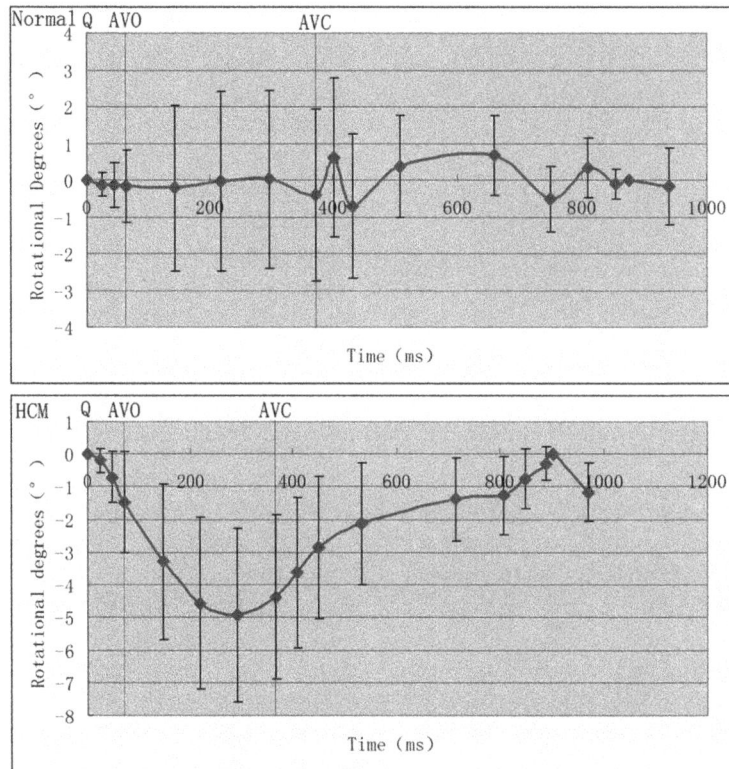

Fig. 3 The curve of the longitudinal rotational degrees in normal subjects and HCM patients at 17 different points in two cardiac cycles

strain of the different myocardial layers can sensitively reflect cardiac systolic function.

The different orientation of the ventricular muscle fibers led to the different motion of the heart. In the short-axis view, when viewed from the apex, the LV apex rotates counterclockwise, whereas the base rotates clockwise in systole period. However, when a normal heart is viewed from the long-axis view, the motion can be described as shortening of its long axis and thickening of its walls [31, 32].

Longitudinal rotation, first discussed by Popovic et al. [31], refers to rotational motion in the longitudinal direction. Some researchers [28, 32] have found longitudinal rotation in patients with dilated cardiomyopathy, primary hypertension, and other heart diseases. In the present study, clockwise longitudinal rotation was found in HCM patents. The curves of normal subjects showed longitudinal rotations <3°, around the zero baseline for a

Table 5 Correlation between IVSD and the longitudinal strain of the subendocardial, midmyocardial and subepicardial layers in HCM patients

	Subendocardial	Midmyocardial	Subepicardial
r-value	0.353	0.407	0.444
p-value	0.035	0.014	0.007

small angle movement. However, in HCM patients, clockwise longitudinal rotation was found in the heart. The segmental rotation motion in HCM patients also differed from that of the healthy control subjects. In the normal subjects, the lateral wall rotated counterclockwise, whereas the septum wall rotated clockwise, the rotation degrees were similar, but the direction was the opposite.

In the HCM patients of the present study, the rotational motion of the septum, apex, and the lateral wall of LV also differed from that of the controls. Differences in the segmental and global longitudinal rotation were associated with the unique distribution of myocardium disarray in the HCM patients. The myocardial hypertrophy and fibrosis of these patients was probably responsible for the global and regional abnormalities of the LV myocardial mechanics. When the heart contracted, the abnormal balance of the various myocardial layers resulted in aberrant differences in rotational degrees and the direction of global longitudinal rotation. We also considered that neural and humoral regulation mechanisms may underlie the orientation of the longitudinal rotation. Further researches are necessary to confirm this hypothesis.

In the present study, the IVSD of the HCM patients was found to correlate positively with the peak

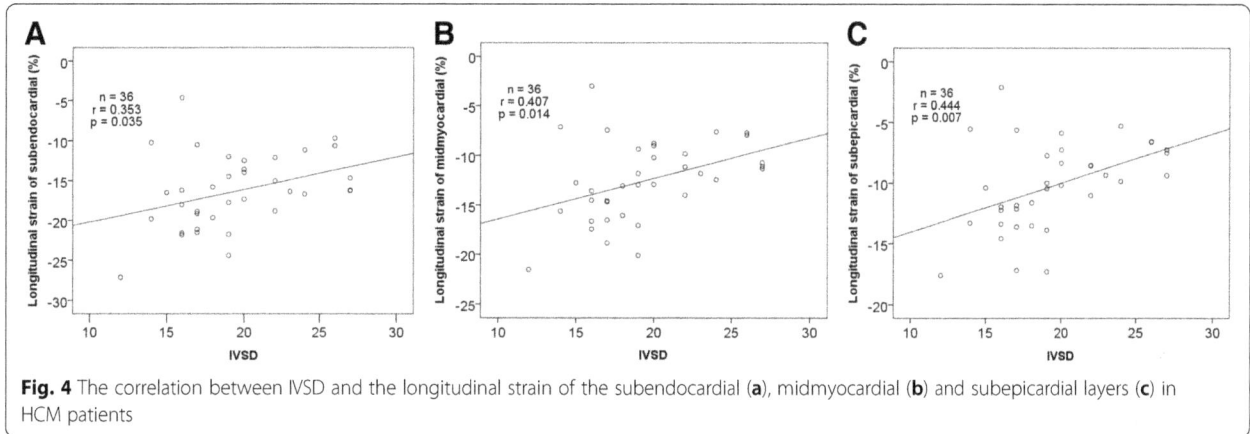

Fig. 4 The correlation between IVSD and the longitudinal strain of the subendocardial (**a**), midmyocardial (**b**) and subepicardial layers (**c**) in HCM patients

longitudinal systolic strain of the subendocardial, mid-myocardial, and subepicardial layers; thickening of the IVSD in HCM patients was consistent with its systolic function. We therefore conclude that obvious thickening of the IVSD reflects impaired longitudinal systolic function.

The ROC analysis for detecting the accuracy of the peak longitudinal systolic strain showed that the area under ROC curve values for subendocardial, midmyocardial and subepicardial layers were 0.923, 0.938, 0.948. The sensitivity was higher for peak longitudinal systolic strain of midmyocardial layer (97.2%) than for the subendocardial and subepicardial layers (94.4% and 91.7%). Specificity was higher for peak longitudinal systolic strain of subepicardial layer (88.9%) than for the subendocardial and midmyocardial layers (80.6% and 83.3%). From ROC analysis, we knew that using 2D–STE for detecting the peak longitudinal systolic strain of HCM is accurately. The results also showed that the LV function was impaired in HCM patients.

Conclusion

Longitudinal function in HCM is damaged, despite normal LVEF. The changes of peak systolic longitudinal strain of the subendocardial, midmyocardial, and subepicardial layers, and the longitudinal rotation detected by 2D–STE can reflect the LV systolic dysfunction in HCM patients. In clinician, early detection of LV dysfunction in HCM patients can make us to understand the pathophysiology of HCM better, and it also can help the physician to have an earlier symptomatic treatment and then compare the efficacy of the different drugs. The peak longitudinal systolic strain of the subendocardial, midmyocardial, and subepicardial layers and the longitudinal rotation (detected by 2D–STE) are very sensitive determinants of systolic function in patients with HCM.

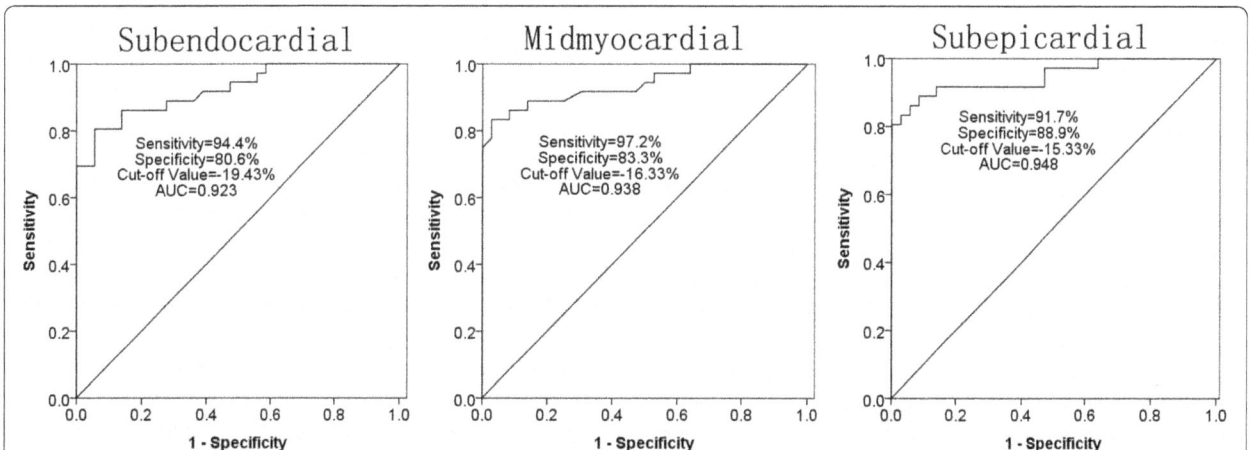

Fig. 5 ROC analysis for detecting the accuracy of the peak longitudinal systolic strain of different myocardial layers in HCM patients. The area under ROC curve values for the subendocardial, midmyocardial and subepicardial layers were 0.923, 0.938, 0.948, respectively. Sensitivity for the subendocardial, midmyocardial and subepicardial layers were 94.4%, 97.2% and 91.7%, respectively. Specificity for the subendocardial, midmyocardial and subepicardial layers were 80.6%, 83.3% and 88.9%, respectively. Cut-off values for the subendocardial, midmyocardial and subepicardial layers were −19.43%, −16.33% and −15.33%, respectively

Table 6 Interobserver and intraobserver reproducibility and repeatability

		Interobserver			Intraobserver		
		HCM	Normal	p-value	HCM	Normal	p-value
Global Strain (%)	subendocardial	−16.94 ± 4.47	−24.08 ± 3.41	< 0.001	−17.63 ± 5.20	−23.88 ± 3.72	< 0.001
	midmyocardial	−13.60 ± 3.90	−21.01 ± 2.99	< 0.001	−14.39 ± 4.56	−20.60 ± 3.34	< 0.001
	subepicardial	−10.98 ± 3.48	−18.43 ± 2.70	< 0.001	−11.76 ± 4.02	−17.86 ± 3.12	< 0.001
Global LR(°)		−4.97 ± 2.66	−0.05 ± 2.44	< 0.001	−4.88 ± 2.59	−0.03 ± 2.39	< 0.001

Limitation

The high standard deviations are indicative of the high variability with this technique - when narrow ROI is chosen to try and assess myocardial layers, higher strain values (more deformation) are recorded and more noise is introduced.

Abbreviations

2D–STE: 2-dimensional speckle tracking echocardiography; HCM: Hypertrophic cardiomyopathy; IVSD: Interventricular septal thickness in end-diastolic period; LAD: Left atrial diameter; LV: Left ventricular; LVEDV: Left ventricular end-diastolic volume; LVEF: Left ventricular ejection fraction; LVESV: Left ventricular end-systolic volume; LVH: Left ventricular hypertrophy; LVPWD: LV posterior wall thickness in end-diastolic period

Acknowledgements

The authors would like to thank the department of Echocardiography, ChangZhou No. 2 People's Hospital Affiliated to NanJing Medical University.

Funding

None.

Authors' contributions

HJ and YZN designed the study and carried out the study, data collection and analysis, HJ wrote and revised the manuscript. FL, RYF and SXT designed part of the experiments, and collected the HCM patients. HJ and SXT performed the statistical analysis. All authors have read and approved the manuscript.

Competing interests

The authors declared no conflict of interest.

References

1. Gersh BJ, MaronBJ BRO, Dearani JA, Fifer MA, Link MS, et al. American College of Cardiology Foundation/American Heart Association task force on practice guidelines; American Association for Thoracic Surgery; American Society of Echocardiography; American Society of Nuclear Cardiology; Heart Failure Society of America; Heart Rhythm Society; Society for Cardiovascular Angiography and Interventions; Society of Thoracic Surgeons. 2011 ACCF/AHA guideline for the diagnosis and treatment of hypertrophic cardiomyopathy: a report of the American College of Cardiology Foundation/American Heart Association task force on practice guidelines. Circulation. 2011;124:e783–831.
2. Maron BJ. Hypertrophic cardiomyopathy: a systematic review. JAMA. 2002; 287:1308–20.
3. Kauer F, van Dalen BM, Michels M, Soliman OI, Vletter WB, van Slegtenhorst M, et al. Diastolic abnormalities in normal phenotype hypertrophic cardiomyopathy gene carriers: a study using speckle tracking echocardiography. Echocardiography. 2013;30:558–63.
4. Hensley N, Dietrich J, Nyhan D, Mitter N, Yee MS, Brady M. Hypertrophic cardiomyopathy: a review. Anesth Analg. 2015;120:554–69.
5. Shah PM, Gramiak R, Kramer DH. Ultrasound localization of left ventricular outflow obstruction in hypertrophic obstructive cardiomyopathy. Circulation. 1969;40:3–11.
6. Nagueh SF, Bierig SM, Budoff MJ, Desai M, Dilsizian V, Eidem B, et al. American Society of Echocardiography; American Society of Nuclear Cardiology; Society for Cardiovascular Magnetic Resonance; Society of Cardiovascular Computed Tomography. American Society of Echocardiography clinical recommendations for multimodality cardiovascular imaging of patients with hypertrophic cardiomyopathy: endorsed by the American Society of Nuclear Cardiology, Society for Cardiovascular Magnetic Resonance, and society of cardiovascular computed tomography. J Am Soc Echocardiogr. 2011;24:473–98.
7. Olivotto I, Maron MS, Autore C, Lesser JR, Rega L, Casolo G, et al. Assessment and significance of left ventricular mass by cardiovascular magnetic resonance in hypertrophic cardiomyopathy. J Am Coll Cardiol. 2008;52:559–66.
8. Yajima R, Kataoka A, Takahashi A, Uehara M, Saito M, Yamaguchi C, et al. Distinguishing focal fibrotic lesions and non-fibrotic lesions in hypertrophic cardiomyopathy by assessment of regional myocardial strain using two-dimensional speckle tracking echocardiography: comparison with multislice CT. Int J Cardiol. 2012;158:423–32.
9. Sun JP, Popovic ZB. Noninvasive quantification of regional myocardial function using Doppler-derived velocity, Displacement,Strain rate, and strain in healthy volunteers: effects of aging. J Am Soc Echocardiogr. 2004;2:132–8.
10. Van de Veire NR, De Sutter J, Bax JJ, Roelandt JR. Technological advances in tissue Doppler imaging echocardiography. Heart. 2008;94:1065–74.
11. Nesbitt GC, Mankad S, Jae KO. Strain imaging in echocardiography: methods and clinical applications. Int J Cardiovasc Imaging. 2009;25:9–22.
12. Notomi Y, Lysyansky P, Setser RM, Shiota T, Popović ZB, Martin-Miklovic MG, et al. Measurement of ventricular torsion by two-dimensional ultrasound speckle tracking imaging. J Am Coll Cardiol. 2005;45:2034–41.
13. Hurlburt HM, Aurigemma GP, Hill JC, Narayanan A, Gaasch WH, Vinch CS, et al. Direct ultrasound measurement of longitudinal, circumferential, and radial strain using 2-dimensional strainimaging in normal adults. Echocardiography. 2007;4:723–31.
14. Sengupta PP, Tajik AJ, Chandrasekaran K, Khandheria BK. Twist mechanics of the left ventricle: principles and application. JACC Cardiovasc Imaging. 2008; 1:366–76.
15. Burns AT, La Gerche A, Prior DL, Macisaac AI. Left ventricular torsion parameters are affected by acute changes in load. Echocardiography. 2010;27:407–14.
16. Gabrielli L, Enríquez A, Córdova S, Yáñez F, Godoy I, Corbalán R. Assessment of left atrial function in hypertrophic cardiomyopathy and athlete's heart: a left atrial myocardial deformation study. Echocardiography. 2012;29:943–9.
17. Helle-Valle T, Crosby J, Edvardsen T, Lyseggen E, Amundsen BH, Smith HJ, et al. New noninvasive method for assessment of left ventricular rotation: speckle tracking echocardiography. Circulation. 2005;112:3149–56.
18. Baccouche H, Maunz M, Beck T, Gaa E, Banzhaf M, Knayer U, et al. Differentiating cardiac amyloidosis and hypertrophic cardiomyopathy by use of three-dimensional speckle tracking echocardiography. Echocardiography. 2012;29:668–77.
19. Urbano Moral JA, Arias Godinez JA, Maron MS, Malik R, Eagan JE, Patel AR, et al. Left ventricular twist mechanics in hypertrophic cardiomyopathy assessed by three-dimensional speckle tracking echocardiography. Am J Cardiol. 2011;108:1788–95.
20. Nemes A, Domsik P, Kalapos A, Gavallér H, Forster T, Sepp R. Quantification of changes in septal strain after alcohol septal ablation in hypertrophic obstructive cardiomyopathy-cases from the three-dimensional speckle

tracking echocardiographic MAGYAR-path study. Echocardiography. 2013;30:E289–91.

21. Urbano-Moral JA, Rowin EJ, Maron MS, Crean A, Pandian NG. Investigation of global and regional myocardial mechanics with 3-dimensional speckle tracking echocardiography and relations to hypertrophy and fibrosis in hypertrophic cardiomyopathy. Circ Cardiovasc Imaging. 2014;7:11–9.

22. Ni XD, Huang J, Hu YP, Xu R, Yang WY, Zhou LM. Assessment of the rotation motion at the papillary muscle short-axis plane with normal subjects by two-dimensional speckle tracking echocardiography: a basic clinical study. PLoS One. 2013;8:e83071.

23. Gustafsson U, Lindqvist P, Mörner S, Waldenström A. Assessment of regional rotation patterns improves the understanding of the systolic and diastolic left ventricular function: an echocardiographic speckle-tracking study in healthy individuals. Eur J Echocardiogr. 2009;10:56–61.

24. van Dalen BM, Soliman OI, Vletter WB, ten Cate FJ, Geleijnse ML. Insights into left ventricular function from the time course of regional and global rotation by speckle tracking echocardiography. Echocardiography. 2009;25:371–7.

25. Xie MY, Yin JB, Lv Q, Wang J. Assessment of the left ventricular systolic function in multi-vessel coronary artery disease with normal wall motion by two-dimensional speckle tracking echocardiography. Eur Rev Med Pharmacol Sci. 2015;19:3928–34.

26. Wang Q, Huang D, Zhang L, Shen D, Ouyang Q, Duan Z, et al. Assessment of myocardial infarct size by three-dimensional and two-dimensional speckle tracking echocardiography: a comparative study to single photon emission computed tomography. Echocardiography. 2015;32:1539–46.

27. Qin C, David Meggo-Quiroz L, Nanda NC, Wang X, Xie M. Early effect of essential hypertension on the left ventricular twist-displacement loop by two-dimensional ultrasound speckle tracking imaging. Echocardiography. 2014;31:631–7.

28. Huang J, Yan ZN, Ni XD, Hu YP, Rui YF, Fan L, et al. Left ventricular longitudinal rotation changes in primary hypertension patients with normal left ventricular ejection fraction detected by two-dimensional speckle tracking echocardiography. J Hum Hypertens. 2016;30:30–4.

29. Popović ZB, Kwon DH, Mishra M, Buakhamsri A, Greenberg NL, Thamilarasan M, et al. Association between regional ventricular function and myocardial fibrosis in hypertrophic cardiomyopathy assessed by speckle tracking echocardiography and delayed hyperenhancement magnetic resonance imaging. J Am Soc Echocardiogr. 2008;21:1299–305.

30. Kofflard MJ, Michels M, Krams R, Kliffen M, Geleijnse ML, Ten Cate FJ, et al. Coronary flow reserve in hypertrophic cardiomyopathy: relation with microvascular dysfunction and pathophysiological characteristics. Neth Heart J. 2007;15:209–15.

31. Popović ZB, Grimm RA, Ahmad A, Agler D, Favia M, Dan G, et al. Longitudinal rotation: an unrecognised motion pattern in patients with dilated cardiomyopathy. Heart. 2007;94:1–6.

32. Huang J, Ni XD, Hu YP, Song ZW, Yang WY, Xu R. Left ventricular longitudinal rotation changes in patients with dilated cardiography detected by two dimensional speckle tracking imaging. Zhonghua Xin Xue Guan Bing Za Zhi. 2011;39:920–4.

23

A case report of myocarditis combined with hepatitis caused by herpes simplex virus

Tetsuya Yamamoto[1], Tsuneaki Kenzaka[1,2]* ⓘ, Masanori Matsumoto[1], Ryo Nishio[1,2], Satoru Kawasaki[1] and Hozuka Akita[1]

Abstract

Background: Viral myocarditis presents with various symptoms, including fatal arrhythmia and cardiogenic shock, and may develop into chronic myocarditis and dilated cardiomyopathy in some patients. We report a case of viral myocarditis and hepatitis caused by herpes simplex virus.

Case presentation: A 20-year-old woman was admitted to our hospital with fever, fatigue, and anorexia. The initial investigation showed elevated liver enzyme levels and elevated creatine phosphokinase, and computed tomography showed diffuse swelling and internal heterogeneous image in the liver. These findings were consistent with acute hepatitis; therefore, we performed a liver biopsy, which showed parenchymal necrosis and lymphocytic infiltration. The night that the liver biopsy was performed, blood pressure gradually decreased and revealed cardiogenic shock. Electrocardiography showed diffuse ST-segment elevation, and echocardiography showed a dilated, spherical ventricle with reduced systolic function and pericardial effusion. An endomyocardial biopsy revealed lymphocyte infiltration of the myocardium, confirming acute myocarditis. After a few days, tests for immunoglobin M and immunoglobin G antibodies against herpes simplex virus were positive.

Conclusions: We presented a rare case of myocarditis combined with hepatitis that was caused by herpes simplex virus. Acute myocarditis can occur concurrently with hepatitis, pancreatitis, nephritis, and encephalitis; thus, determining the presence of other infectious lesions is necessary to provide appropriate treatment for the patient.

Keywords: Myocarditis, Hepatitis, Herpes simplex virus, Case report

Background

Myocarditis can present with various symptoms, ranging from mild dyspnea to chest pain, cardiogenic shock, and fatal arrhythmia. The main cause of myocarditis is current or recent viral infection [1]. Enteroviruses, specifically Coxsackievirus (CV) group B serotypes, have traditionally been perceived as the predominant viral cause [2], although adenoviruses, parvovirus B19, and human herpes virus 6 can also cause myocarditis [3–5]. In contrast, herpes simplex virus (HSV) rarely causes acute myocarditis. A few case reports described that viral myocarditis may be combined with hepatitis, pancreatitis, nephritis, and encephalitis [6–8].

We encountered a case of combined myocarditis and hepatitis caused by HSV infection.

Case presentation

A 20-year-old woman, who had an unremarkable medical history and was immunocompetent, was admitted to another hospital due to fever, fatigue, and anorexia, and she was administered acetaminophen and antibiotics. She also experienced vomiting, as well as systemic myalgia 5 days after admission causing an inability to move.

* Correspondence: smile.kenzaka@jichi.ac.jp
[1]Department of Internal Medicine, Hyogo Prefectural Kaibara Hospital, 5208-1, Kaibara, Kaibara-cho, Tanba, Hyogo 669-3395, Japan
[2]Division of Community Medicine and Career Development, Kobe University Graduate School of Medicine, 2-1-5, Arata-cho, Hyogo-ku, Kobe, Hyogo 652-0032, Japan

Her condition was worsening, and she was transferred to our hospital 7 days after her initial admission. Upon admission, her liver enzyme and creatine phosphokinase (CPK or CK) levels were high. She had no history of jaundice, pruritus, clay stools, melena, hematemesis, abdominal distension, or altered sensorium. She reported only an occasional small amount of ethanol intake and had not had sexual intercourse. The patient denied intake of indigenous medicine or intoxication. The patient did not report any past major surgeries, blood transfusions, or intravenously injected drug abuse prior to onset of the disease. Additionally, she did not report any history of diabetes, hypertension, tuberculosis, thyroid disease, trauma, exposure to industrial toxins or radiation, blood or blood component therapy, bleeding disorders, promiscuity, or similar complaints in the family or neighborhood.

Upon admission, her vital signs were as follows: body temperature, 37.2 °C; blood pressure, 110/72 mmHg; pulse, 75 beats/min; respiratory rate, 20 breaths/min; and oxygen

Table 1 Laboratory data upon admission

Parameter	Recorded value	Standard value
White blood cell count	10,060/μL	4500–7500/μL
Neutrophils	56.9%	
Hemoglobin	16.4 g/dL	11.3–15.2 g/dL
Hematocrit	47.6%	36–45%
Platelet count	12.6×10^4/μL	$13–35 \times 10^3$/μL
International normalized ratio	1.19	0.80–1.20
Activated partial thromboplastin time	33.4 s	26.9–38.1 s
C-reactive protein	1.52 mg/L	≤1.0 mg/L
Total protein	6.8 g/dL	6.9–8.4 g/dL
Albumin	4.0 g/dL	3.9–5.1 g/dL
Total bilirubin	0.8 mg/dL	0.2–1.2 mg/dL
Aspartate aminotransferase	2082 U/L	11–30 U/L
Alanine aminotransferase	1824 U/L	4–30 U/L
LDH	4191 U/L	109–216 U/L
LDH-1	12.9%	
LDH-2	15.2%	
LDH-3	13.3%	
LDH-4	18.2%	
LDH-5	38.7%	
CK	3753 U/L	40–150 U/L
CK-MM	99.4%	
CK-MB	0.6%	
Blood urea nitrogen	38.8 mg/dL	8–20 mg/dL
Creatinine	0.8 mg/dL	0.63–1.03 mg/dL
Sodium	134 mEq/L	136–148 mEq/L
Potassium	5.2 mEq/L	3.6–5.0 mEq/L
Chloride	106 mEq/L	98–108 mEq/L
Glucose	108 mg/dL	70–109 mg/dL
pH	7.474	7.350–7.450
Partial pressure of carbon dioxide	34.9 mmHg	35.0–45.0 mmHg
Bicarbonate ion	25.1 mEq/L	23.0–28.0 mEq/L
Lactic acid	3.04 mmol/L	0.44–1.78 mmol/L
Anion gap	11.9 mEq/L	10.0–14.0 mEq/L

LDH lactate dehydrogenase, *CK* creatine phosphokinase, *CK-MM* CK in the skeletal muscle, *CK-MB* CK in the blood

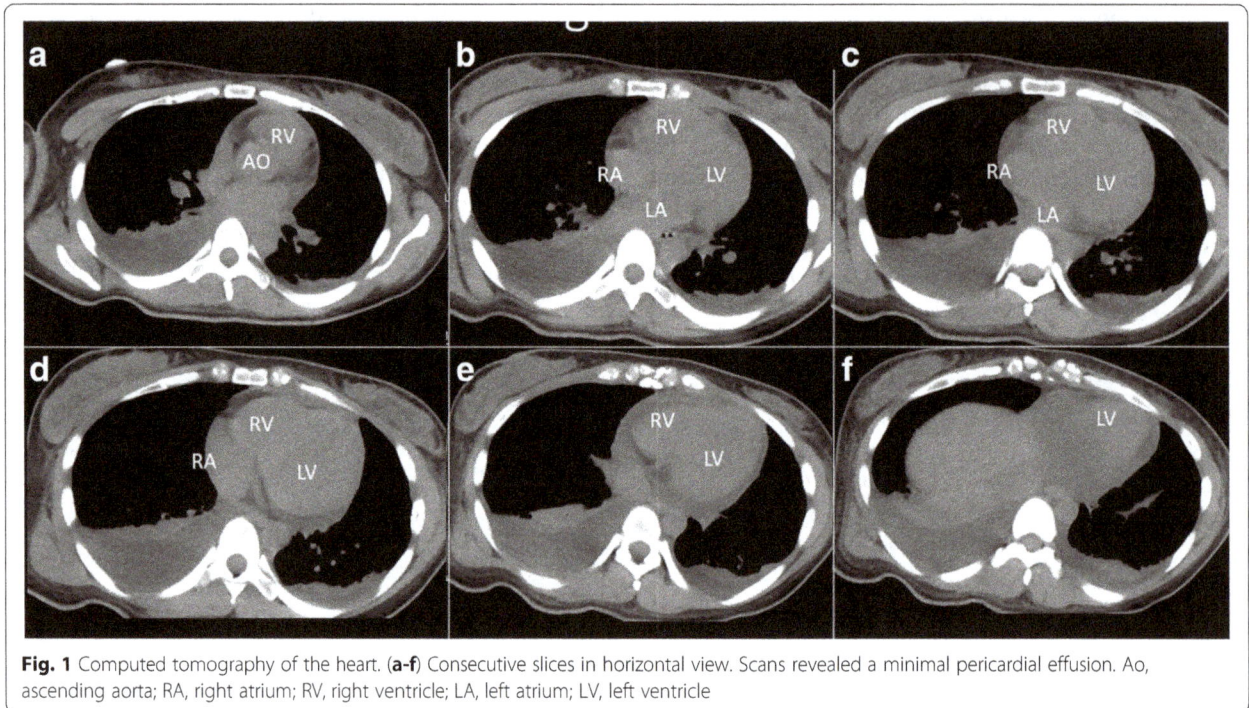

Fig. 1 Computed tomography of the heart. (**a-f**) Consecutive slices in horizontal view. Scans revealed a minimal pericardial effusion. Ao, ascending aorta; RA, right atrium; RV, right ventricle; LA, left atrium; LV, left ventricle

saturation, 98% on room air. A physical examination revealed mild enlargement of the liver, no pitting edema in both legs, and no coarse crackles over the lung fields. Laboratory findings are presented in Table 1.

Additionally, a chest radiography showed absence of pulmonary congestion, pleural effusion, and cardiomegaly. Electrocardiography was not performed on admission. Computed tomography of the chest (Fig. 1) and abdomen revealed minimal pericardial effusion, diffuse swelling, and an internal heterogeneous image in the

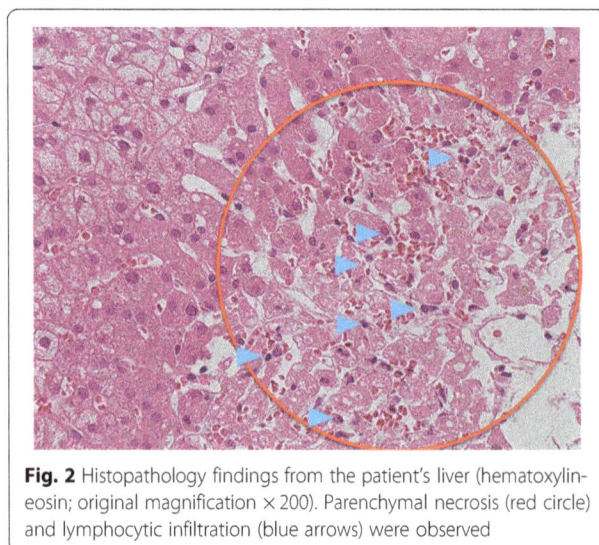

Fig. 2 Histopathology findings from the patient's liver (hematoxylin-eosin; original magnification × 200). Parenchymal necrosis (red circle) and lymphocytic infiltration (blue arrows) were observed

liver. These findings were compatible with acute hepatitis; therefore, we did not examine for cardiac function despite the presentation of pericardial effusion.

On the second day of hospitalization, we performed a liver biopsy, which showed parenchymal necrosis and lymphocytic infiltration (Fig. 2). On that same night, the patient was hypotensive, with a blood pressure of 80/65 mmHg, and her heart rate was elevated (113 beats/min). Physical examination revealed cyanosis of the lips, distended external jugular veins, pretibial edema in both legs, and coarse crackles over the lower bilateral lung fields.

Electrocardiography showed diffuse ST-segment elevation (Fig. 3). Her troponin I, CK level in the blood (CK-MB), and brain natriuretic peptide (BNP) were elevated (troponin T, 0.879 ng/mL [normal value: ≤0.016 ng/mL]; CK-MB, 253 U/L [normal value: ≤5 U/L]; BNP, 1513 pg/mL [normal value: ≤18.4 pg/mL]). Chest radiography showed a normal cardiac size, pulmonary congestion, and pleural effusion in the right lung only (Fig. 4). Echocardiography showed a dilated, spherical ventricle with reduced systolic function (left ventricle ejection fraction [LVEF], 17%) and pericardial effusion (Fig. 5).

Cardiac catheterization on day 3 revealed high pulmonary capillary wedge pressure (22 mmHg) and a low cardiac index (2.0 L/min/m^2). Coronary angiography showed no abnormalities. Endomyocardial biopsy (EMB) was performed via the right internal jugular vein, and five specimens were obtained from the right ventricle

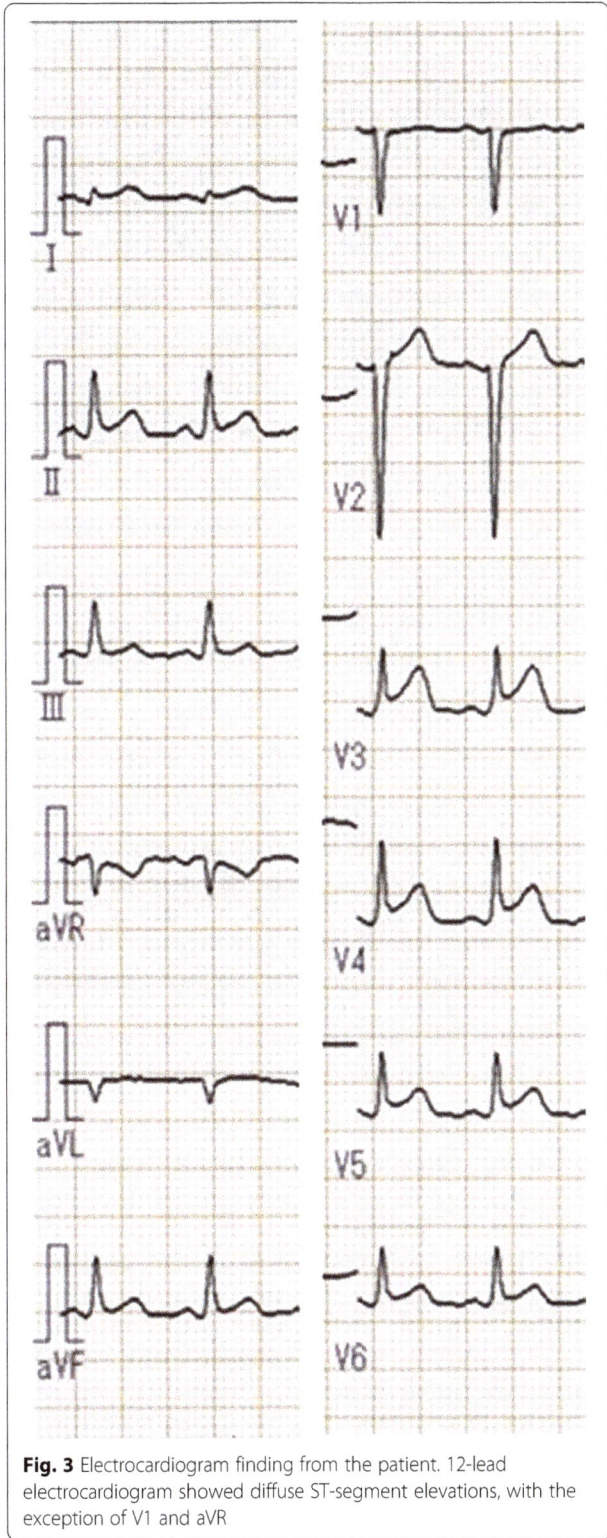

Fig. 3 Electrocardiogram finding from the patient. 12-lead electrocardiogram showed diffuse ST-segment elevations, with the exception of V1 and aVR

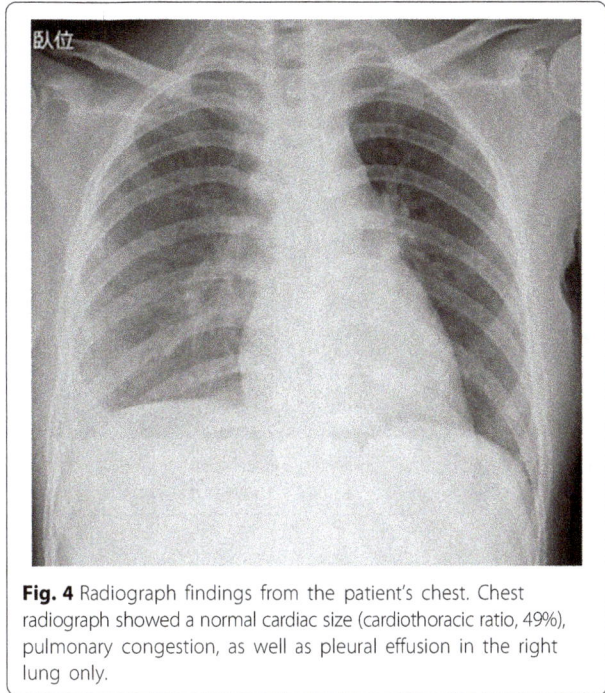

Fig. 4 Radiograph findings from the patient's chest. Chest radiograph showed a normal cardiac size (cardiothoracic ratio, 49%), pulmonary congestion, as well as pleural effusion in the right lung only.

intravenous administration of dobutamine (4 μg/kg/min) was started on day 3. The patient's systolic blood pressure increased to approximately 100 mmHg and stabilized, and dobutamine administration was gradually tapered off. On day 10, echocardiography showed normalization of LVEF to 71%, dobutamine was stopped, and laboratory findings were almost normalized as follows: CPK, 143 U/L (standard values: 40–150 U/L); aspartate aminotransferase (AST), 36 U/L (standard values: 11–30 U/L); and alanine aminotransferase (ALT), 278 U/L (standard values: 4–30 U/L). Laboratory findings on day 18 were normalized as follows: CPK, 123 U/L; AST, 18 U/L; ALT, 21 U/L, and BNP, 18 pg/mL. She was eventually discharged on day 19 of her hospital stay.

One serum sample for viral serological testing was collected before the EMBs were obtained. Follow-up serum samples were collected between 2 weeks, 1 month, and 6 months after the initial serum sample. The presence of HSV-specific immunoglobulin M (IgM) was detected upon admission to our hospital, increased at 2 weeks, and returned to normal 6 months later. Additionally, HSV-specific immunoglobulin G (IgG) increased from hospital admission to 2 weeks (Table 2). Other viral serologic tests, including HIV, were negative (Table 3). Based on this finding, we diagnosed the patient with acute myocarditis combined with hepatitis arising from HSV infection.

Discussion and conclusions

We described a rare case of combined myocarditis and hepatitis caused by HSV infection. To the best of

side of the interventricular septum. Endomyocardial biopsy findings showed lymphocyte infiltration of the myocardium and intranuclear inclusions, which was confirmed as acute myocarditis (Fig. 6). In response,

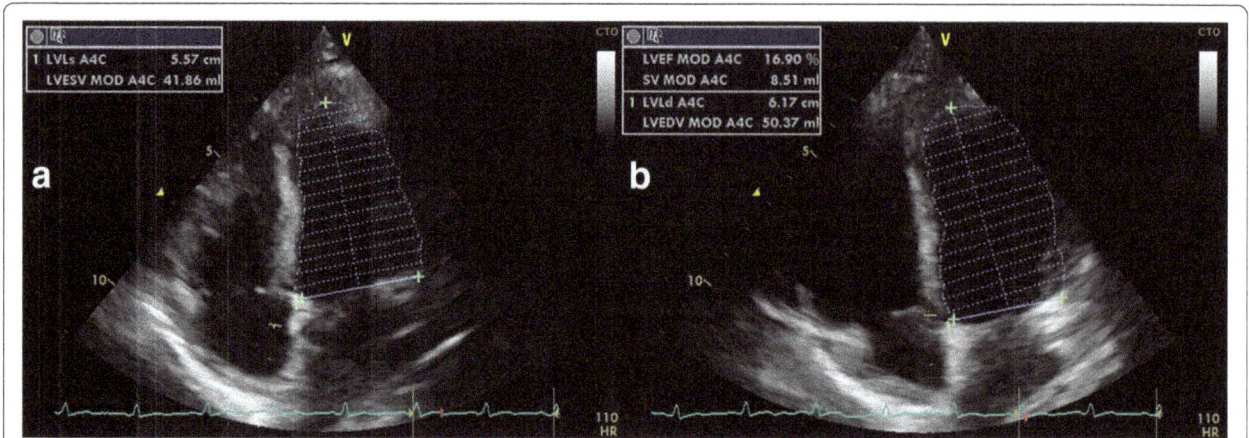

Fig. 5 Echocardiographic findings via apical four chamber views showing (**a**) end-systolic and (**b**) end-diastolic volumes. The echocardiography showed a dilated, spherical ventricle with reduced systolic function (left ventricle ejection fraction, 17%) and pericardial effusion

our knowledge, this is the first case of combined myocarditis and hepatitis arising from HSV infection. In our case, both heart and liver biopsies were completed, and lymphocytic infiltration was detected in both biopsies.

Herpes simplex virus hepatitis is an uncommon complication of HSV infection, often leading to acute liver failure (ALF). It is thought to represent less than 1% of all ALF cases, and less than 2% of all viral causes of ALF [9]. Additionally, 24% of HSV hepatitis cases were considered immunocompetent. The remaining patients were either pregnant (23%) or immunocompromised from a previous solid organ, hematopoietic cell transplantation (30%), or immunosuppressive agent (23%) [10]. Symptoms are transient and mild in immunocompetent patients, and serious or fatal in immunocompromised patients [11].

Herpes simplex virus-induced myocarditis is also uncommon. Bowles et al. reported that polymerase chain reactions were positive for HSV in 5 of 624

(0.8%) samples obtained from patients with myocarditis [12]. It has been reported that viral myocarditis may be combined with hepatitis, pancreatitis, nephritis, and encephalitis, but the majority of these reports used postmortem biopsies [6–8]. In our case, both heart and liver biopsies were completed, and lymphocytic infiltration was observed in both biopsies. Moreover, the pathological findings of the EMB specimen did not indicate ischemic hepatitis. We performed a biopsy from multiple organs of the patient, whereas previous reports generally obtained a pathology specimen via necropsy examination. Therefore, reports that obtained a pathology specimen during the patient's lifetime were rare. Although we could not confirm HSV in our pathological examination, it was serologically apparent that HSV was the cause of the infection.

It is often believed that liver enzyme elevation in a patient with myocarditis stems from ischemic hepatitis. In most cases, we cannot perform liver biopsy because of the patient's systemic condition and coagulation disorder; however, we must not forget that in a few instances, hepatitis is combined with myocarditis. Acute myocarditis may be combined with hepatitis, pancreatitis, nephritis, and encephalitis; therefore, it is important to determine whether other infectious lesions are present.

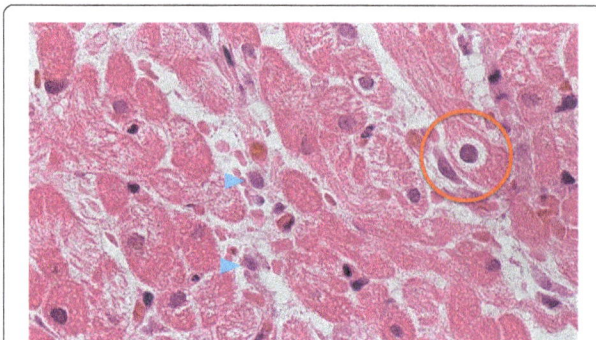

Fig. 6 Endomyocardial biopsy (hematoxylin-eosin; original magnification × 400). Lymphocyte infiltration of the myocardium and intranuclear inclusions (red circle) were observed

Table 2 Clinical course of herpes simplex virus-specific immunoglobulin M and immunoglobulin G

	Standard value	Admission	2 week	1 month	6 month
HSV-IgM	0.7	11.72	13.27	10.06	0.20
HSV-IgG	1.9	8.0	19.4	20.6	12.0

HSV herpes simplex virus, *IgM* immunoglobin M, *IgG* immunoglobin G

Table 3 Laboratory data for hepatitis and causative infection agent

T-SPOT	Negative
Antinuclear antibody	40
Anti-M2 Ab	Negative
HBs Ag	Negative
Anti-HBs Ab	Negative
Anti-HBc Ab	Negative
Anti-HCV Ab	Negative
HAV-IgM	0.16
HAV-IgG	0.2
HEV-IgA	Negative
EBVCA-IgM	0.0
EBVCA-IgG	3.3
EBNA-IgG	2.1
HSV-IgM	11.72
HSV-IgG	8.0
CMV-IgM	0.16
CMV-IgG	0.2
PVB19-IgM	Negative
Coxsackievirus	Negative
Adenovirus 3	Negative
Adenovirus 7	Negative
Influenza A/B antigen	Negative
Anti-HIV Ag/Ab	Negative

Ab antibody, *CMV* cytomegalovirus, *EBNA* Epstein–Barr nuclear antigen, *EBVCA* Epstein-Barr virus capsid antigen, *HAV* hepatitis A virus, *HBc Ab* hepatitis B core antibody, *HEV* hepatitis E virus, *HBs AG* hepatitis B surface antigen, *HIV* human immunodeficiency virus, *HSV* herpes simplex virus, *IgA, IgG, IgM* immunoglobulin A, G, M; PVB19, parvovirus B19

In conclusion, we presented a rare case of myocarditis combined with hepatitis that was caused by HSV infection. Acute myocarditis can have concurrence with hepatitis, pancreatitis, nephritis, and encephalitis; thus, determining the presence of other infectious lesions is necessary to provide appropriate treatment for the patient.

Abbreviations
ALF: Acute liver failure; ALT: Alanine aminotransferase; AST: Aspartate aminotransferase; BNP: Brain natriuretic peptide; CK-MB: CK level in the blood; CPK or CK: Creatine phosphokinase; CV: Coxsackievirus; EMB: Endomyocardial biopsy; HSV: Herpes simplex virus; IgG: Immunoglobulin G; IgM: Immunoglobulin M; LDH: Lactate dehydrogenase; LVEF: Left ventricle ejection fraction

Authors' contributions
TY managed the case and redaction and correction of the manuscript. TK assisted with redaction, correction, and reconstruction of the manuscript. MM, RN, and SK also assisted with clinical management of the case and correction of the manuscript. HA assisted with manuscript correction and redaction of comments from the illustrations. All authors read and approved the final manuscript.

Competing interests
The authors declare that they have no competing interests.

References
1. Cooper LT Jr. Myocarditis. N Engl J Med. 2009;360:1526–38.
2. Magnani JW, Dec GW. Myocarditis: current trends in diagnosis and treatment. Circulation. 2006;113:876–90.
3. Feldman AM, McNamara D. Myocarditis. N Engl J Med. 2000;343:1388–98.
4. Dec GW Jr, Palacios IF, Fallon JT, Aretz HT, Mills J, Lee DC, et al. Active myocarditis in the spectrum of acute dilated cardiomyopathies. Clinical features, histologic correlates, and clinical outcome. N Engl J Med. 1985;312: 885–90.
5. Mahrholdt H, Wagner A, Deluigi CC, Kispert E, Hager S, Meinhardt G, et al. Presentation, patterns of myocardial damage, and clinical course of viral myocarditis. Circulation. 2006;114:1581–90.
6. Smith WG, Coxsackie B. Myopericarditis in adults. Am Heart J. 1970;80:34–46.
7. Akuzawa N, Harada N, Hatori T, Imai K, Kitahara Y, Sakurai S, et al. Myocarditis, hepatitis, and pancreatitis in a patient with coxsackievirus A4 infection: a case report. Virol J. 2014;11:3.
8. Martin AB, Webber S, Fricker FJ, Jaffe R, Demmler G, Kearney D, et al. Acute myocarditis. Rapid diagnosis by PCR in children. Circulation. 1994;90:330–9.
9. Schiødt FV, Davern TJ, Shakil AO, McGuire B, Samuel G, Lee WM. Viral hepatitis-related acute liver failure. Am J Gastroenterol. 2003;98:448–53.
10. Norvell JP, Blei AT, Jovanovic BD, Levitsky J. Herpes simplex virus hepatitis: an analysis of the published literature and institutional cases. Liver Transpl. 2007;13:1428–34.
11. Miyagawa K, Shibata M, Kumei S, Matsuhashi T, Hiura M, Abe S, et al. A case of resolved hepatitis B who was observed HBV viremia transiently during HSV hepatitis immediately after steroid pulse therapy. Kanzo. 2014;55:51–6.
12. Bowles NE, Ni J, Kearney DL, Pauschinger M, Schultheiss HP, McCarthy R, et al. Detection of viruses in myocardial tissues by polymerase chain reaction. Evidence of adenovirus as a common cause of myocarditis in children and adults. J Am Coll Cardiol. 2003;42:466–72.

24

Clinical outcomes associated with catecholamine use in patients diagnosed with Takotsubo cardiomyopathy

Uzair Ansari[1,3]* ⓘ, Ibrahim El-Battrawy[1,2], Christian Fastner[1], Michael Behnes[1], Katherine Sattler[1], Aydin Huseynov[1], Stefan Baumann[1], Erol Tülümen[1], Martin Borggrefe[1,2] and Ibrahim Akin[1,2]

Abstract

Background: Recent hypotheses have suggested the pathophysiological role of catecholamines in the evolution of the Takotsubo syndrome (TTS). The extent of cardiac and circulatory compromise dictates the use of some form of supportive therapy. This study was designed to investigate the clinical outcomes associated with catecholamine use in TTS patients.

Methods: Our institutional database constituted a collective of 114 patients diagnosed with TTS between 2003 and 2015. The study-patients were subsequently classified into two groups based on the need for catecholamine support during hospital stay (catecholamine group $n = 93$; 81%, non-catecholamine group = 21; 19%). The primary end-point of our study was all-cause mortality.

Results: Patients receiving catecholamine support showed higher grades of circulatory and cardiac compromise (left ventricular ejection fraction (LVEF) 39.6% vs. 32.7%, p-value < 0.01) and the course of disease was often complicated by the occurrence of different TTS-associated complications. The in-hospital mortality (3.2% vs. 28.5%, $p < 0.01$), 30-day mortality (17.2% vs. 51.4%, $p < 0.01$) as well as long-term mortality (38.7% vs. 80.9%, $p < 0.01$) was significantly higher in the group of patients receiving catecholamine support. A multivariate Cox regression analysis attributed EF $\leq 35\%$ (HR 3.6, 95% CI 1.6–8.1; $p < 0.01$) and use of positive inotropic agents (HR 2.2, 95% CI 1.0–4.8; p 0.04) as independent predictors of the adverse outcome.

Conclusion: Rates of in-hospital events and short- as well as long-term mortality were significantly higher in TTS patients receiving catecholamine support as compared to the other study-patients. These results need further evaluation in pre-clinical and clinical trials to determine if external catecholamines contribute to an adverse clinical outcome already compromised by the initial insult.

Keywords: Takotsubo cardiomyopathy, Cardiogenic shock, Heart failure, Catecholamines

Background

The Takotsubo Syndrome (TTS) is as an acute and usually reversible from of heart failure characterized by a transient dysfunction of the left ventricle [1, 2]. The TTS patient presents with clinical features such as acute chest pain and dyspnea, bearing some similarity to the patient presenting with an acute myocardial infarction or an acute coronary syndrome (ACS) [3]. An increase in cardiac troponin and creatine kinase levels as well as electrocardiogram (ECG) changes on admission suggesting ST-segment elevation in precordial leads adds to the confusion in early diagnosis. The absence of significant coronary stenosis on coronary angiography, which could correlate with this presentation, and the history of an emotional or physical trigger, leads to the potential diagnosis of TTS [3, 4]. This non-ischemic syndrome has also alternatively been labeled as a stress- or stress-induced cardiomyopathy, an apical ballooning syndrome, or 'broken heart syndrome' [4–8].

---

* Correspondence: uzair.ansari@umm.de

[1]First Department of Medicine, University Medical Center Mannheim, University of Heidelberg, Mannheim, Germany

[3]First Department of Medicine, University Medical Center Mannheim, Theodor-Kutzer-Ufer 1-3, 68167 Mannheim, Germany

Full list of author information is available at the end of the article

The classical pattern of left ventricular (LV) morphology in TTS, present in almost 50–80% of all patients, is the apical variant, which is characterized by apical ballooning of the LV at end-systole. Other morphological presentations include those defined by a predominantly hypokinetic circumferential base (inverted Takotsubo variant), or a hypokinetic circumferential mid ventricle (mid LV variant), or demonstrating focal variations [9–13].

The pathophysiology of TTS has been well-debated, however is still poorly described. The influence of an acute catecholaminergic surge contributing to some form of myocardial stunning has been hypothesized by several researchers [14]. Stressful triggers could potentially contribute to an increased hypothalamic-pituitary-adrenal axis (HPA) gain and catecholamine release. This resulting catecholamine surge possibly directs a pathological response from the cardiovascular as well the sympathetic nervous system and serves as the basis for the evolution of TTS [15, 16].

This interesting correlate, naturally, has far-reaching clinical implications. The therapeutic use of catecholamines has been routinely advocated in cases of circulatory compromise, however, its use in the setting of TTS could have potential drawbacks. Extrapolating this thought, our study attempts to explore the hither to poorly understood pathophysiological mechanisms involved in the TTS and determine if external catecholamines contribute to an adverse clinical outcome already compromised by the initial insult.

Methods

Study design and population characteristics

This study incorporated a population subset derived from a patient collective diagnosed with TTS at the University Medical Centre Mannheim, Germany between January 2003 and September 2015. A total of 114 patients were included consecutively to this monocentric and observational study designed for retrospective data analysis. All these patients were essentially diagnosed with the TTS on hospital admission, and their presenting features met the conditions set out by the modified Mayo Clinic Criteria [17]. These criteria essentially highlight the transient wall motion abnormality in the LV mid-segments with or without apical involvement; describe regional wall motion abnormalities that extend beyond a single epicardial vascular distribution; and define an event that occurs frequently, but not always in the wake of a successful trigger. Additionally, these salient criteria mandate the effective rule-out of occlusive coronary disease; focuses on the appearance of new ECG pathologies, which mimic ACS or modest elevations in cardiac troponin levels; and underlines the prerequisite absence of diseases like pheochromocytoma and myocarditis in the patient.

Patients with co-existing occlusive coronary artery disease as well as those exhibiting wall-motion abnormalities corresponding to any single coronary vessel territory were excluded from this study. A total of 18 patients with uncertain TTS, with no record of coronary angiography or echocardiography results, were excluded from this study. The relevant clinical data of each study-patient was ascertained and compiled in a database with significant aspects of their medical history, laboratory work-up and medical/surgical therapy efficiently earmarked for future reference. Additional parameters outlined for evaluation included duration of hospital stay, need for monitoring and care in the ICU (intensive care unit), use of invasive or non-invasive ventilation, inotropic support, temporary pacing, and demand for renal replacement therapy. Essential diagnostic workup including a routine ECG, echocardiography (to evaluate LV, RV function and wall-motion abnormalities), and a coronary and LV angiography (to rule out occlusive coronary artery disease) was performed on all patients. A consolidated review of this data was conducted by two independent cardiologists and once the diagnosis of TTS was reaffirmed, the study-patients were subsequently classified into two groups based on the need for catecholamine support during hospital stay. A consortium diagram to explain the population recruitment has been outlined in Fig. 1.

The primary end-point of our study was all-cause mortality as assessed by chart review and/or telephonic review. If medical records, treating physicians or relatives were unable to provide further information concerning the circumstances of death, it was defined as death due to unknown cause.

The research conduct corresponded to the principles outlined in the declaration of Helsinki and was approved by the medical ethics committee of the Faculty of Medicine in Mannheim, University of Heidelberg, Germany.

Statistics

Statistical analyses were performed using SPSS Version 22 (SPSS Inc., Chicago, Illinois). Data is presented here as means ± SD for continuous variables with a normal distribution, median (interquartile range) for continuous variables with a non-normal distribution, and as frequency (%) for categorical variables. The Kolmogorov–Smirnov test was used to assess normal distribution. Student's t-test and the Mann–Whitney U-test were used to compare continuous variables with normal and non-normal distributions, respectively. The chi-squared-test or Fisher's exact test was used to compare categorical variables. The log-rank test was used to compare the survival curves between the two patient groups classified as per catecholamine use. p-values < 0.10 on univariate analysis were further evaluated via the Cox multivariate

132 patients received the diagnosis Takotsubo syndrome (TTS)
between 2003-2015 at Institution of Medical Faculty Mannheim

Clinical Profile   In-hospital complications

18 patients with uncertain TTS were excluded

114 patients were included in 5 years follow-up analysis

114 patients were included in Kaplan-Meier

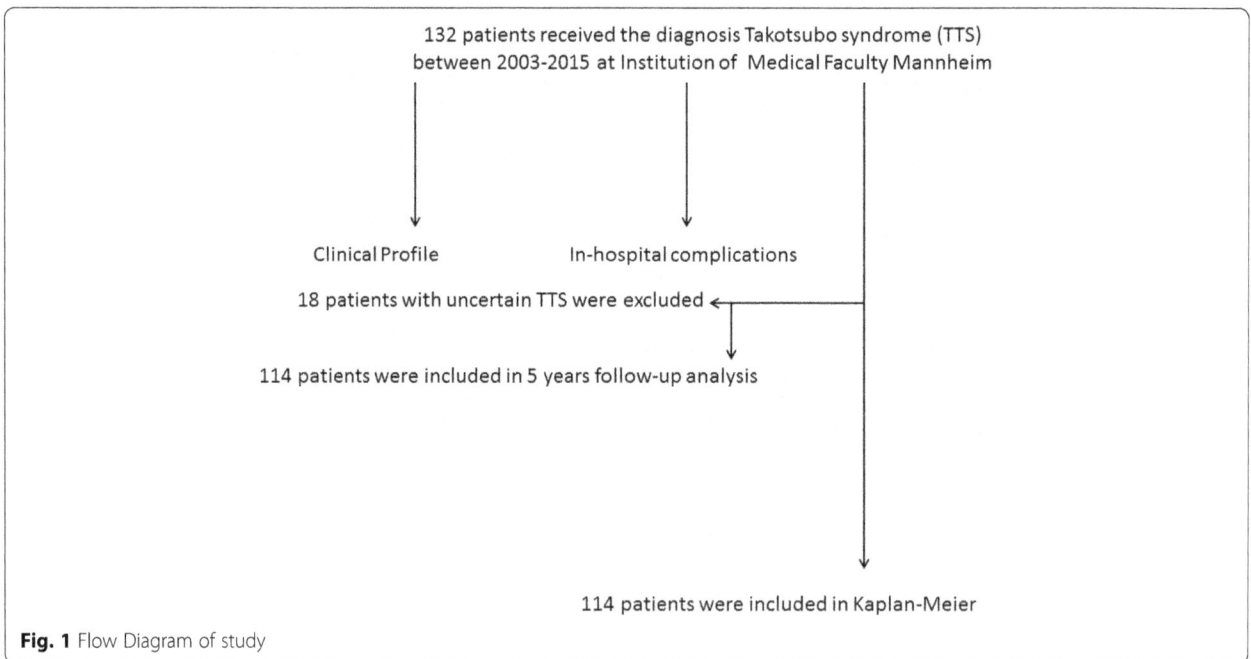

Fig. 1 Flow Diagram of study

regression to define independent risk factors for the respective end-point. A two-tailed p-value of < 0.05 was considered statistically significant.

Results

Baseline characteristics

The baseline characteristics of the 114 patients included in this study have been referenced in Table 1.

A detailed analysis of available data revealed an insignificant demographic distribution, with age and gender variables expressed almost similarly in both patient groups. Chest pain was interestingly more pronounced in the hemodynamically stable patient (55.9%, $n = 52$, vs. 28.5%, $n = 6$, $p = 0.03$) as compared to those requiring some form of catecholamine support. The clinical parameters used to ascertain patient status, such as systolic blood pressure (134.96 ± 28.41 mmHg vs. 116.25 ± 42.3 mmHg, $p = 0.01$) and heart rate (98.1 ± 27.6 bpm vs. 110.9 ± 22.7 bpm, $p = 0.03$), expectedly showed variation between the two groups, wherein lower blood pressure values and mild tachycardia was frequently observed among patients requiring catecholamine support.

Diagnostic parameters

The initial diagnostic work-up, detailed with an electrocardiogram, suggested catecholamine-support-free patients recorded significantly longer QTc-Interval's as opposed to the hemodynamically unstable catecholamine therapy-dependent patient (484.49 ± 50.83 ms vs. 455.30 ± 52.82 ms, $p = 0.02$). Other diagnostic parameters like echocardiographic estimates of left-ventricular ejection fraction revealed a comparatively lower degree

of compromise in cardiac function among patients not requiring external catecholamines (index LVEF measurements $39.67 \pm 9.12\%$ vs. $32.76 \pm 9.09\%$, $p < 0.01$). Similarly, lower index troponin-I levels were documented in this group (3.20 ± 4.41 U/l vs. 6.57 ± 8.46 U/l, $p = 0.01$). Right ventricular involvement was less pronounced in the non-catecholamine support patient-group (18.2%, $n = 17$ vs. 42.85%, $n = 9$, $p = 0.02$).

In-hospital outcome

Data detailing in-hospital events and treatment strategies adopted for our study population suggested that patients suffering from hemodynamic compromise and requiring catecholamine support had a significantly increased incidence of life-threatening arrhythmias (33.3%, $n = 7$ vs. 6.4%, $n = 6$, $p < 0.01$) as well as cardiogenic shock (85.7%, $n = 18$ vs. 4.3%, $n = 4$, $p < 0.01$) and often required admission to an intensive care unit with longer stays (9.5 ± 11.3 days vs. 3.2 ± 3.5 days, $p < 0.01$). Rates of in-hospital death were higher among patients receiving catecholamine support (28.5%, n = 6 vs. 3.2%, $n = 3$, $p < 0.01$). Non-invasive positive pressure ventilation, endotracheal intubation and cardiopulmonary resuscitation procedures were practised significantly more often in patients constituting this group, Table 2.

Long-term follow-up

TTS patients receiving catecholamine support registered significantly higher 30-day mortality rates as compared to the clinically stable patient (57.14%, $n = 12$ vs.17.2%, $n = 16$, $p < 0.01$). Furthermore, these patients showed an ongoing increased risk of death beyond the first 30-days

Table 1 Baseline characteristics of 114 patients initially presenting with TTC

Variables	No catecholamines (n = 93)	catecholamines (n = 21)	p value*
Demographics			
Age, mean ± SD	67.65 ± 11.00	65.00 ± 12.30	0.33
Male, n (%)	13 (13.97)	6 (28.57)	0.11
Symptoms, n (%)			
Dyspnoe	34 (36.55)	9 (42.85)	0.62
Chest pain	52 (55.91)	6 (28.57)	**0.03**
Clinic parameter			
Systolic BP, mmHg	134.96 ± 28.41	116.25 ± 42.32	**0.01**
Diastolic BP, mmHg	78.41 ± 13.67	66.55 ± 31.22	**0.03**
Heart rate, bpm	98.17 ± 27.64	110.95 ± 22.79	**0.05**
ECG Data, n (%)			
ST-segment elevation	27 (29.03)	7 (33.33)	0.79
Inversed T-Waves	83 (89.24)	19 (90.47)	0.74
PQ-interval	160.67 ± 27.97	160.00 ± 34.38	0.92
QTc (ms), mean ± SD	484.49 ± 50.83	455.30 ± 52.82	**0.02**
Stress factor, n (%)			
Emotional sress	28 (30.10)	2 (9.52)	**0.05**
Physical stress	50 (53.76)	14 (66.66)	0.33
Laboratory values, mean ± SD			
Troponin I (U/L)	3.20 ± 4.41	6.57 ± 8.46	**0.01**
Creatine phosphatkinase (U/L)	721.11 ± 2900.64	323.74 ± 469.71	0.55
CKMB	37.44 ± 65.08	31.00 ± 23.56	0.77
C-Reactive protein (mg/l)	42.63 ± 64.25	80.30 ± 126.15	0.06
Hemoglobin	12.10 ± 1.99	12.29 ± 2.08	0.70
Creatinine (mg/dl)	1.14 ± 0.76	1.19 ± 0.50	0.79
GFR < 60 ml/min	25 (26.88)	7 (33.33)	0.59
Echocardiography data, n (%)			
LV EF %	39.67 ± 9.12	32.76 ± 9.09	**< 0.01**
Follow-up LV EF %	55.23 ± 7.54	48.63 ± 14.90	**< 0.01**
Apical ballooning	64 (68.81)	18 (85.71)	0.15
Mitral regurgation	50 (53.76)	10 (47.61)	0.63
Tricspid regurgation	42 (45.16)	7 (33.33)	0.46
RV-Involvement	17 (18.27)	9 (42.85)	**0.02**
Medical history, n (%)			
Smoking	30 (32.25)	6 (28.57)	0.80
Diabetes mellitus	22 (23.65)	4 (19.04)	0.64
Obesity (BMI > 25 kg/m²)	27 (29.03)	4 (19.04)	0.75
Hypertension	54 (58.06)	12 (57.14)	1.00
COPD	19 (20.43)	7 (33.33)	0.25
Atrial fibrillation	15 (16.12)	6 (28.57)	0.21
Coronary artery disease	16 (17.20)	6 (28.57)	0.23

Table 1 Baseline characteristics of 114 patients initially presenting with TTC *(Continued)*

Variables	No catecholamines (n = 93)	catecholamines (n = 21)	p value*
History of malignancy	13 (13.97)	3 (14.28)	0.97
Drugs on admission, n (%)			
Beta-blocker	32 (34.40)	3 (14.28)	0.06
ACE inhibitor	30 (32.25)	5 (23.80)	0.45
ASS	24 (25.80)	5 (23.80)	0.87
Anticoagulation	7 (7.52)	0 (0)	0.19

*p values for the comparison between *group 1* and *group 2*; *SD* Standard deviation, *ECG* Electrocardiogram, *EF* Ejection fraction, *BMI* body-mass-index, *COPD* Chronic obstructive pulmonary disease, *ACE* Angiotensin-convetring-enzyme
EFhochversusnichthoch*Katecholaminpflichtigkeit: 0.000
The bolded indication highlight significant values

after hospital admission resulting in considerably higher long-term mortality-rates (80.95%, $n = 17$ vs. 38.70%, $n = 36$, $p < 0.01$); Table 3, Fig. 2. In a Cox univariate analysis EF ≤35% (HR 4.8, 95% CI 2.2–104; $p < 0.01$), male gender (HR 2.6, 95% CI 1.2–5.7; p 0.01) and use of positive inotropic agents (HR 3.9, 95% CI 1.9–7.9; $p < 0.01$) were associated with an adverse outcome. In comparison, a multivariate Cox regression analysis attributed EF ≤ 35% (HR 3.6, 95% CI 1.6–8.1; $p < 0.01$) and use of positive inotropic agents (HR 2.2, 95% CI 1.0–4.8; p 0.04) as independent predictors of the adverse outcome, Table 4. The various causes of death have been illustrated in Table 5.

Discussion

The principal foundation of this study was to determine the role and influence of catecholamine therapy in the treatment of the hemodynamically unstable TTS patient. At the outset, patients receiving catecholamine support showed

Table 2 In-hospital events and treatment strategy

Variables	No catecholamines (n = 93)	catecholamines (n = 21)	p value*
Life-threatening arrhythmia	6 (6.45)	7 (33.33)	**< 0.01**
NPPV and intubation	21 (22.5)	18 (85.7)	**< 0.01**
Resuscitation	3 (3.22)	6 (28.57)	**< 0.01**
Defibrillator-Implantation	1 (1.0)	1 (4.7)	0.33
VA-ECMO	0 (0)	1 (4.7)	0.18
Admission to ICU, length of stay	3.24 ± 3.59	9.57 ± 11.32	**< 0.01**
In-hospital death	3 (3.2)	6 (28.5)	**< 0.01**
Thromboembolic events	10 (10.75)	4 (19.04)	0.29
Acquired Long QTs	61 (65.59)	12 (57.14)	0.41
Cardiogenic Shock	4 (4.30)	18 (85.71)	**< 0.01**

*p values for the comparison between *no catecholamines* and catecholamines; *NPPV* Noninvasive positive pressure ventilation, *VA-ECMO* Veno-arterial extracorporal membrane oxygenation, *ICU* Intermediate care unit
The bolded indication highlight significant values

Table 3 Outcome (mortality) in TTS patients

Variables	No catecholamines (n = 93)	catecholamines (n = 21)	Relative risk (95% CI)	p value *
In-hospital mortality	3 (3.22)	6 (28.57)	(1.0–6.5)	< 0.01
30-day mortality	3 (2.15)	6 (28.57)	(1.0–6.5)	< 0.01
1-year mortality	6 (6.45)	8 (38.09)	(1.1–3.7)	< 0.01
2-year mortality	11 (11.82)	10 (47.61)	(1.1–2.5)	< 0.01
3-year mortality	12 (12.90)	11 (52.38)	(1.1–2.5)	< 0.01
4-year mortality	18 (19.35)	11 (52.38)	(1.0–1.9)	< 0.01
Long-term mortality	20 (21.50)	13 (61.90)	(1.1–2.0)	< 0.01

*p values for the comparison between no catecholamines and catecholamines

higher degrees of circulatory and cardiac compromise, and the course of disease was often complicated by the occurrence of different TTS-associated complications. This group of patients also demonstrated poorer in-hospital outcomes and had higher long-term mortality rates as compared to the group of patients not receiving any catecholamine support therapy. It could therefore be inferred that circulatory support in the form of catecholamines entails a poorer outcome for the TTS patient. A pertinent question arises when debating the role of catecholamines exacerbating the mortality risk in such a clinical scenario solely on the basis of the pathophysiology of the syndrome. All patients, irrelevant of diagnosis, requiring catecholamine support constitute a clinically compromised group, however, do TTS patients in circulatory or cardiac shock suffer from additional drawbacks due to this line of management? Our results indicate that contemporary circulatory support drugs like catecholamines additionally exacerbates the risk of mortality in a TTS patient. This study is probably the first of many to follow, that has attempted to express this distinct correlation. Although, many studies have attributed some form of

catecholamine toxicity leading to the pathophysiological evolution of TTS, we shall explore this line of discussion further, considering the potential impact on current treatment strategies.

A detailed research of recently published literature highlights the several hypotheses which have been postulated to explain the pathogenesis of TTS. These mechanisms essentially entail the possibility of coronary microvascular dysfunction, coronary artery spasm, catecholamine-induced myocardial stunning, acute LV outflow obstruction, acute increased ventricular afterload, myocardial microinfarction or abnormalities in cardiac fatty acid metabolism influencing the development of TTS [15].

A common link serving these several theories can be construed with the consistent demonstration of some form of microvascular dysfunction among all TTS patients. The research work conducted by Uchida et al. could successfully exhibit the presence of extensive endothelial apoptosis in myocardial biopsies [18] while Afonso et al. demonstrated circulatory disturbances in myocardial contrast echocardiography [19].

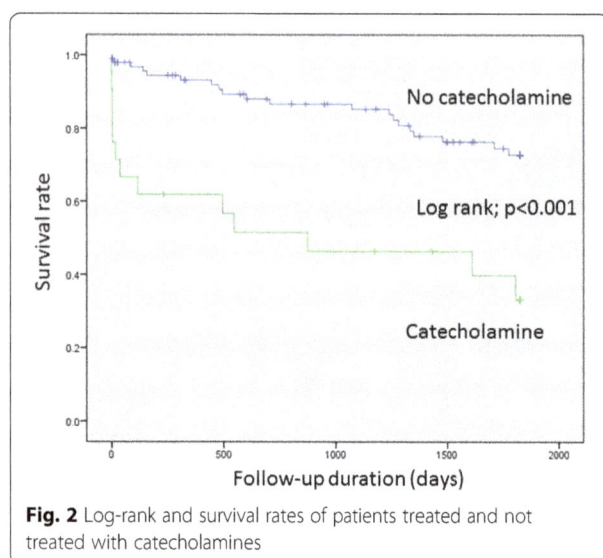

Fig. 2 Log-rank and survival rates of patients treated and not treated with catecholamines

Table 4 Multivariate analysis for the end point (all-cause mortality)

	Univariate analysis			Multivariate analysis[a]		
	HR	95% CI	P-value	HR	95% CI	P-value
Male	2.6	1.2–5.7	**0.01**	1.8	0.8–4.0	0.14
EF ≤ 35%	4.8	2.2–104	**< 0.01**	3.6	1.6–8.1	**< 0.01**
Emotionalerstress	0.4	0.1–1.1	0.10			
Inotropic drugs	3.9	1.9–7.9	**< 0.01**	2.2	1.0–4.8	**0.04**
Diabetes mellitus Typ II	1.0	0.7–1.4	0.81			
Hypertension	0.9	0.7–1.2	0.64			
Apical ballooning	1.1	0.8–1.4	0.39			
History of cancer	1.7	0.7–4.2	0.21			
Smoking	0.7	0.3–1.6	0.49			

HR hazard ratio, EF ejection fraction, CRP c-reactive protein, GFR glomerular filtration rate
[a]Only the following variables with significant effects in univariate analysis were analyzed by multivariate Cox regression: Male, EF ≤ 35%, Inotropic drugs
The bolded indication highlight significant values

Table 5 All-Cause of death

In-hospital mortality

1. Cardiac cause including cardiogenic shock and life-threatening arrhythmia ($n = 6$)
2. Malignoma ($n = 1$)
3. Neurological cause ($n = 2$)

Out of hospital mortality

1. Cardiac cause including cardiogenic shock and life-threatening arrhythmia ($n = 4$)
2. Malignoma ($n = 6$)
3. Sepsis ($n = 4$)
4. Kidney failure ($n = 2$)
5. Pulmonary cause ($n = 2$)
6. Unknown cause ($n = 6$)

Abnormalities associated with endothelium dependent vasodilatation, excessive vasoconstriction and impairment of myocardial perfusion have been associated with coronary microvascular dysfunction seen in TTS patients [20]. The additional demonstration of regional contraction band necrosis, inflammatory cell inflammation and localised fibrosis, all attributed to direct catecholamine toxicity, further corroborates this theory [17, 21]. Interesting results interpreted from the research of Morel et al. suggested that an increase in C-reactive protein levels and white blood cell counts corresponded to increased levels of catecholamines in TTS patients [22]. The raised levels could in theory initiate a systemic inflammation mediated by cytokines like TNF-alpha and interleukin-6, explaining the observation of myocardial oedema in cardiac MRI [23]. In animal models of TTS, as prepared by Paur et al., the use of high bolus doses of catecholamines has simulated LV apical ballooning [24]. Additional studies by Wittstein et al., proving increased levels of circulating catecholamines in TTS patients as compared to those with myocardial infarction, as well as the theory of "stimulus trafficking" (involving a switch in intracellular signal trafficking from Gs protein to Gi protein) proposed by Lyon et al. have all given credence to the hypothesised pathogenic role of catecholamines in the development of TTS [24–26].

Although, these above-mentioned studies effectively hint at a definitive pathophysiological role played by catecholamines in the evolution of the syndrome, they fall short of explaining the potential effects of exogenous catecholamines in exacerbating a case of existing TTS.

A detailed analysis of our published research in this respect revealed that in-hospital events as well as short- and long-term mortality rates among TTS patients diagnosed with a significantly reduced LVEF on admission were significantly higher [27, 28]. We also showed that rates of in-hospital events and short- as well as long-term mortality rates were significantly higher in TTS patients suffering from arrhythmias such as atrial fibrillation [29, 30]. Although, such clinical scenarios do place the TTS patient at the worse end of the spectrum, it does not effectively explain the additional deleterious effects observed when patients received exogenous catecholamines as a form of therapy. An extrapolation of our data suggests reduced LVEF and use of positive inotropic agents as independent predictors of adverse outcome. A plausible explanation for this observation is perhaps the reactivation of catecholamine receptors or their downstream molecular pathways in the acute phase of TTS, which exacerbates the effects of the syndrome.

Our study has significant clinical implications. The essential role of catecholamines in the treatment of circulatory compromise has been consistently validated in the past, however, its use in TTS patients is now certainly questionable. Considering the pathophysiology of the syndrome, it would be pertinent to avoid any sort of catecholamine therapy for such patients. The Heart Failure Association of the European Society of Cardiology has recommended the avoidance or withdrawal of exogenous catecholamines as they could probably prolong or exacerbate the acute phase of the syndrome by activation of catecholamine receptors or their downstream molecular pathways [31]. It is for this reason that experts have suggested the early use of left ventricular assist device (LVAD) or extracorporeal membrane oxygenation (ECMO) as a bridge to recovery in highly unstable patients. Although treatment with levosimendan in this scenario is controversial, the absence of mechanical support may necessitate its use in certain scenarios [15].

This study clearly highlights the pitfalls associated with catecholamine use in patients suffering from circulatory compromise. The observation that most patients did not noticeably profit from this line of management and consistently suffered from poorer clinical outcomes with higher long-term mortality rates cements further support to recently postulated hypotheses and current recommendations for clinical management.

Study limitations

This study was limited by its single-center retrospective observational study design, which included patients admitted over the period of 13 years. There was insufficient data detailing the proposed limits and quantified catecholamine doses used in these patients, furthermore, preventing the definitive assessment of the prognostic impact of different treatment strategies such as ECMO and intra-aortic balloon pump (IABP).

Conclusion

This study equivocally suggests that TTS patients receiving catecholamine therapy show higher grades of circulatory and cardiac compromise, have poorer in-hospital outcomes and demonstrate higher long-term mortality rates in comparison to patients not receiving any form of catecholamine support. Although, these patients could in effect be suffering from a severe form of TTS, the interplay between the several mechanisms involved in the pathogenesis of this syndrome dictates the planning of therapeutic strategies precluding exogenous catecholamine use.

Abbreviations
ACS: Acute Coronary Syndrome; ECMO: Extracorporeal membrane oxygenation; HPA: Hypothalamic-pituitary-adrenal axis; IABP: Intra-aortic balloon pump; ICU: Intensive care unit; LV: Left ventricle; LVAD: Left ventricular assist device; LVEF: Left ventricular ejection fraction; RV: Right ventricle; TTS: Takotsubo Syndrome

Acknowledgements
Not applicable.

Funding
Not applicable.

Authors' contributions
UA and IEB conceived the study, participated in its design and coordination, participated in data analysis and interpretation and helped to draft and revise the manuscript for important intellectual content. CF participated in the study design and coordination, data acquisition and analysis and helped to draft the manuscript for important intellectual content. MBe participated in the study design and coordination, data acquisition and analysis and helped to draft the manuscript for important intellectual content. KS participated in the study design and coordination, as well as data analysis and revised the manuscript. SB helped to draft and revise the manuscript for important intellectual content after critically analysing and interpreting the data. AH helped to draft and revise the manuscript for important intellectual content after critically analysing and interpreting the data. ET participated in the study design and coordination, as well as data analysis and revised the manuscript. MBo participated in the study design and coordination, as well as data acquisition and revised the manuscript for important intellectual content. IA conceived the study, participated in its design and coordination, participated in data analysis and interpretation and helped to draft and revise the manuscript for important intellectual content. All authors read and approved the final manuscript.

Competing interests
The authors declare that they have no competing interests.

Author details
[1]First Department of Medicine, University Medical Center Mannheim, University of Heidelberg, Mannheim, Germany. [2]DZHK (German Center for Cardiovascular Research) partner site Mannheim, Mannheim, Germany. [3]First Department of Medicine, University Medical Center Mannheim, Theodor-Kutzer-Ufer 1-3, 68167 Mannheim, Germany.

References
1. Hurst RT, Prasad A, Askew JW III, Sengupta PP, Tajik AJ. Takotsubo cardiomyopathy: a unique cardiomyopathy with variable ventricular morphology. JACC Cardiovasc Imaging. 2010;3:641–9.
2. Medeiros K, O'Connor MJ, Baicu CF, et al. Systolic and diastolic mechanics in stress cardiomyopathy. Circulation. 2014;129:1659–67.
3. Prasad A. Apical ballooning syndrome: an important differential diagnosis of acute myocardial infarction. Circulation. 2007;115:e56–9.
4. Maron BJ, Towbin JA, Thiene G, Antzelevitch C, Corrado D, Arnett D, Moss AJ, Seidman CE, Young JB. Contemporary definitions and classification of the cardiomyopathies: an American Heart Association scientific statement from the council on clinical cardiology, heart failure and transplantation committee; quality of care and outcomes research and functional genomics and translational biology interdisciplinary working groups; and council on epidemiology and prevention. Circulation. 2006;113:1807–16.
5. Sharkey SW, Lesser JR, Maron MS, Maron BJ. Why not just call it takotsubo cardiomyopathy: a discussion of nomenclature. J Am Coll Cardiol. 2011;57:1496–7.
6. El-Battrawy I, Behnes M, Ansari U, Hillenbrand D, Haghi D, Hoffmann U, Akin I. Comparison and outcome analysis of patients with apical and non-apical takotsubo cardiomyopathy. QJM: An International Journal of Medicine. 2016;1–6.
7. Owa M, Aizawa K, Urasawa N, Ichinose H, Yamamoto K, Karasawa K, Kagoshima M, Koyama J, Ikeda S. Emotional stress-induced 'ampulla cardiomyopathy': discrepancy between the metabolic and sympathetic innervation imag- ing performed during the recovery course. Jpn Circ J. 2001;65:349–52.
8. Mukherjee A, Sunkel-Laing B, Dewhurst N. 'Broken heart' syndrome in Scotland: a case of Takotsubo cardiomyopathy in a recently widowed lady. Scott Med J. 2013;58:e15–9.
9. Haghi D, Athanasiadis A, Papavassiliu T, Suselbeck T, Fluechter S, Mahrholdt H, Borggrefe M, Sechtem U. Right ventricular involvement in Takotsubo cardiomyopathy. Eur Heart J. 2006;27:2433–9.
10. Kurowski V, Kaiser A, von Hof K, Killermann DP, Mayer B, Hartmann F, Schunkert H, Radke PW. Apical and midventricular transient left ventricular dysfunction syndrome (tako-tsubo cardiomyopathy): frequency, mechanisms, and prognosis. Chest. 2007;132:809–16.
11. Ennezat PV, Pesenti-Rossi D, Aubert JM, Rachenne V, Bauchart JJ, Auffray JL, Logeart D, Cohen-Solal A, Asseman P. Transient left ventricular basal dysfunction without coronary stenosis in acute cerebral disorders: a novel heart syndrome (inverted Takotsubo). Echocardiography. 2005;22:599–602.
12. Van deWalle SO, Gevaert SA, Gheeraert PJ, De Pauw M, Gillebert TC. Transient stress-induced cardiomyopathy with an 'inverted takotsubo' contractile pattern. Mayo Clin Proc. 2006;81:1499–502.
13. Cacciotti L, Camastra GS, Beni S, Giannantoni P, Musaro S, Proietti I, De Angelis L, Semeraro R, Ansalone GA. New variant of Tako-tsubo cardiomyopathy: transient mid-ventricular ballooning. J Cardiovasc Med. 2007;8:1052–4.
14. Templin C, Ghadri JR, Diekmann J, Napp LC, Bataiosu DR, Jaguszewski M, Lüscher TF. Clinical features and outcomes of Takotsubo (stress) cardiomyopathy. N Engl J Med. 2015;373(10):929–38.
15. Lyon AR, Bossone E, Schneider B, Sechtem U, Citro R, Underwood SR, Omerovic E. Current state of knowledge on Takotsubo syndrome: a position statement from the taskforce on Takotsubo syndrome of the heart failure Association of the European Society of cardiology. Eur J Heart Fail. 2016;18(1):8–27.
16. Wittstein IS, Thiemann DR, Lima JAC, Baughman KL, Schulman SP, Gerstenblith G, Wu KC, Rade JJ, Bivalacqua TJ, Champion HC. Neurohumoral features of myocardial stunning due to sudden emotional stress. N Engl J Med. 2005;352:539–48.
17. Khullar M, Datta BN, Wahi PL, Chakravarti RN. Catecholamine-induced experimental cardiomyopathy - a histopathological, histochemical and ultrastructural study. Indian Heart J 1989; 41: 307–313 [PMID: 2599540].
18. Uchida Y, Egami H, Uchida Y, Sakurai T, Kanai M, Shirai S, Nakagawa O, Oshima T. Possible participation of endothelial cell apoptosis of coronary microvessels in the genesis of Takotsubo cardiomyopathy. Clin Cardiol. 2010;33
19. Afonso L, Bachour K, Awad K, Sandidge G. Takotsubo cardiomyopathy: pathogenetic insights and myocardial perfusion kinetics using myocardial contrast echocardiography. Eur J Echocardiogr. 2008;9:849–54.
20. Galiuto L, De Caterina AR, Porfidia A, Paraggio L, Barchetta S, Locorotondo G, Rebuzzi AG, Crea F. Reversible coronary microvascular dysfunction: a common pathogenetic mechanism in apical ballooning or Tako-Tsubo syndrome. Eur Heart J 2010; 31: 1319–1327 [PMID: 20215125 https://doi.org/10.1093/ eurheartj/ehq039.
21. Nef HM, Möllmann H, Kostin S, Troidl C, Voss S, Weber M, Dill T, Rolf A, Brandt R, Hamm CW, Elsässer A. Takotsubo cardiomyopathy: intra-individual structural analysis in the acute phase and after functional recovery. Eur

Heart J 2007; 28: 2456–2464 [PMID: 17395683 https://doi.org/10.1093/ eurheartj/ ehl570].

22. Morel O, Sauer F, Imperiale A, Cimarelli S, Blondet C, Jesel L, Trinh A, De Poli F, Ohlmann P, Constantinesco A, Bareiss P. Importance of inflammation and neurohumoral activation in Takotsubo cardiomyopathy. J Card Fail 2009; 15: 206–213 [PMID: 19327622 https://doi.org/10.1016/j.cardfail.2008.10.031].

23. Avegliano G, Huguet M, Costabel JP, Ronderos R, Bijnens B, Kuschnir P, Thierer J, Tobón-Gomez C, Martinez GO, Frangi A. Morphologic pattern of late gadolinium enhancement in Takotsubo cardiomyopathy detected by early cardiovascular magnetic resonance. Clin Cardiol 2011; 34: 178–182 [PMID: 21400545 https://doi.org/10.1002/clc.20877.

24. Paur H, Wright PT, Sikkel MB, Tranter MH, Mansfield C, O'Gara P, et al. High levels of circulating epinephrine trigger apical cardiodepression in a β2-adrenergic receptor/Gi-dependent manner: a new model of Takotsubo cardiomyopathy. Circulation. 2012;126:697–706.

25. Lyon AR, Rees PSC, Prasad S, Poole-Wilson PA, Harding SE. Stress (Takotsubo) cardiomyopathy—a novel pathophysiological hypothesis to explain catecholamine-induced acute myocardial stunning. Nat Clin Pract CardiovascMed. 2008;5:22–9.

26. Scantlebury D, Prasad A. Diagnosis of Takotsubo cardiomyopathy. Circ J. 2014;78(9):2129–39.

27. El-Battrawy I, Ansari U, Lang S, Behnes M, Schramm K, Fastner C, Zhou X, Kuschyk J, Tülümen E, Röger S, et al. Impact and management of left ventricular function on the prognosis of Takotsubo syndrome. Eur J Clin Investig. 2017;47:477–85.

28. Becher T, El-Battrawy I, Baumann S, Fastner C, Behnes M, Loßnitzer D, Elmas E, Hoffmann U, Papavassiliu T, Kuschyk J, et al. Characteristics and long-term outcome of right ventricular involvement in Takotsubo cardiomyopathy. Int J Cardiol. 2016;220:371–5.

29. El-Battrawy I, Lang S, Ansari U, Tülümen E, Schramm K, Fastner C, Zhou X, Hoffmann U, Borggrefe M, Akin I. Prevalence of malignant arrhythmia and sudden cardiac death in takotsubo syndrome Borggrefe, M., Akin, I. Prevalence of malignant arrhythmia and sudden cardiac death in takotsubo syndrome and its management. EP Europace. 2017. https://doi.org/10.1093/ europace/eux073

30. El-Battrawy I, Lang S, Ansari U, Tülümen E, Schramm K, Fastner C, Zhou X, Hoffmann U, Borggrefe M, Akin I. Prevalence of malignant arrhythmia and sudden cardiac death in takotsubo syndrome and its management. EP Europace. 2017;

31. Redmond M, Knapp C, Salim M, Shanbhag S, Jaumdally R. Use of vasopressors in Takotsubo cardiomyopathy: a cautionary tale. Br J Anaesth. 2013;110:487–8.

25

Current status and strategies of long noncoding RNA research for diabetic cardiomyopathy

Tarun Pant[1,6], Anuradha Dhanasekaran[6], Juan Fang[3], Xiaowen Bai[4,5], Zeljko J. Bosnjak[1,5], Mingyu Liang[5] and Zhi-Dong Ge[2*] (iD)

Abstract

Long noncoding RNAs (lncRNAs) are endogenous RNA transcripts longer than 200 nucleotides which regulate epigenetically the expression of genes but do not have protein-coding potential. They are emerging as potential key regulators of diabetes mellitus and a variety of cardiovascular diseases. Diabetic cardiomyopathy (DCM) refers to diabetes mellitus-elicited structural and functional abnormalities of the myocardium, beyond that caused by ischemia or hypertension. The purpose of this review was to summarize current status of lncRNA research for DCM and discuss the challenges and possible strategies of lncRNA research for DCM. A systemic search was performed using PubMed and Google Scholar databases. Major conference proceedings of diabetes mellitus and cardiovascular disease occurring between January, 2014 to August, 2018 were also searched to identify unpublished studies that may be potentially eligible. The pathogenesis of DCM involves elevated oxidative stress, myocardial inflammation, apoptosis, and autophagy due to metabolic disturbances. Thousands of lncRNAs are aberrantly regulated in DCM. Manipulating the expression of specific lncRNAs, such as *H19*, *metastasis-associated lung adenocarcinoma transcript 1*, and *myocardial infarction-associated transcript,* with genetic approaches regulates potently oxidative stress, myocardial inflammation, apoptosis, and autophagy and ameliorates DCM in experimental animals. The detail data regarding the regulation and function of individual lncRNAs in DCM are limited. However, lncRNAs have been considered as potential diagnostic and therapeutic targets for DCM. Overexpression of protective lncRNAs and knockdown of detrimental lncRNAs in the heart are crucial for defining the role and function of lncRNAs of interest in DCM, however, they are technically challenging due to the length, short life, and location of lncRNAs. Gene delivery vectors can provide exogenous sources of cardioprotective lncRNAs to ameliorate DCM, and CRISPR–Cas9 genome editing technology may be used to knockdown specific lncRNAs in DCM. In summary, current data indicate that LncRNAs are a vital regulator of DCM and act as the promising diagnostic and therapeutic targets for DCM.

Keywords: Long noncoding RNAs, Diabetic cardiomyopathy, H19, MALAT1, MIAT, SENCR, MT-LIPCAR

Background

Diabetic cardiomyopathy (DCM) refers to diabetes-associated changes in the structure and function of the myocardium that are not directly attributable to other confounding factors such as coronary heart disease or hypertension [1]. It is estimated that DCM occurs in approximately 12% of diabetic patients [2]. DCM is associated with the development of overt heart failure and

worse prognosis of diabetic patients [3, 4]. A strategy for prevention and treatment in order to improve the prognosis of DCM has not been established [5–7].

Long noncoding RNAs (lncRNAs) are RNA transcripts longer than 200 nucleotides which, although not having the function of direct coding proteins, can regulate the expression of genes at transcriptional, post-transcriptional, and translational levels [8]. Over the past decade, lncRNAs have received widespread attention as potentially new and crucial players of biological regulation [9, 10]. Their cell-type and tissue-specific expression in health and cardiovascular disease provides the avenue for the

* Correspondence: Wilson.ge99@gmail.com
[2]Department of Ophthalmology, Stanford School of Medicine, 1651 Page Mill Road, Stanford, CA 94304, USA
Full list of author information is available at the end of the article

diagnosis and treatment of cardiovascular disease [11, 12]. Emerging studies find that lncRNAs are aberrantly regulated in DCM, and impacting the expression of specific lncRNAs is capable of regulating the pathophysiological process of DCM [13–15]. Although the detailed data regarding the role of specific lncRNAs in DCM are limited, they are increasingly identified as a vital regulator of DCM in experimental animals. To get insight into current status of lncRNA research for DCM, we used PubMed and Google Scholar databases to search systemically the published articles that are involved in lncRNAs and DCM. Major conference proceedings of diabetes mellitus and cardiovascular disease occurring between January, 2014 to August, 2018 were also searched to identify unpublished studies that may be potentially eligible. Based on the data obtained from these databases, we present an overview of lncRNA research for DCM. We also discuss the challenges and possible strategies of lncRNAs as diagnostic and therapeutic targets for DCM.

Diabetes-induced cardiac damage

Diabetes mellitus affects the heart through various mechanisms including metabolic disturbance (suppressed glucose oxidation, enhanced fatty acid metabolism, hyperinsulinemia, insulin resistance, accumulation of advanced glycation end-products, etc.), subcellular component abnormalities, microvascular impairment, and autonomic dysfunction [16, 17]. Eventually myocardium develops local inflammation, coronary arterial endothelial dysfunction, necrosis, apoptosis, autophagy, fibrosis, atherosclerosis, steatosis, and ventricular hypertrophy (Fig. 1) [18, 19]. These pathological changes in the structure, morphology, and function of the heart develop in diabetic patients, especially patients with type 2 diabetes mellitus (T2DM), even without the presence of ischemic heart disease and hypertension, termed diabetic cardiomyopathy (DCM) [1]. It is estimated that DCM occurs in approximately 12% of diabetic patients [2]. Clinical studies indicate that DCM increases the risk of overt heart failure and worsens the prognosis in diabetic patients [3, 4].

Animal models of DCM are critically important for us to advance the understanding of pathogenic mechanisms of DCM and discover new diagnostic and therapeutic targets for DCM. Over the past thirty years, investigators have developed many rodent models of diabetes mellitus and DCM [19, 20]. They are able to provide many advantages in the availability of adequate healthy controls and the absence of confounding factors such as marked differences in age, concomitant pathologies, and pharmacological treatments. Among these models, streptozotocin (STZ)-induced cardiomyopathy of type 1 diabetes mellitus (T1DM) and leptin receptor deficient (db/db)- or leptin deficient (ob/ob)-cardiomyopathy of T2DM are frequently used in the study of lncRNAs [5, 20, 21].

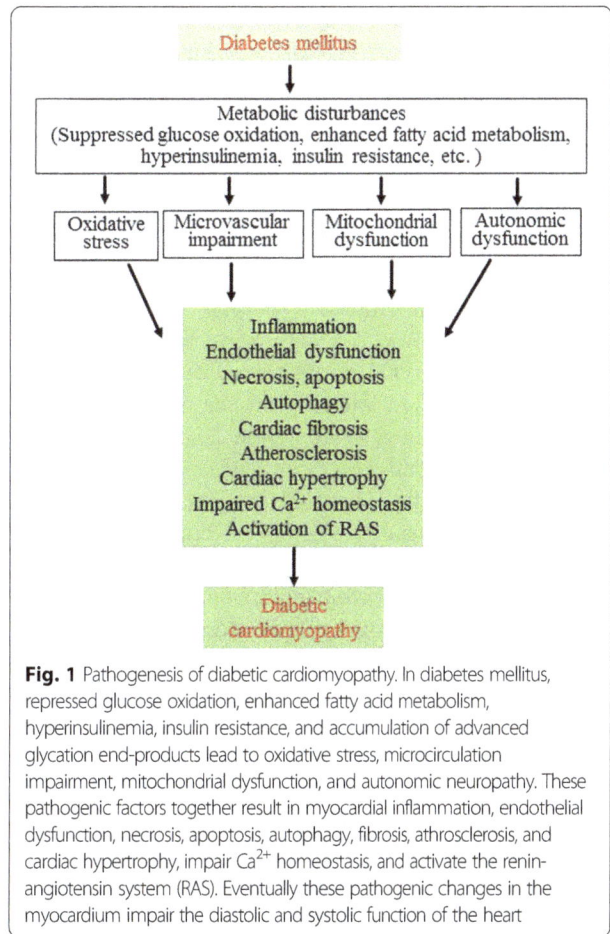

Fig. 1 Pathogenesis of diabetic cardiomyopathy. In diabetes mellitus, repressed glucose oxidation, enhanced fatty acid metabolism, hyperinsulinemia, insulin resistance, and accumulation of advanced glycation end-products lead to oxidative stress, microcirculation impairment, mitochondrial dysfunction, and autonomic neuropathy. These pathogenic factors together result in myocardial inflammation, endothelial dysfunction, necrosis, apoptosis, autophagy, fibrosis, athrosclerosis, and cardiac hypertrophy, impair Ca^{2+} homeostasis, and activate the renin-angiotensin system (RAS). Eventually these pathogenic changes in the myocardium impair the diastolic and systolic function of the heart

LncRNAs in the heart

LncRNAs represent one of the most prominent but least understood transcriptome in the heart. According to the NONCODE database (http:www.noncode.org/, version 5), there are 172,216 and 131,697 lncRNA transcripts for humans and mice, respectively. Thousands of lncRNAs have been identified to express abundantly in the myocardial tissues [22–24]. Many of these lncRNAs are dynamically transcribed during the development, differentiation, and maturation of cardiac myocytes [25–27].

LncRNAs have been known to control and regulate the expression of broad ranges of genes in cardiomyocytes [28, 29]. Similar to protein-coding RNAs, individual lncRNAs have specific subcellular distribution that is critical for their functions [30, 31]. Some lncRNAs are enriched in the nucleus and are involved in regulating nuclear processes, such as DNA replication-associated biological processes, mRNA transcription, and RNA processing [23, 32]. In the nucleus, lncRNAs can interact with DNA to form RNA-DNA complexes to reprogram gene expression, act as molecular scaffold, activate or suppress transcription [33, 34]. Other lncRNAs are enriched in the cytoplasm where they can impact protein localization or modulate mRNA stability and translation [35]. LncRNAs can also bind mRNA transcripts to either stabilize or promote translation, cause steric hindrance to block translation (e.g., acting as decoys), regulate RNA splicing and stability, and act as a sponge for microRNAs [36–38]. In the cytoplasm, lncRNAs can interact with proteins to mediate protein trafficking and signaling and impact the function of bound proteins [39].

LncRNA-mediated regulation of gene expression in the heart has been known to involve a variety of mechanisms [40, 41]. Some lncRNAs (for example, cardiac-specific lncRNA *Myheart*) can interact with chromatin remodeling factors to reprogram gene expression [28]. Some lncRNAs (e.g., the lncRNA *Braveheart*) can guide chromatin-modifying complexes to their required genomic destination and serve as docking stations for complex recruitment (acting as scaffolding) [42]. Certain lncRNAs (e.g., the cardiac-enriched lncRNA *Upperhad*) activate transcription of certain genes by guiding transcription factors to their promoters [43, 44]. Particular lncRNAs (e.g., the lncRNA *cardiac autophagy inhibitory factor*) are capable of suppressing transcription by sequestering transcription factors [45]. Some lncRNAs (e.g., the lncRNA *myocardial infarction-associated transcript* [*MIAT*]) can bind to complementary microRNAs (e.g., microRNA-24) via base pairing to sequester them (acting as "microRNA sponges") [46]. Various lncRNAs (e.g., the lncRNA *metastasis-associated lung adenocarcinoma transcript 1* [*MALAT1*]) can interact with mRNA to regulate their translation and splicing [47, 48]. Other lncRNAs (e.g., *cardiac autophagy inhibitory factor*) can interact with proteins to mediate their trafficking and signaling and regulate the function of bound proteins [45].

LncRNAs play crucial roles in various cardiac diseases [38, 45, 49, 50]. LncRNAs can be targeted to change the physiological function of cardiac myocytes [51, 52]. In cardiac disease, lncRNAs are regulated in a cell type/tissue-specific manner [53, 54]. Manipulating the expression of specific lncRNAs with genetic and pharmacological approaches impacts the severity of myocardial ischemia/reperfusion injury, cardiac hypertrophy, heart failure, and diabetic vascular complications. Thus, certain lncRNAs that are conserved in the heart may have therapeutic potential on various heart diseases [12, 14, 55]. Moreover, some circulating lncRNAs have been proposed to be the biomarker of cardiac disease [56].

Regulation and function of specific lncRNAs in DCM
Specific lncRNAs have been identified to express differentially in the heart with DCM [15, 37, 57, 58]. The aberrant expression of specific lncRNAs is associated with the pathophysiological process of DCM, such as oxidative stress, inflammation, apoptosis, myocardial fibrosis, and autophagy (Fig. 2) [15, 37, 57, 58]. Manipulating

specific lncRNAs to alter their expression is able to ameliorate DCM [37, 57, 58]. Despite the limited data regarding the regulation and function of specific lncRNAs in DCM, lncRNAs are considered as a promising target/candidate for the treatment and diagnosis of DCM. In this section, we discuss several of the lncRNAs that may have a good potential as a target/candidate for the treatment and diagnosis of DCM (Table 1).

H19
H19 is a 2.3-kb lncRNA which is transcribed from H19/insulin-like growth factor-II (IGF2) genomic imprinted cluster located on human chromosome 11p15.5 (syntenic to mouse chromosome 7) [59]. *H19* and IGF2 genes are expressed in a monoallelic fashion from the maternal and paternal chromosomes, respectively [60, 61]. *H19* is transcribed by a polymerase II [62]. *H19* transcripts start from the blastocyst stage and reach a high level in the tissues of endodermal, mesodermal, and ectodermal origins [63]. After the birth, *H19* expression will be inhibited in most of mammalian tissues [64]. However, *H19* remains in high accumulation in mature myocardium of both mice and humans possibly due to enhanced RNA stabilization during cardiomyocyte differentiation [65]. Both primary sequence and secondary structures of *H19* show a great extent of conservation among mammals [66].

H19 has recently been identified as an important regulator of the cardiomyopathy of T1DM in experimental rats [57, 58]. Sprague-Dawley rats injected with STZ developed the cardiomyopathy of T1DM with decreased expression of cardiac *H19* [57, 58]. Overexpression of *H19* in myocardial tissues caused decreases in oxidative stress, inflammation, apoptosis, and autophagy, leading to the amelioration of DCM [57, 58].

H19 serves as template for microRNA-675 expression from H19 first exon [67, 68]. Since microRNA-675 has multiple targets in diverse signaling pathways, *H19* is able to regulate a number of biological processes via microRNA-675. For example, the *H19*/microRNA-675 reduces high glucose-induced apoptosis by targeting voltage-dependent anion channel 1 which is a critical protein required for the mitochondria-mediated apoptosis [58, 69]. In addition, by down-regulating GTP-binding protein Di-Ras-3, the *H19*/microRNA-675 promotes the phosphorylation of the mechanistic target of rapamycin and inhibits activated autophagy in cardiomyocytes exposed to high glucose [57]. Another pattern of *H19* exerting its function is through interacting with proteins and microRNAs. H19 is capable of being folded into a special secondary structure, which allows it to serve as a platform and collect relative proteins [70]. Multiple proteins have been identified to associate with H19, including the RNA binding proteins, KH-type splicing regulatory proteins, inner membrane protease 1,

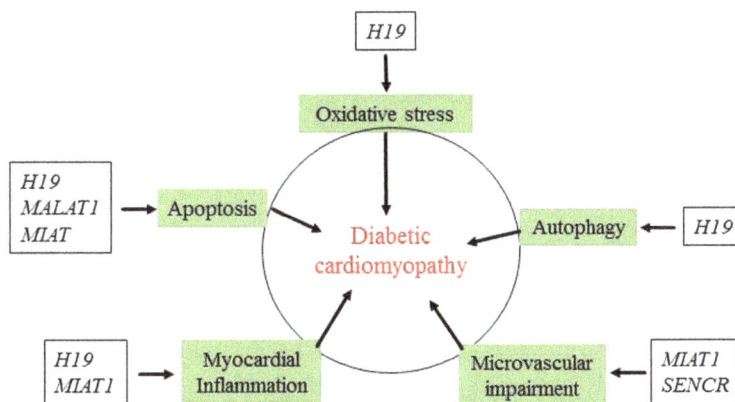

Fig. 2 Long noncoding RNAs (lncRNAs) impact the pathophysiological process of diabetic cardiomyopathy. Long noncoding RNAs are regulated in diabetic cardiomyopathy. Changes in the expression of long noncoding RNAs in myocardial tissues influence oxidative stress, myocardial inflammation, cardiomyocyte apoptosis, autophagy, and microvascular impairments. *MALAT1: metastasis-associated lung adenocarcinoma transcript 1; MIAT: myocardial infarction-associated transcript; MT-LIPCAR: the mitochondrially encoded long non-coding cardiac associated RNA; SENCR: smooth muscle and endothelial cell-enriched migration/differentiation-associated long noncoding RNA*

the Hu family of RNA-binding proteins, heterogeneous nuclear ribonucleoprotein U, polypyrimidine tract-binding protein 1, the DNA/chromatin modification factors, S-adenyl-L-homocysteine hydrolase, polycomb repressive complex 2, p53, and isoleucyl tRNA synthetase of mitochondria [68]. These proteins are actively involved in a wide variety of physiological and pathological processes, such as RNA metabolism, gene transcription, and epigenetic modification [68]. MicroRNAs are another group of partners that are essential for H19 to exert its function. It is evident that *H19* interacts with Let-7, microRNA-138, microRNA-200a, microRNA-106a, and microRNA-141 [68].

IGF2 proteins are an important growth factor during pregnancy, where they promote both fetal and placental growth [71, 72]. However, the overexpression of IGF2 and its receptors in acute hyperglycemia and diabetes is associated with the progression of DCM by triggering cardiac hypertrophy and apoptosis [73]. The effect of *H19* overexpression on the levels of myocardial IGF2 in adults remains unclear. In embryos, the overexpression of *H19* results in a decrease in IGF2 expression due to a *cis* effect of the *H19* locus on the adjacent IGF2 gene [74]. It is reasonably believed that IGF2 levels are decreased too in *H19*-overexpressing animals, and decreased IGF2 contributes to the beneficial effects of *H19* overexpression on DCM.

In summary, cardiac *H19* is downregulated in DCM, and transgenic overexpression of *H19* improves DCM by attenuation of myocardial oxidative stress, inflammation, apoptosis, and autophagy.

MALAT1

MALAT1 is a nuclear transcript localized to the nuclear speckles, a nuclear domain for storage and/or the sites of pre-mRNA splicing [75]. Pre-mRNAs splicing is a pivotal step between transcription and translation of most eukaryotic mRNAs [76]. *MALAT1* interacts with several serine/arginine proteins, such as serine/arginine-rich splicing factors and spliceosomal proteins, to regulate pre-mRNA splicing [77–79]. In addition, *MALAT1* is involved in nuclear organization and epigenetic modulation of gene expression [80, 81]. *MALAT1* was abundantly expressed in cardiac myocytes and highly conserved across mammalian species [82, 83]. In the rat cardiomyopathy of T1DM induced by streptozotocin, MALAT1 in myocardial tissues was up-regulated [15, 84]. The knockdown of *MALAT1* with the small interfering RNA to

Table 1 Regulation and function of specific long noncoding RNA in DCM

LncRNAs	Models	Species	Regulation during DCM	Function in DCM	References
H19	STZ-included T1DM	Rats	Down	Suppress oxidative stress, inflammation, apoptosis, and autophagy	[57, 58]
MALAT1	STZ-included T1DM	Rats	Up	Suppress inflammation and apoptosis	[15, 84]
MIAT	STZ-included T1DM	Rats	Up	Decrease apoptosis	[37]
SENCR	db/db T2DM	Mice	Down	Promote proliferation and migration of smooth muscle cells	[87]
MT-LIPCAR	T2DM	Humans	Down	Not available	[13]

DCM diabetic cardiomyopathy, LncRNAs long noncoding RNAs, STZ streptozocin, MALAT1 metastasis-associated lung adenocarcinoma transcript 1, MIAT myocardial infarction-associated transcript, SENCR smooth muscle and endothelial cell-enriched migration/defferentiation-associated long noncoding RNA, MT-LIPCAR the mitochondrially encoded long non-coding cardiac associated RNA

attenuate the expression of *MALAT1* in diabetic hearts significantly attenuated inflammation and apoptosis and improved DCM [15, 84]. Thus, the upregulation of *MALAT1* represents a critical pathogenic mechanism for DCM.

In short, cardiac *MALAT1* is upregulated in DCM, and the knockdown of *MALAT1* improves DCM by attenuation of myocardial inflammation and apoptosis.

MIAT

MIAT is first identified to be associated with myocardial infarction in a genome-wide association study in 2006 [85]. Before that, *MIAT* was also known as *RNCR2, 2 AK02836* or *GOMAFU*. *MIAT* may function as a competing endogenous RNA to upregulate the expression of death-associated protein kinase-2 by sponging miR-22-3p, which consequently leads to the apoptosis of cardiac myocytes [37]. Like *MALAT1*, the expression of cardiac *MIAT* was significantly upregulated in Sprague-Dawley rats with the cardiomyopathy of T1DM [37]. The knockdown of *MIAT* with *MIAT*-shRNA resulted in improvement of DCM and reduction of apoptosis of cardiac myocytes [37]. The inhibitory effect of *MIAT* knockdown on apoptosis is attributed to a decrease in the expression of death-associated protein kinase-2. Taken together, the upregulation of cardiac *MIAT* contributes to the pathogenesis of DCM.

Smooth muscle and endothelial cell-enriched migration/ differentiation-associated long noncoding RNA (SENCR)

SENCR is a vascular cell-enriched lncRNA [86]. It promotes the proliferation and migration of smooth muscle cells through regulation of forkhead box protein O1 and transient receptor potential cation channel 6. However, *SENCR* was down-regulated in T2DM db/db mice and in vascular smooth muscle cells exposed to high glucose [87]. The overexpression of *SENCR* reversed the inhibitory effect of high glucose on the proliferation and migration of mouse vascular smooth muscle cells. Both clinical and experimental studies indicate that impaired vascular smooth muscle cells by diabetes and high glucose contribute to the increased incidence of DCM [88]. Although there are no reports about the direct impacts of *SENCR* on DCM, the downregulation of cardiac *SENCR* may contribute to the pathogenesis of DCM.

The mitochondrially encoded long non-coding cardiac associated RNA (MT-LIPCAR)

MT-LIPCAR (*uc022bqs.1*, Gene ID: 103504742*)* is a 781-nucleotide lncRNA which is possibly transcribed from mitochondrial DNA [89]. It can cross the membrane barrier and is released into the circulation. Although there are a large number of RNase in plasma [90], *MT-LIPCAR* is stable in blood serum/plasma [13,

49, 91]. Recently, de Gonzalo-Calvo et al. analyzed lncRNAs derived from the serum of 48 patients with cardiomyopathy of T2DM and 12 healthy volunteers [13]. *MT-LIPCAR* levels in plasma were positively associated with left ventricular diastolic dysfunction. Moreover, *MT-LIPCAR* was strongly correlated with waist circumference, plasma fasting insulin, subcutaneous fat volume, and high-density lipoproteins-C. Collectively, *MT-LIPCAR* may be an independent predictor of diastolic dysfunction in T2DM patients with DCM [13].

In the clinic, the specific diagnosis of DCM is difficult, since the patients are asymptomatic in the early and middle stages and may concomitantly suffer from ischemic heart disease or hypertension during the late stage [7, 92, 93]. The significant increase in the levels of specific lncRNAs in serum/plasma of patients with DCM, such as *MT-LIPCAR*, could make lncRNAs specific biomarkers for the diagnosis and prognosis of DCM. A clinical trial recently suggests that *MT-LIPCAR* in plasma may serve as a promising biomarker of DCM [13]. The value of *MT-LIPCAR* and other circulating lncRNAs as diagnostic and prognostic markers in DCM needs to be validated. Large multicenter randomized, controlled trials with *MT-LIPCAR* need to be conducted in patients with DCM.

Antisense non-coding RNA in the INK4 locus (ANRIL)

ANRIL [alias *cyclin dependent kinase inhibitor 2B antisense RNA 1 (CDKN2B-AS1)* and *P15 antisense RNA (P15AS)*] is a 3.8 kb lncRNA transcribed from the short arm of human chromosome 9 on p21.3 [94]. *ANRIL* and the adjacent protein coding genes, *cyclin dependent kinase inhibitor 2A (CDKN2A)* and *cyclin dependent kinase inhibitor 2B (CDKN2B)*, locate on chromosome 9p21 [95]. The *CDKN2A* gene encodes several transcripts/ proteins, the p16 protein of which functions as inhibitors of cyclin-dependent kinase 4 [96, 97]. The *CDKN2B* gene encodes cyclin-dependent kinase 4 inhibitor B that functions as a cell growth regulator that control cell cycle G1 progression [98]. *ANRIL is an antisense of the CDKN2B gene and* is transcribed by RNA polymerase II and spliced into multiple linear and circular isoforms in a tissue-specific manner [99]. *ANRIL* is capable of recruiting polycomb group proteins to modify the epigenetic chromatin state and binding to a site or sequence to regulate gene expression [100]. It is well known to know that single nucleotide polymorphisms in the human chromosome 9p21 locus are associated with diabetes, cardiovascular disease, and multiple cancers [101–106]. Recent studies have identified *ANRIL* as a highly susceptible region for T2DM, coronary artery disease, and hypertension [107]. Although there is no report regarding the role of *ANRIL* in DCM, it is reasonably believed that *ANRIL* might be involved in the pathogenesis of DCM.

In summary, ANRIL is a potential candidate that is associated with the pathogenesis of DCM.

Challenges and potential strategies of lncRNA research for DCM

LncRNAs may be a promising target and/or candidate as biomarkers of DCM diagnosis and for the treatment of DCM. However, at present the function and regulation of thousands of lncRNAs in DCM are still ambiguous. Recently, we performed a systemic microarray-based analysis of the cardiac expression profiles of lncRNAs in T2DM db/db mice on a genetic background of C57BL/6 mice with and without DCM. Among the 23,578 lncRNAs identified, 1479 were differentially expressed in the myocardium of db/db mice between with DCM and without DCM [108]. These results suggest that at least 1479 lncRNAs might be involved in DCM in obese type 2 db/db mice. Determining the individual functionality of these lncRNAs is important for good understanding of cardiac developmental biology and DCM. For the study of individual lncRNAs in DCM, the following questions should be considered: Do lncRNAs contribute to the pathogenesis of DCM? How stable are the lncRNAs in circulation? Is their stability altered in diabetes mellitus and cardiac dysfunction? Are lncRNAs toxic? What are the pharmacokinetics of the lncRNAs? Answering these questions will be important as we study the individual lncRNAs and their role in diagnosis and treatment of DCM.

Some lncRNAs are protective to DCM, such as *H19*. These lncRNAs are down-regulated in DCM [57], and their overexpression in the heart is considered as a therapeutic strategy for DCM [58]. Owing to the length of lncRNA molecules their overexpression in cardiomyocytes is a complicated matter. Moreover, the long modified transcript is difficult to cross the membrane barrier. Thus, its efficient in vivo delivery would be difficult. Recent studies have reported that gene delivery vectors are capable of provide exogenous expression of the desired lncRNAs [38]. Utilization of gene delivery vectors, like engineered adeno-associated virus, is an alternative approaches to increase the expression of protective lncRNAs in the heart to ameliorate DCM.

Up-regulation of detrimental lncRNAs in DCM, such as *MALAT1* and *MIAT*, could make them promising therapeutics targets for DCM [109]. However, in vivo inhibition of detrimental lncRNAs is a challenge mainly due to their short half live as they are easily degraded by nucleases in bio fluids and the length of lncRNA transcripts. At present, the approaches which are used to manipulate lncRNAs in vivo include mainly the use of small interfering RNAs, antisense oligonucleotides, and

the 5′ and 3′ end-modified antisense oligonucleotides, GapmeRs [53, 110]. Each of these approaches have their own advantages and disadvantages. Small interfering RNAs specifically bind to complementary sequences and inhibit the expression of lncRNA targets [111, 112]. Antisense oligonucleotides are capable of targeting specific genes or transcripts directly through Watson-Crick base pairing, and they thus can reduce the levels of lncRNAs of interest [113]. Locked nucleic acid GapmeRs can modulate target lncRNA expression, block lncRNA activity, or induce enzyme-mediated degradation [53, 114]. Despite the potential therapeutic value of small interfering RNAs, antisense oligonucleotides, and GapmeRs in treating human disease, the effects of these approaches may have varied efficacy within the cell due to poor accessibility. Many studies have made use of antisense oligonucleotides to knockdown lncRNAs successfully for functional studies in mice or rats [115–117]. Compared with small interfering RNAs, antisense oligonucleotides are able be a better approach since cytoplasmic lncRNAs are efficiently ablated using small interfering RNA. To inhibit upregulated lncRNAs that show co-localization, the hybrid approach works the best [111].

Some lncRNAs are refractory to inhibition by either antisense oligonucleotides or small interfering RNAs. This may be related to the subcellular localization of the lncRNAs, which is not accessible to either RNase H or the interfering RNA machinery [111]. Another cause may be that the lncRNAs are highly structured or blocked due to excessive protein binding or hybridizing to other cellular nucleic acids. To overcome these hurdles, it is necessary to produce a high-throughput method to delete lncRNAs. Emerging studies suggest that CRISPR–Cas9 genome editing technology is able to quickly and effectively delete lncRNAs [118, 119]. Despite no reports about the utilization of CRISPR–Cas9 genome editing technology in DCM, this technology is a potential tool to delete the lncRNAs of interest and modulate the expression of lncRNAs in DCM.

In short, both overexpression of protective lncRNAs and knockdown of detrimental lncRNAs in the heart are crucial for defining the role and function of the lncRNAs of interest in DCM. Either approach is technically challenging due to the length, short life, and location of the lncRNAs of interest. In addition to traditional utilization of small interfering RNAs, antisense oligonucleotides, and GapmeRs to inhibit the lncRNAs of interest, CRISPR–Cas9 genome editing technology is a potential tool to knockdown specific lncRNAs.

Conclusions

LncRNAs play vital roles in the pathogenesis of DCM. Manipulating specific lncRNAs with pharmacological and genetic approaches to alter their expression impacts the development of DCM. In spite of limited data of specific lncRNAs in DCM, they are the potential targets/candidates for DCM. The future research needs to elucidate the regulation, function, and action mechanisms of more lncRNAs in the pathogenesis of DCM to search potential targets/candidates as diagnostic biomarkers of DCM and potential treatment of DCM.

Abbreviations

ANRIL: Antisense non-coding RNA in the INK4 locus; DCM: Diabetic cardiomyopathy; IGF2: Insulin-like growth factor-II; lncRNAs: Long noncoding RNAs; MALAT1: Metastasis-associated lung adenocarcinoma transcript; MIAT: Myocardial infarction-associated transcript; MT-LIPCAR: The mitochondrially encoded long non-coding cardiac associated RNA; SENCR: Smooth muscle and endothelial cell-enriched migration/differentiation-associated long noncoding RNA; STZ: Streptozotocin; T1DM: Type 1 diabetes mellitus; T2DM: Type 2 diabetes mellitus

Acknowledgements
None.

Funding
This work was supported, in part, by a National Institutes of Health research grant P01GM 066730 (to Dr. Bosnjak) from the United States Public Health Services, Bethesda, Maryland, USA. The funding body had no role in the design of the study, collection, analysis, and interpretation of data, and in writing the manuscript.

Authors' contributions
ZDG, ZJB, ML, and TP conceived the original idea. TP and JF collected and prepared the literature. ZDG, ZJB, ML, AD, and XB contributed to interpretation of the literature. ZDG and TP reviewed the literature and wrote the original manuscript. All authors read, discussed, and revised the initial manuscript and contributed to the final manuscript. All authors read and approved the final manuscript.

Competing interests
The authors declare that they have no competing interests.

Author details
[1]Department of Medicine, Medical College of Wisconsin, 8701 Watertown Plank Road, Milwaukee, WI 53226, USA. [2]Department of Ophthalmology, Stanford School of Medicine, 1651 Page Mill Road, Stanford, CA 94304, USA. [3]Department of Pediatrics, Medical College of Wisconsin, 8701 Watertown Plank Road, Milwaukee, WI 53226, USA. [4]Department of Cell Biology, Neurology & Anatomy, Medical College of Wisconsin, 8701 Watertown Plank Road, Milwaukee, WI 53226, USA. [5]Department of Physiology, Medical College of Wisconsin, 8701 Watertown Plank Road, Milwaukee, WI 53226, USA. [6]Centre for Biotechnology, Anna University, Chennai, Tamil Nadu, India.

References
1. Jia G, Hill MA, Sowers JR. Diabetic cardiomyopathy: an update of mechanisms contributing to this clinical entity. Circ Res. 2018;122:624–38.
2. Trachanas K, Sideris S, Aggeli C, Poulidakis E, Gatzoulis K, Tousoulis D, Kallikazaros I. Diabetic cardiomyopathy: from pathophysiology to treatment. Hell J Cardiol. 2014;55:411–21.
3. Qazi MU, Malik S. Diabetes and cardiovascular disease: original insights from the Framingham heart study. Glob Heart. 2013;8:43–8.
4. Marcinkiewicz A, Ostrowski S, Drzewoski J. Can the onset of heart failure be delayed by treating diabetic cardiomyopathy? Diabetol Metab Syndr. 2017;9:21.
5. Baumgardt SL, Paterson M, Leucker TM, Fang J, Zhang DX, Bosnjak ZJ, Warltier DC, Kersten JR, Ge ZD. Chronic co-administration of sepiapterin and L-citrulline ameliorates diabetic cardiomyopathy and myocardial ischemia/reperfusion injury in obese type 2 diabetic mice. Circ Heart Fail. 2016;9:e002424.
6. Gilca GE, Stefanescu G, Badulescu O, Tanase DM, Bararu I, Ciocoiu M. Diabetic cardiomyopathy: current approach and potential diagnostic and therapeutic targets. J Diabetes Res. 2017;2017:1310265.
7. Lorenzo-Almoros A, Tunon J, Orejas M, Cortes M, Egido J, Lorenzo O. Diagnostic approaches for diabetic cardiomyopathy. Cardiovasc Diabetol. 2017;16:28.
8. Kopp F, Mendell JT. Functional classification and experimental dissection of long noncoding RNAs. Cell. 2018;172:393–407.
9. Lee JT. Epigenetic regulation by long noncoding RNAs. Science. 2012;338:1435–9.
10. Kataoka M, Wang DZ. Non-coding RNAs including mirnas and lncrnas in cardiovascular biology and disease. Cell. 2014;3:883–98.
11. Haemmig S, Feinberg MW. Targeting lncRNAs in cardiovascular disease: options and expeditions. Circ Res. 2017;120:620–3.
12. Sallam T, Sandhu J, Tontonoz P. Long noncoding RNA discovery in cardiovascular disease: decoding form to function. Circ Res. 2018;122:155–66.
13. de Gonzalo-Calvo D, Kenneweg F, Bang C, Toro R, van der Meer RW, Rijzewijk LJ, Smit JW, Lamb HJ, Llorente-Cortes V, Thum T. Circulating long-non coding RNAs as biomarkers of left ventricular diastolic function and remodelling in patients with well-controlled type 2 diabetes. Sci Rep. 2016;6:37354.
14. Boon RA, Jae N, Holdt L, Dimmeler S. Long noncoding RNAs: from clinical genetics to therapeutic targets? J Am Coll Cardiol. 2016;67:1214–26.
15. Zhang M, Gu H, Chen J, Zhou X. Involvement of long noncoding RNA MALAT1 in the pathogenesis of diabetic cardiomyopathy. Int J Cardiol. 2016;202:753–5.
16. DeFronzo RA, Ferrannini E, Groop L, Henry RR, Herman WH, Holst JJ, Hu FB, Kahn CR, Raz I, Shulman GI, Simonson DC, Testa MA, Weiss R. Type 2 diabetes mellitus. Nat Rev Dis Primers. 2015;1:15019.
17. Lee WS, Kim J. Diabetic cardiomyopathy: where we are and where we are going. Korean J Intern Med. 2017;32:404–21.
18. Miki T, Yuda S, Kouzu H, Miura T. Diabetic cardiomyopathy: pathophysiology and clinical features. Heart Fail Rev. 2013;18:149–66.
19. Fuentes-Antras J, Picatoste B, Gomez-Hernandez A, Egido J, Tunon J, Lorenzo O. Updating experimental models of diabetic cardiomyopathy. J Diabetes Res. 2015;2015:656795.
20. Wu HE, Baumgardt SL, Fang J, Paterson M, Liu Y, Du J, Shi Y, Qiao S, Bosnjak ZJ, Warltier DC, Kersten JR, Ge ZD. Cardiomyocyte GTP cyclohydrolase 1 protects the heart against diabetic cardiomyopathy. Sci Rep. 2016;6:27925.
21. Ge ZD, Li Y, Qiao S, Bai X, Warltier DC, Kersten JR, Bosnjak ZJ, Liang M. Failure of isoflurane cardiac preconditioning in obese type 2 diabetic mice involves aberrant regulation of microRNA-21, endothelial nitric-oxide synthase, and mitochondrial complex I. Anesthesiology. 2018;128:117–29.
22. Kurian L, Aguirre A, Sancho-Martinez I, Benner C, Hishida T, Nguyen TB, Reddy P, Nivet E, Krause MN, Nelles DA, Rodriguez Esteban C, Campistol JM, Yeo GW, Izpisua Belmonte JC. Identification of novel long noncoding RNAs underlying vertebrate cardiovascular development. Circulation. 2015;131:1278–90.
23. Touma M, Kang X, Zhao Y, Cass AA, Gao F, Biniwale R, Coppola G, Xiao X, Reemtsen B, Wang Y. Decoding the long noncoding RNA during cardiac maturation: a roadmap for functional discovery. Circ Cardiovasc Genet. 2016;9:395–407.
24. Tang Z, Wu Y, Yang Y, Yang YT, Wang Z, Yuan J, Yang Y, Hua C, Fan X, Niu G, Zhang Y, Lu ZJ, Li K. Comprehensive analysis of long non-coding RNAs highlights their spatio-temporal expression patterns and evolutional conservation in sus scrofa. Sci Rep. 2017;7:43166.
25. He C, Hu H, Wilson KD, Wu H, Feng J, Xia S, Churko J, Qu K, Chang HY, Wu JC. Systematic characterization of long noncoding RNAs reveals the contrasting coordination of cis- and trans-molecular regulation in human fetal and adult hearts. Circ Cardiovasc Genet. 2016;9:110–8.
26. Li Y, Zhang J, Huo C, Ding N, Li J, Xiao J, Lin X, Cai B, Zhang Y, Xu J. Dynamic organization of lncRNA and circular RNA regulators collectively controlled cardiac differentiation in humans. EBioMedicine. 2017;24:137–46.

27. Beermann J, Kirste D, Iwanov K, Lu D, Kleemiss F, Kumarswamy R, Schimmel K, Bar C, Thum T. A large shRNA library approach identifies lncRNA Ntep as an essential regulator of cell proliferation. Cell Death Differ. 2018;25:307–18.

28. Chang CP, Han P. Epigenetic and lncRNA regulation of cardiac pathophysiology. Biochim Biophys Acta. 2016;1863:1767–71.

29. Li Y, Du W, Zhao R, Hu J, Li H, Han R, Yue Q, Wu R, Li W, Zhao J. New insights into epigenetic modifications in heart failure. Front Biosci. 2017;22:230–47.

30. Wilk R, Hu J, Blotsky D, Krause HM. Diverse and pervasive subcellular distributions for both coding and long noncoding RNAs. Genes Dev. 2016;30:594–609.

31. Chen LL. Linking long noncoding RNA localization and function. Trends Biochem Sci. 2016;41:761–72.

32. Sun X, Han Q, Luo H, Pan X, Ji Y, Yang Y, Chen H, Wang F, Lai W, Guan X, Zhang Q, Tang Y, Chu J, Yu J, Shou W, Deng Y, Li X. Profiling analysis of long non-coding RNAs in early postnatal mouse hearts. Sci Rep. 2017;7:43485.

33. Quinn JJ, Ilik IA, Qu K, Georgiev P, Chu C, Akhtar A, Chang HY. Revealing long noncoding RNA architecture and functions using domain-specific chromatin isolation by RNA purification. Nat Biotechnol. 2014;32:933–40.

34. Dykes IM, Emanueli C. Transcriptional and post-transcriptional gene regulation by long non-coding RNA. Genomics Proteomics Bioinformatics. 2017;15:177–86.

35. Kretz M, Siprashvili Z, Chu C, Webster DE, Zehnder A, Qu K, Lee CS, Flockhart RJ, Groff AF, Chow J, Johnston D, Kim GE, Spitale RC, Flynn RA, Zheng GX, Aiyer S, Raj A, Rinn JL, Chang HY, Khavari PA. Control of somatic tissue differentiation by the long non-coding RNA TINCR. Nature. 2013;493:231–5.

36. Matkovich SJ, Edwards JR, Grossenheider TC, de Guzman Strong C, Dorn GW. Epigenetic coordination of embryonic heart transcription by dynamically regulated long noncoding RNAs. Proc Natl Acad Sci U S A. 2014;111:12264–9.

37. Zhou X, Zhang W, Jin M, Chen J, Xu W, Kong X. LncRNA MIAT functions as a competing endogenous RNA to upregulate DAPK2 by sponging miR-22-3p in diabetic cardiomyopathy. Cell Death Dis. 2017;8:e2929.

38. Lv L, Li T, Li X, Xu C, Liu Q, Jiang H, Li Y, Liu Y, Yan H, Huang Q, Zhou Y, Zhang M, Shan H, Liang H. The lncRNA Plscr4 controls cardiac hypertrophy by regulating miR-214. Mol Ther Nucleic Acids. 2018;10:387–97.

39. Liu Y, Zhou D, Li G, Ming X, Tu Y, Tian J, Lu H, Yu B. Long non coding RNA-UCA1 contributes to cardiomyocyte apoptosis by suppression of p27 expression. Cell Physiol Biochem. 2015;35:1986–98.

40. Rayner KJ, Liu PP. Long noncoding RNAs in the heart: the regulatory roadmap of cardiovascular development and disease. Circ Cardiovasc Genet. 2016;9:101–3.

41. Schmitz SU, Grote P, Herrmann BG. Mechanisms of long noncoding RNA function in development and disease. Cell Mol Life Sci. 2016;73:2491–509.

42. Xue Z, Hennelly S, Doyle B, Gulati AA, Novikova IV, Sanbonmatsu KY, Boyer LA. A G-rich motif in the lncRNA Braveheart interacts with a zinc-finger transcription factor to specify the cardiovascular lineage. Mol Cell. 2016;64:37–50.

43. Wamstad JA, Alexander JM, Truty RM, Shrikumar A, Li F, Eilertson KE, Ding H, Wylie JN, Pico AR, Capra JA, Erwin G, Kattman SJ, Keller GM, Srivastava D, Levine SS, Pollard KS, Holloway AK, Boyer LA, Bruneau BG. Dynamic and coordinated epigenetic regulation of developmental transitions in the cardiac lineage. Cell. 2012;151:206–20.

44. Anderson KM, Anderson DM, McAnally JR, Shelton JM, Bassel-Duby R, Olson EN. Transcription of the non-coding RNA upperhand controls hand2 expression and heart development. Nature. 2016;539:433–6.

45. Liu CY, Zhang YH, Li RB, Zhou LY, An T, Zhang RC, Zhai M, Huang Y, Yan KW, Dong YH, Ponnusamy M, Shan C, Xu S, Wang Q, Zhang J, Wang K. LncRNA CAIF inhibits autophagy and attenuates myocardial infarction by blocking p53-mediated myocardin transcription. Nat Commun. 2018;9:29.

46. Qu X, Du Y, Shu Y, Gao M, Sun F, Luo S, Yang T, Zhan L, Yuan Y, Chu W, Pan Z, Wang Z, Yang B, Lu Y. MIAT is a pro-fibrotic long non-coding RNA governing cardiac fibrosis in post-infarct myocardium. Sci Rep. 2017;7:42657.

47. Wang K, Long B, Zhou LY, Liu F, Zhou QY, Liu CY, Fan YY, Li PF. CARL lncRNA inhibits anoxia-induced mitochondrial fission and apoptosis in cardiomyocytes by impairing miR-539-dependent PHB2 downregulation. Nat Commun. 2014;5:3596.

48. Zhang G, Sun H, Zhang Y, Zhao H, Fan W, Li J, Lv Y, Song Q, Zhang M, Shi H. Characterization of dysregulated lncRNA-mRNA network based on ceRNA hypothesis to reveal the occurrence and recurrence of myocardial infarction. Cell Death Discov. 2018;4:35.

49. Zhang Z, Gao W, Long QQ, Zhang J, Li YF, Liu DC, Yan JJ, Yang ZJ, Wang LS. Increased plasma levels of lncRNA H19 and LIPCAR are associated with increased risk of coronary artery disease in a chinese population. Sci Rep. 2017;7:7491.

50. Piccoli MT, Gupta SK, Viereck J, Foinquinos A, Samolovac S, Kramer FL, Garg A, Remke J, Zimmer K, Batkai S, Thum T. Inhibition of the cardiac fibroblast-enriched lncRNA MEG3 prevents cardiac fibrosis and diastolic dysfunction. Circ Res. 2017;121:575–83.

51. Ounzain S, Burdet F, Ibberson M, Pedrazzini T. Discovery and functional characterization of cardiovascular long noncoding RNAs. J Mol Cell Cardiol. 2015;89:17–26.

52. Devaux Y, Zangrando J, Schroen B, Creemers EE, Pedrazzini T, Chang CP, Dorn GW, Thum T, Heymans S. Long noncoding RNAs in cardiac development and ageing. Nat Rev Cardiol. 2015;12:415–25.

53. Leti F, DiStefano JK. Long noncoding RNAs as diagnostic and therapeutic targets in type 2 diabetes and related complications. Genes. 2017;8.

54. Leung A, Natarajan R. Long noncoding RNAs in diabetes and diabetic complications. Antioxid Redox Signal. 2017.

55. Lorenzen JM, Thum T. Long noncoding RNAs in kidney and cardiovascular diseases. Nat Rev Nephrol. 2016;12:360–73.

56. Viereck J, Thum T. Circulating noncoding RNAs as biomarkers of cardiovascular disease and injury. Circ Res. 2017;120:381–99.

57. Zhuo C, Jiang R, Lin X, Shao M. LncRNA H19 inhibits autophagy by epigenetically silencing of DIRAS3 in diabetic cardiomyopathy. Oncotarget. 2017;8:1429–37.

58. Li X, Wang H, Yao B, Xu W, Chen J, Zhou X. LncRNA H19/miR-675 axis regulates cardiomyocyte apoptosis by targeting VDAC1 in diabetic cardiomyopathy. Sci Rep. 2016;6:36340.

59. Gabory A, Jammes H, Dandolo L. The H19 locus: role of an imprinted non-coding RNA in growth and development. BioEssays. 2010;32:473–80.

60. Bartolomei MS, Zemel S, Tilghman SM. Parental imprinting of the mouse H19 gene. Nature. 1991;351:153–5.

61. DeChiara TM, Robertson EJ, Efstratiadis A. Parental imprinting of the mouse insulin-like growth factor II gene. Cell. 1991;64:849–59.

62. Pachnis V, Belayew A, Tilghman SM. Locus unlinked to alpha-fetoprotein under the control of the murine raf and Rif genes. Proc Natl Acad Sci U S A. 1984;81:5523–7.

63. Davis RL, Weintraub H, Lassar AB. Expression of a single transfected cDNA converts fibroblasts to myoblasts. Cell. 1987;51:987–1000.

64. Lustig O, Ariel I, Ilan J, Lev-Lehman E, De-Groot N, Hochberg A. Expression of the imprinted gene H19 in the human fetus. Mol Reprod Dev. 1994;38:239–46.

65. Milligan L, Antoine E, Bisbal C, Weber M, Brunel C, Forne T, Cathala G. H19 gene expression is up-regulated exclusively by stabilization of the RNA during muscle cell differentiation. Oncogene. 2000;19:5810–6.

66. Smits G, Mungall AJ, Griffiths-Jones S, Smith P, Beury D, Matthews L, Rogers J, Pask AJ, Shaw G, VandeBerg JL, McCarrey JR, Consortium S, Renfree MB, Reik W, Dunham I. Conservation of the H19 noncoding RNA and H19-IGF2 imprinting mechanism in therians. Nat Genet. 2008;40:971–6.

67. Huang Y, Zheng Y, Jia L, Li W. Long noncoding RNA H19 promotes osteoblast differentiation via TGF-β1/SMAD3/HDAC signaling pathway by deriving miR-675. Stem Cells. 2015;33:3481–92.

68. Zhang L, Zhou Y, Huang T, Cheng AS, Yu J, Kang W, To KF. The interplay of lncRNA-H19 and its binding partners in physiological process and gastric carcinogenesis. Int J Mol Sci. 2017;18.

69. Shimizu S, Matsuoka Y, Shinohara Y, Yoneda Y, Tsujimoto Y. Essential role of voltage-dependent anion channel in various forms of apoptosis in mammalian cells. J Cell Biol. 2001;152:237–50.

70. Matouk IJ, Mezan S, Mizrahi A, Ohana P, Abu-Lail R, Fellig Y, Degroot N, Galun E, Hochberg A. The oncofetal H19 RNA connection: hypoxia, p53 and cancer. Biochim Biophys Acta. 2010;1803:443–51.

71. DeChiara TM, Efstratiadis A, Robertson EJ. A growth-deficiency phenotype in heterozygous mice carrying an insulin-like growth factor II gene disrupted by targeting. Nature. 1990;345:78–80.

72. Baker J, Liu JP, Robertson EJ, Efstratiadis A. Role of insulin-like growth factors in embryonic and postnatal growth. Cell. 1993;75:73–82.

73. Feng CC, Pandey S, Lin CY, Shen CY, Chang RL, Chang TT, Chen RJ, Viswanadha VP, Lin YM, Huang CY. Cardiac apoptosis induced under high glucose condition involves activation of IGF2r signaling in H9C2 cardiomyoblasts and streptozotocin-induced diabetic rat hearts. Biomed Pharmacother. 2018;97:880–5.

74. Gabory A, Ripoche MA, Le Digarcher A, Watrin F, Ziyyat A, Forne T, Jammes H, Ainscough JF, Surani MA, Journot L, Dandolo L. H19 acts as a trans regulator of the imprinted gene network controlling growth in mice. Development. 2009;136:3413–21.

75. Spector DL, Lamond AI. Nuclear speckles. Cold Spring Harb Perspect Biol. 2011;3.

76. Kornblihtt AR, Schor IE, Allo M, Dujardin G, Petrillo E, Munoz MJ. Alternative splicing: a pivotal step between eukaryotic transcription and translation. Nat Rev Mol Cell Biol. 2013;14:153–65.

77. Yoshimoto R, Mayeda A, Yoshida M, Nakagawa S. MALAT1 long non-coding RNA in cancer. Biochim Biophys Acta. 2016;1859:192–9.

78. Tripathi V, Ellis JD, Shen Z, Song DY, Pan Q, Watt AT, Freier SM, Bennett CF, Sharma A, Bubulya PA, Blencowe BJ, Prasanth SG, Prasanth KV. The nuclear-retained noncoding RNA MALAT1 regulates alternative splicing by modulating SR splicing factor phosphorylation. Mol Cell. 2010;39:925–38.

79. Gu J, Xia Z, Luo Y, Jiang X, Qian B, Xie H, Zhu JK, Xiong L, Zhu J, Wang ZY. Spliceosomal protein U1A is involved in alternative splicing and salt stress tolerance in arabidopsis thaliana. Nucleic Acids Res. 2018;46:1777–92.

80. Engreitz JM, Sirokman K, McDonel P, Shishkin AA, Surka C, Russell P, Grossman SR, Chow AY, Guttman M, Lander ES. RNA-RNA interactions enable specific targeting of noncoding RNAs to nascent pre-mRNAs and chromatin sites. Cell. 2014;159:188–99.

81. Luan W, Li L, Shi Y, Bu X, Xia Y, Wang J, Djangmah HS, Liu X, You Y, Xu B. Long non-coding RNA MALAT1 acts as a competing endogenous rna to promote malignant melanoma growth and metastasis by sponging miR-22. Oncotarget. 2016;7:63901–12.

82. Ji P, Diederichs S, Wang W, Boing S, Metzger R, Schneider PM, Tidow N, Brandt B, Buerger H, Bulk E, Thomas M, Berdel WE, Serve H, Muller-Tidow C. MALAT-1, a novel noncoding RNA, and thymosin β4 predict metastasis and survival in early-stage non-small cell lung cancer. Oncogene. 2003;22:8031–41.

83. Hutchinson JN, Ensminger AW, Clemson CM, Lynch CR, Lawrence JB. Chess a. a screen for nuclear transcripts identifies two linked noncoding RNAs associated with sc35 splicing domains. BMC Genomics. 2007;8:39.

84. Zhang M, Gu H, Xu W, Zhou X. Down-regulation of lncRNA MALAT1 reduces cardiomyocyte apoptosis and improves left ventricular function in diabetic rats. Int J Cardiol. 2016;203:214–6.

85. Ishii N, Ozaki K, Sato H, Mizuno H, Saito S, Takahashi A, Miyamoto Y, Ikegawa S, Kamatani N, Hori M, Saito S, Nakamura Y, Tanaka T. Identification of a novel non-coding RNA, MIAT, that confers risk of myocardial infarction. J Hum Genet. 2006;51:1087–99.

86. Bell RD, Long X, Lin M, Bergmann JH, Nanda V, Cowan SL, Zhou Q, Han Y, Spector DL, Zheng D, Miano JM. Identification and initial functional characterization of a human vascular cell-enriched long noncoding RNA. Arterioscler Thromb Vasc Biol. 2014;34:1249–59.

87. Zou ZQ, Xu J, Li L, Han YS. Down-regulation of SENCR promotes smooth muscle cells proliferation and migration in db/db mice through up-regulation of Foxo1 and TRPC6. Biomed Pharmacother. 2015;74:35–41.

88. Riches K, Angelini TG, Mudhar GS, Kaye J, Clark E, Bailey MA, Sohrabi S, Korossis S, Walker PG, Scott DJ, Porter KE. Exploring smooth muscle phenotype and function in a bioreactor model of abdominal aortic aneurysm. J Transl Med. 2013;11:208.

89. Dorn GW 2nd. LIPCAR: a mitochondrial lnc in the noncoding RNA chain? Circ Res. 2014;114:1548–50.

90. Arita T, Ichikawa D, Konishi H, Komatsu S, Shiozaki A, Shoda K, Kawaguchi T, Hirajima S, Nagata H, Kubota T, Fujiwara H, Okamoto K, Otsuji E. Circulating long non-coding RNAs in plasma of patients with gastric cancer. Anticancer Res. 2013;33:3185–93.

91. Kumarswamy R, Bauters C, Volkmann I, Maury F, Fetisch J, Holzmann A, Lemesle G, de Groote P, Pinet F, Thum T. Circulating long noncoding RNA, LIPCAR, predicts survival in patients with heart failure. Circ Res. 2014;114:1569–75.

92. Aneja A, Tang WH, Bansilal S, Garcia MJ, Farkouh ME. Diabetic cardiomyopathy: insights into pathogenesis, diagnostic challenges, and therapeutic options. Am J Med. 2008;121:748–57.

93. Seferovic PM, Paulus WJ. Clinical diabetic cardiomyopathy: a two-faced disease with restrictive and dilated phenotypes. Eur Heart J. 2015;36(27):1718 1727a-27c.

94. Yu W, Gius D, Onyango P, Muldoon-Jacobs K, Karp J, Feinberg AP, Cui H. Epigenetic silencing of tumour suppressor gene p15 by its antisense RNA. Nature. 2008;451:202–6.

95. Holdt LM, Sass K, Gabel G, Bergert H, Thiery J, Teupser D. Expression of chr9p21 genes CDKN2B (p15ink4b), CDKN2A (p16ink4a, p14ARF) and MTAP in human atherosclerotic plaque. Atherosclerosis. 2011;214:264–70.

96. Nobori T, Miura K, Wu DJ, Lois A, Takabayashi K, Carson DA. Deletions of the cyclin-dependent kinase-4 inhibitor gene in multiple human cancers. Nature. 1994;368:753–6.

97. Kamb A, Gruis NA, Weaver-Feldhaus J, Liu Q, Harshman K, Tavtigian SV, Stockert E, Day RS, Johnson BE, Skolnick MH. A cell cycle regulator potentially involved in genesis of many tumor types. Science. 1994;264:436–40.

98. Hannon GJ, Beach D. p15INK4B is a potential effector of TGF-1β-induced cell cycle arrest. Nature. 1994;371:257–61.

99. Kong Y, Hsieh CH, Alonso LC. ANRIL: a lncRNA at the CDKN2A/bb locus with roles in cancer and metabolic disease. Front Endocrinol. 2018;9:405.

100. Yap KL, Li S, Munoz-Cabello AM, Raguz S, Zeng L, Mujtaba S, Gil J, Walsh MJ, Zhou MM. Molecular interplay of the noncoding RNA ANRIL and methylated histone H3 lysine 27 by polycomb CBX7 in transcriptional silencing of INK4a. Mol Cell. 2010;38:662–74.

101. McPherson R, Pertsemlidis A, Kavaslar N, Stewart A, Roberts R, Cox DR, Hinds DA, Pennacchio LA, Tybjaerg-Hansen A, Folsom AR, Boerwinkle E, Hobbs HH, Cohen JC. A common allele on chromosome 9 associated with coronary heart disease. Science. 2007;316:1488–91.

102. Helgadottir A, Thorleifsson G, Manolescu A, Gretarsdottir S, Blondal T, Jonasdottir A, Sigurdsson A, Baker A, Palsson A, Masson G, Gudbjartsson DF, Magnusson KP, Andersen K, Levey AI, Backman VM, Matthiasdottir S, Jonsdottir T, Palsson S, Einarsdottir H, Gunnarsdottir S, Gylfason A, Vaccarino V, Hooper WC, Reilly MP, Granger CB, Austin H, Rader DJ, Shah SH, Quyyumi AA, Gulcher JR, Thorgeirsson G, Thorsteinsdottir U, Kong A, Stefansson K. A common variant on chromosome 9p21 affects the risk of myocardial infarction. Science. 2007;316:1491–3.

103. Samani NJ, Erdmann J, Hall AS, Hengstenberg C, Mangino M, Mayer B, Dixon RJ, Meitinger T, Braund P, Wichmann HE, Barrett JH, Konig IR, Stevens SE, Szymczak S, Tregouet DA, Iles MM, Pahlke F, Pollard H, Lieb W, Cambien F, Fischer M, Ouwehand W, Blankenberg S, Balmforth AJ, Baessler A, Ball SG, Strom TM, Braenne I, Gieger C, Deloukas P, Tobin MD, Ziegler A, Thompson JR, Schunkert H. Genomewide association analysis of coronary artery disease. N Engl J Med. 2007;357:443–53.

104. Kojima Y, Downing K, Kundu R, Miller C, Dewey F, Lancero H, Raaz U, Perisic L, Hedin U, Schadt E, Maegdefessel L, Quertermous T, Leeper NJ. Cyclin-dependent kinase inhibitor 2b regulates efferocytosis and atherosclerosis. J Clin Invest. 2014;124:1083–97.

105. Campa D, Pastore M, Gentiluomo M, Talar-Wojnarowska R, Kupcinskas J, Malecka-Panas E, Neoptolemos JP, Niesen W, Vodicka P, Delle Fave G, Bueno-de-Mesquita HB, Gazouli M, Pacetti P, Di Leo M, Ito H, Kluter H, Soucek P, Corbo V, Yamao K, Hosono S, Kaaks R, Vashist Y, Gioffreda D, Strobel O, Shimizu Y, Dijk F, Andriulli A, Ivanauskas A, Bugert P, Tavano F, Vodickova L, Zambon CF, Lovecek M, Landi S, Key TJ, Boggi U, Pezzilli R, Jamroziak K, Mohelnikova-Duchonova B, Mambrini A, Bambi F, Busch O, Pazienza V, Valente R, Theodoropoulos GE, Hackert T, Capurso G, Cavestro GM, Pasquali C, Basso D, Sperti C, Matsuo K, Buchler M, Khaw KT, Izbicki J, Costello E, Katzke V, Michalski C, Stepien A, Rizzato C, Canzian F. Functional single nucleotide polymorphisms within the cyclin-dependent kinase inhibitor 2a/2b region affect pancreatic cancer risk. Oncotarget. 2016;7:57011–20.

106. Campa D, Capurso G, Pastore M, Talar-Wojnarowska R, Milanetto AC, Landoni L, Maiello E, Lawlor RT, Malecka-Panas E, Funel N, Gazouli M, De Bonis A, Kluter H, Rinzivillo M, Delle Fave G, Hackert T, Landi S, Bugert P, Bambi F, Archibugi L, Scarpa A, Katzke V, Dervenis C, Lico V, Furlanello S, Strobel O, Tavano F, Basso D, Kaaks R, Pasquali C, Gentiluomo M, Rizzato C, Canzian F. Common germline variants within the CDKN2A/2B region affect risk of pancreatic neuroendocrine tumors. Sci Rep. 2016;6:39565.

107. Rahimi E, Ahmadi A, Boroumand MA, Mohammad Soltani B, Behmanesh M. Association of ANRIL expression with coronary artery disease in type 2 diabetic patients. Cell J. 2018;20:41–5.

108. Pant T, Dhanasekaran A, Bosnjak ZJ, Ge ZD. Microarray analysis of long

noncoding RNAs in the heart and plasma of type 2 diabetic db/db mice. FASEB J. 2018;32:A580.517.

109. Zur Bruegge J, Einspanier R, Sharbati S. A long journey ahead: long non-coding RNAs in bacterial infections. Front Cell Infect Microbiol. 2017;7:95.

110. Adams BD, Parsons C, Walker L, Zhang WC, Slack FJ. Targeting noncoding RNAs in disease. J Clin Invest. 2017;127:761–71.

111. Lennox KA, Behlke MA. Cellular localization of long non-coding RNAs affects silencing by RNAi more than by antisense oligonucleotides. Nucleic Acids Res. 2016;44:863–77.

112. Prabhakar B, Zhong XB, Rasmussen TP. Exploiting long noncoding RNAs as pharmacological targets to modulate epigenetic diseases. Yale J Biol Med. 2017;90:73–86.

113. Zhou T, Kim Y, MacLeod AR. Targeting long noncoding RNA with antisense oligonucleotide technology as cancer therapeutics. Methods Mol Biol. 2016; 1402:199–213.

114. Amodio N, Stamato MA, Juli G, Morelli E, Fulciniti M, Manzoni M, Taiana E, Agnelli L, Cantafio MEG, Romeo E, Raimondi L, Caracciolo D, Zuccala V, Rossi M, Neri A, Munshi NC, Tagliaferri P, Tassone P. Drugging the lncRNA MALAT1 via LNA gapmeR ASO inhibits gene expression of proteasome subunits and triggers anti-multiple myeloma activity. Leukemia. 2018.

115. Micheletti R, Plaisance I, Abraham BJ, Sarre A, Ting CC, Alexanian M, Maric D, Maison D, Nemir M, Young RA, Schroen B, Gonzalez A, Ounzain S, Pedrazzini T. The long noncoding RNA WISPER controls cardiac fibrosis and remodeling. Sci Transl Med. 2017;9.

116. Li DY, Busch A, Jin H, Chernogubova E, Pelisek J, Karlsson J, Sennblad B, Liu S, Lao S, Hofmann P, Backlund A, Eken SM, Roy J, Eriksson P, Dacken B, Ramanujam D, Dueck A, Engelhardt S, Boon RA, Eckstein HH, Spin JM, Tsao PS, Maegdefessel L. H19 induces abdominal aortic aneurysm development and progression. Circulation. 2018. https://doi.org/10.1161/CIRCULATIONAHA.117.032184.

117. d'Ydewalle C, Ramos DM, Pyles NJ, Ng SY, Gorz M, Pilato CM, Ling K, Kong L, Ward AJ, Rubin LL, Rigo F, Bennett CF, Sumner CJ. The antisense transcript SMN-AS1 regulates SMN expression and is a novel therapeutic target for spinal muscular atrophy. Neuron. 2017;93:66–79.

118. Zhu S, Li W, Liu J, Chen CH, Liao Q, Xu P, Xu H, Xiao T, Cao Z, Peng J, Yuan P, Brown M, Liu XS, Wei W. Genome-scale deletion screening of human long non-coding RNAs using a paired-guide RNA CRISPR-CAS9 library. Nat Biotechnol. 2016;34:1279–86.

119. Aparicio-Prat E, Arnan C, Sala I, Bosch N, Guigo R, Johnson R. DECKO: Single-oligo, dual-crispr deletion of genomic elements including long non-coding RNAs. BMC Genomics. 2015;16:846.

26

Takotsubo cardiomyopathy in a patient with ileus

Chen-Yu C. Guo[1] and Nan-Sung Chou[2*] (iD)

Abstract

Background: Takotsubo cardiomyopathy (TCM) is a form of stress-induced cardiomyopathy featured by the dilatation of the apex of the left ventricle during systole. Whereas the pathogenesis of this disorder is not well understood, it usually occurs after an emotional or physical stress such as acute asthma, surgery, chemotherapy, and stroke. However, its occurrence in ileus patients is rarely reported. We hereby report probably the first case of TCM after ileus in the literature and discuss its implications.

Case presentation: An 85-year-old man was brought to the Emergency Department due to vomiting, abdominal pain, and no stool passages for 2 days. His abdomen was markedly distended, and ileus pattern was observed in the plain film of abdomen. Electrocardiogram showed right axis deviation, poor R-wave progression, and diffuse ST-segment elevation in the anterior leads, and cardiomegaly was observed by roentgenogram. A ventriculography showed an ejection fraction of 33% and confirmed the apical dilation consistent with TCM. He was treated with medication and discharged without remarkable adverse events. A follow-up transthoracic echocardiogram 4 months later showed normalization of his left ventricular systolic functions.

Conclusion: The precise mechanisms of the development of TCM are still unknown, but it is widely believed that it is triggered by the catecholamine surge produced in response to stress. This case demonstrated that such a stress can be of various forms, including ileus and other conditions that may lead to severe abdominal pain, and highlight the importance of awareness in diagnosing this rare but potentially lethal condition.

Keywords: Takotsubo cardiomyopathy, Ileus, Stress, Ventricular dilatation, Ventriculography, Case report

Background

Takotsubo cardiomyopathy (TCM) is a form of stress-induced cardiomyopathy, featured by the dilatation of the apex of the left ventricle during systole. It was first described in the English language in 1991 [1] and was given the name because of the dilatation of the left ventricular apex that leads to the appearance of a Japanese octopus trap (takotsubo) [2]. The pathogenesis of this disorder is not well understood, but a preceding emotional or physical stress is a unique feature, with approximately two-thirds of cases having associated identifiable acute stressors [3–5]. Such physical stressors include acute asthma, surgery, chemotherapy, and stroke [6]. However, to our knowledge, its occurrence in ileus patients has not been reported. We hereby report a case

of TCM in a patient with paralytic ileus and discuss its implications.

Case presentation

An 85-year-old man with diabetes, hypertension, and chronic obstructive pulmonary disease was brought by ambulance to the Emergency Department with the chief complaints of vomiting, abdominal pain, and no stool passages for 2 days. Physical examination revealed labored breathing. Patient also demonstrated peritoneal signs, including muscle guarding and rebounding tenderness. Bowel sounds were absent, but cardiac sounds were normal without rub, murmur, or gallop. Upper and lower extremity pulses were intact and symmetric. His initial electrocardiogram (ECG) showed normal sinus rhythm with right axis deviation, poor R-wave progression, and diffuse ST-segment elevation in the anterior leads (Fig. 1). A roentgenogram demonstrated marked cardiomegaly (Fig. 2). Laboratory data

* Correspondence: nansongchou23@gmail.com
[2]Department of Surgery, Madou Sin-Lau Hospital, 20 Lingzilin, Tainan 72152, Taiwan
Full list of author information is available at the end of the article

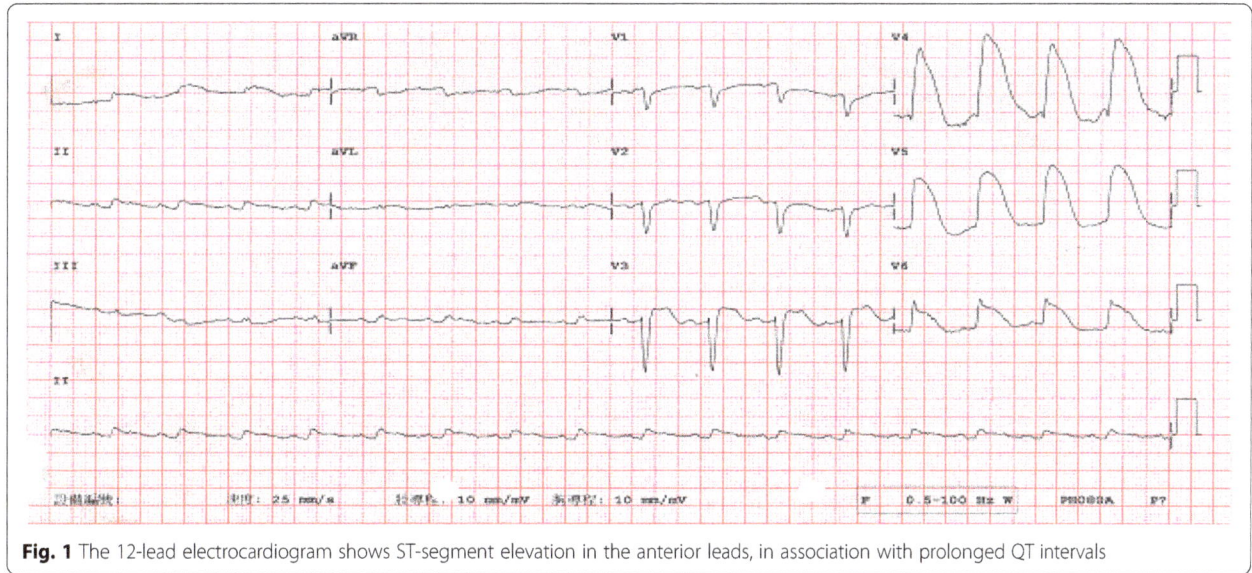

Fig. 1 The 12-lead electrocardiogram shows ST-segment elevation in the anterior leads, in association with prolonged QT intervals

revealed a hemoglobin level of 11.7 g/dL, a hematocrit level of 34.5%, a potassium level of 4.2 mEq/L, a creatine kinase level of 342 U/L, a creatine kinase MB fraction of 23.7 ng/mL, a relative index of 13.2%, and a troponin I level of 8.10 ng/mL. Results of the initial arterial blood gas analysis with the use of 10 L nonrebreathing mask were as follows: pH, 7.30; carbon dioxide tension, 45 mmHg; oxygen tension, 75 mmHg; base excess, −4; and oxygen saturation, 90%. On presentation, the patient's vital signs and cardiopulmonary examination were normal. His abdomen was markedly distended, and ileus pattern was illustrated in the plain film of abdomen (Fig. 3).

As laparotomy was suggested by a surgeon who was consulted in the intensive care unit, the patient received pre-anesthesia assessment. On the basis of the recommendation from a cardiologist who performed the assessment, the patient underwent left heart catheterization on the second day of hospitalization, which failed to show a significant obstruction in any coronary distribution (Fig. 4). Ventriculography estimated an ejection fraction of 33% and confirmed apical dilation consistent with TCM (Fig. 5). The patient was medically managed and discharged without adverse events. A follow-up transthoracic echocardiogram 4 months later showed normalization of his left ventricular systolic function.

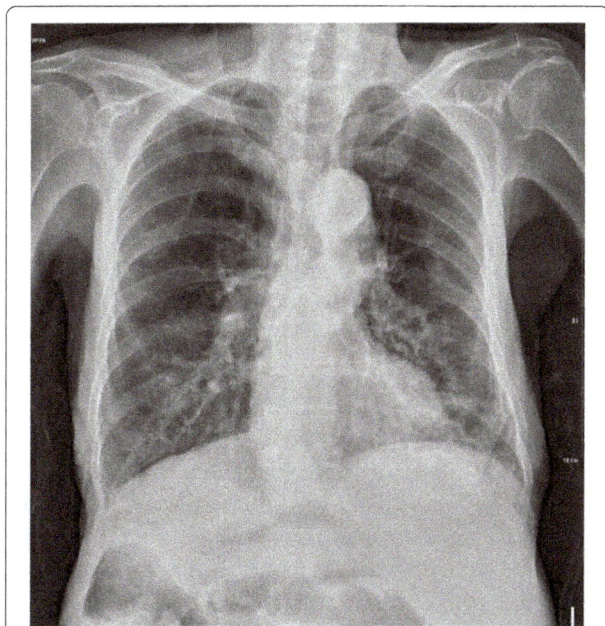

Fig. 2 Prominent left heart border without marked cardiomegaly

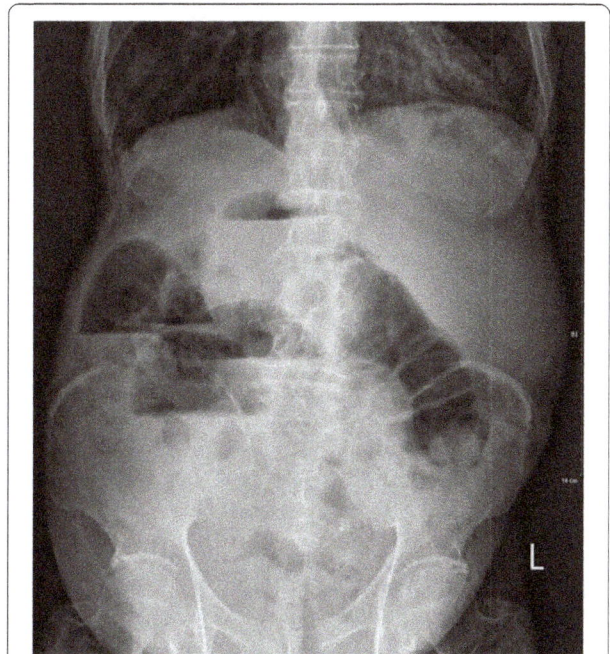

Fig. 3 Multiple air-fluid levels suggesting bowel obstruction

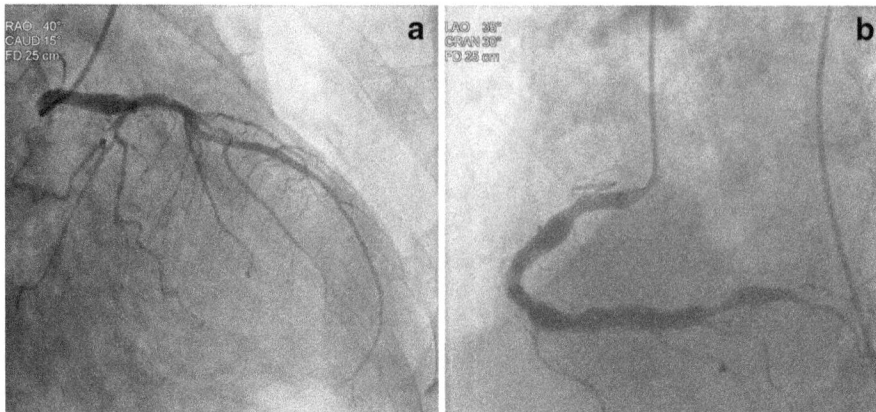

Fig. 4 Coronary angiography of the patient showing no significant obstructions: (**a**) left coronary angiography and (**b**) right coronary angiography

The CARE guidelines were followed in this report.

Discussion and conclusions

Over 90% of TCM cases are observed in postmenopausal women [7], and clinical manifestations of TCM may range from asymptomatic ECG abnormalities and non-specific systemic symptoms, to heart failure, cardiogenic shock, and sudden death. We report an uncommon case of a male patient with TCM accompanied by paralytic ileus. The diagnosis of TCM in this patient was confirmed by the elevated troponin I level (8.10 ng/mL), elevated ST-segment with prolonged QT interval, and unique cardiac imaging that showed left ventricular ballooning. Although the precise mechanisms behind TCM are unclear, it is generally believed that this disorder is triggered by the catecholamine surge produced during the body's sympathetic response to stress. This is

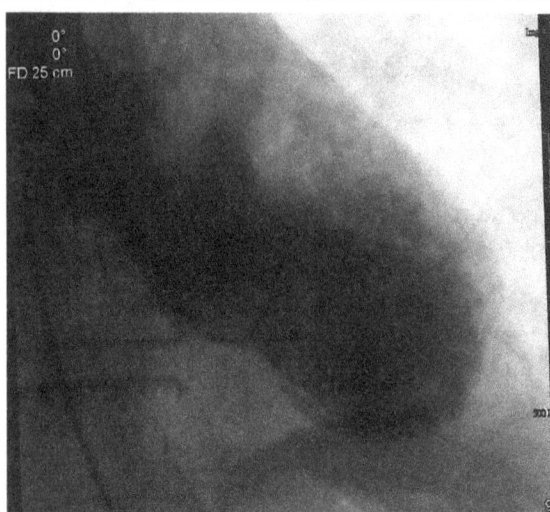

Fig. 5 Left heart catheterization showing persistent left ventricle apical hypokinesis with systolic ballooning

evidenced by the fact that a preceding emotional or physical stress is a unique feature of TCM, with approximately two-thirds of cases having associated, identifiable acute stressors [3–6]. Elevated catecholamine levels and reversible left ventricle ballooning have also been observed in a rat model of immobilization-induced stress [8], and cases of pheochromocytoma with the presentation of TCM confirmed through ventriculography or echocardiography have been reported [7, 9, 10]. Patients with TCM were found to have a higher prevalence of neurologic and psychiatric disorders [11], and psychopathological traits such as neuroticism, depression, and anxiety may persist even after recovery [12].

The physical stressors that can induce TCM include acute asthma attack, surgery, chemotherapy, stroke, car accident, suicide attempt, etc. [6, 7, 10, 13]. Various gastrointestinal symptoms such as acute cholecystitis, vomiting, and diarrhea are considered possible triggers for TCM [7, 14]. In fact, a review of 3719 patients in Japan found that 57 (1.5%) of them had acute gastrointestinal diseases [14]. However, paralytic or any kind of ileus is not specifically listed as one of them [7]. Furthermore, using "Takotsubo cardiomyopathy" combining "ileus," "intestine," "colon," or "gastrointestinal" as key words to search the literature indexed in PubMed, we did not find any previous reports on cases associated with ileus, while a single report specifically on a diarrhea-related case was found [15]. Because the ileus was resolved without any surgical interventions, many acute disorders and conditions that might act as a stressor triggering TCM in this patient can be generally ruled out. As the patient's history did not reveal any other remarkable triggers for TCM, we believe that the ileus caused by stool impaction, and the abdominal pain occurred subsequently, acting as a stressor for developing TCM. It is possible that acute reduction of cardiac output due to foregoing TCM deteriorates the bowel movement, which in turn leads to ileus. However, the initial presentation of this patient was ileus, and the typical symptoms of TMC such as chest discomfort were developed after admission to the hospital. In addition, he did not have history of obvious bowel dysfunction before this episode. Therefore, we believe ileus was more likely to be the cause instead of the consequence of TCM in this case.

Given the nonspecific symptoms and signs, a high clinical index of suspicion is essential for prompt diagnosis of TCM, a rare but potentially fatal disorder. One of the indices of suspicion is either emotional or physical stimulus that is stressful for the patient. This case suggests that ileus, and probably severe abdominal pain caused by other etiologies, can be added to the list of stress triggers that can cause TCM and alarm clinicians.

Acknowledgements
None.

Funding
There was no funding received for this manuscript.

Authors' contributions
Both authors have participated in the preparation, writing, and review of the manuscript. Both authors have read and approved the final manuscript.

Competing interests
The authors declare that they have no competing interests.

Author details
[1]Lewis Katz School of Medicine, Temple University, 3500 N. Broad Street, Philadelphia, PA 19140, USA. [2]Department of Surgery, Madou Sin-Lau Hospital, 20 Lingzilin, Tainan 72152, Taiwan.

References
1. Dote K, Sato H, Tateishi H, Uchida T, Ishihara M. Myocardial stunning duo to simultaneous multi-vessel coronary spasms: a review of 5 cases. J Cardiol. 1991;21:203–14.
2. Bybee KA, Kara T, Prasad A, Lerma A, Barsness GW, Wright RS, et al. Systematic review: transient left apical ballooning: a syndrome that mimics ST-segment elevation myocardial infarction. Ann Intern Med. 2004;141:858–65.
3. Nef HM, Mollmann H, Akashi YJ, Hamm CW. Mechanisms of stress (takotsubo) cardiomyopathy. Nat Rev Cardiol. 2010;7:187–93.
4. Wittstein IS, Thiemann DR, Lima JA, Baughman KL, Schulman SP, Gerstenblith G, et al. Neurohumoral features of myocardial stunning duo to sudden emotional stress. N Engl J Med. 2005;352:539.
5. Lyon AR, Rees PS, Prasad S, Poole-Wilson PA, Harding SE. Stress (takotsubo) cardiomyopathy—a novel pathophysiological hypothesis to explain catecholamine-induced acute myocardial stunning. Nat Clin Pract Cardiovasc Med. 2008;5:22–9.
6. Paur H, Wright PT, Sikkel MB, Tranter MH, Mansfield C, O'Gara P, et al. High levels of circulating epinephrine trigger apical cardiodepression in a bete2-adrenoceptor/gi-dependent manner: a new model of takotsubo cardiomyopathy. Circulation. 2012;126:697–706.
7. Lyon AR, Bossone E, Schneider B, Sechtem U, Citro R, Underwood SR, et al. Current state of knowledge on Takotsubo syndrome: a position statement from the taskforce on Takotsubo syndrome of the heart failure Association of the European Society of cardiology. Eur J Heart Fail. 2016;18:8–27.
8. Ueyama T. Emotional stress-induced takotsubo cardiomyopathy: animal model and molecular mechanism. Ann N Y Acad Sci. 2004;1018:437.
9. Chiang Y-L, Chen P-C, Lee C-C, Chua S-K. Adrenal pheochromocytoma presenting with takotsubo-pattern cardiomyopathy and acute heart failure: a case report and literature review. Medicine. 2016;36(e4846):95.
10. Gervais MK, Gagnon A, Henri M, Bendavid Y. Pheochromocytoma presenting as inverted Takotsubo cardiomyopathy: a case report and review of the literature. J Cardiovasc Med. 2015;16:S113–7.
11. Templin C, Ghadri JR, Diekmann J, Napp LC, Bataiosu DR, Jaguszewski M, et al. Clinical features and outcomes of takotsubo (stress) cardiomyopathy. N Engl J Med. 2015;373:929–38.
12. Christensen TE, Bang LE, Holmvang L, Hasbak P, Kjær A, Bech P, et al. Neuroticism, depression and anxiety in takotsubo cardiomyopathy. BMC Cardiovasc Disord. 2016;16:118.
13. Schlossbauer SA, Ghadri JR, Cammann VL, Maier W, Lüscher TF, Templin C. A broken heart in a broken car. Cardiol J. 2016;23:352–4.
14. Isogai T, Yasunaga H, Matsui H, Tanaka H, Ueda T, Horiguchi H, et al. Out-of-hospital versus in-hospital Takotsubo cardiomyopathy: analysis of 3719 patients in the diagnosis procedure combination database in Japan. Int J Cardiol. 2014;176:413–7.
15. Michel J, Pegg T, Porter D, Fisher N. Atypical variant stress (Takotsubo) cardiomyopathy associated with gastrointestinal illness: rapid normalisation of LV function. N Z Med J. 2012;125:85–7.

27

Takotsubo cardiomyopathy complicated with apical thrombus formation on first day of the illness

H. M. M. T. B. Herath[1*], S. P. Pahalagamage[1], Laura C. Lindsay[2], S. Vinothan[1], Sampath Withanawasam[1], Vajira Senarathne[1] and Milinda Withana[1]

Abstract

Background: Takotsubo cardiomyopathy is characterized by transient systolic dysfunction of the apical and mid segments of the left ventricle in the absence of obstructive coronary artery disease. Intraventricular thrombus formation is a rare complication of Takotsubo cardiomyopathy and current data almost exclusively consists of isolated case reports and a few case series. Here we describe a case of Takotsubo cardiomyopathy with formation of an apical thrombus within 24 h of symptom onset, which has been reported in the literature only once previously, to the best of our knowledge. We have reviewed the available literature that may aid clinicians in their approach to the condition, since no published guidelines are available.

Case presentation: A 68-year-old Sri Lankan female presented to a local hospital with chest pain. Electrocardiogram (ECG) showed ST elevation, and antiplatelets, intravenous streptokinase and a high dose statin were administered. Despite this ST elevation persisted; however the coronary angiogram was negative for obstructive coronary artery disease. Echocardiogram revealed hypokinesia of the mid and apical segments of the left ventricle with typical apical ballooning and a sizable apical thrombus. She had recently had a viral infection and was also emotionally distressed as her sister was recently diagnosed with a terminal cancer. A diagnosis of Takotsubo cardiomyopathy was made and anticoagulation was started with heparin and warfarin. The follow up echocardiogram performed 1 week later revealed a small persistent thrombus, which had completely resolved at 3 weeks.

Conclusion: Though severe systolic dysfunction is observed in almost all the patients with Takotsubo cardiomyopathy, intraventricular thrombus formation on the first day of the illness is rare. The possibility of underdiagnosis of thrombus can be prevented by early echocardiogram in Takotsubo cardiomyopathy. The majority of reports found in the literature review were of cases that had formed an intraventriclar thrombus within the first 2 weeks, emphasizing the importance of follow up echocardiography at least 2 weeks later. The management of a left ventricular thrombus in Takotsubo cardiomyopathy is controversial and in most cases warfarin and heparin were used for a short duration.

Keywords: Takotsubo cardiomyopathy, Early left ventricular thrombus, Streptokinase, Case report

* Correspondence: tharukaherath11@gmail.com
[1]National Hospital, Colombo, Sri Lanka
Full list of author information is available at the end of the article

Background

Takotsubo cardiomyopathy (TCM) or stress-induced cardiomyopathy is characterized by transient systolic dysfunction of the apical and mid segments of the left ventricle in the absence of obstructive coronary artery disease. In the typical type of stress-induced cardiomyopathy, contractility of the mid and apical segments of the left ventricle is depressed and there is balloon-like appearance of the distal ventricle with systole. TCM is much more common in postmenopausal women and is frequently triggered by unexpected emotional or physical stress [1]. Exaggerated sympathetic stimulation [2], catecholamine excess [3], coronary artery spasm and micro vascular dysfunction have been postulated as possible mechanisms in Takotsubo cardiomyopathy. It is a transient disorder and resolves with conservative treatment and supportive therapy. Intraventricular thrombus formation is a rare complication of Takotsubo cardiomyopathy and current data almost exclusively consist of isolated case reports and a few case series. In one case series, only 5 out of 95 patients (5.3%) with TCM developed left ventricular apical thrombus [4].

Here we describe a case of a postmenopausal female who presented with TCM who was initially treated as acute ST segment elevation myocardial infarction (STEMI). Despite administration of streptokinase and enoxaparin, a large left ventricular clot was found on the transthoracic echocardiogram (TTE) performed within 24 h. Rapid development of an apical thrombus within 24 h in TCM is rarely reported in literature and here we illustrate the importance of follow up TTE in these patients to recognize this complication. We also focus on the case reports of TCM complicated with intraventricular thrombus formation with regards to management,

since no treatment guidelines are available and only the previous case reports and case series can be used to guide management.

Case presentation

A 68-year-old Sri Lankan female (BMI 24.3 kg/ m^2) was admitted to a local hospital, complaining of sudden onset severe retrosternal chest pain with autonomic symptoms. Electrocardiogram (ECG) showed ST segment elevations in leads LI, aVL, LII, LIII, aVF and V2 to V6 (Fig. 1). A diagnosis of acute STEMI was made and oral Aspirin 300 mg, Clopidogrel 300 mg, Atorvastatin 40 mg and intravenous streptokinase 1.5 MU were administered 2 h after the onset of chest pain followed by subcutaneous enoxaparin. The patient's chest pain resolved, but due to persistent ST elevation on ECG, the patient was transferred to our cardiology unit for further management. She had been diagnosed with hypertension for 6 months and routine TTE performed 3 months previously showed normal ejection fraction and contractility. One week before this episode, she had 2 days of fever that was managed as viral illness at a local hospital. She was also emotionally stressed because her sister was recently diagnosed with a terminal cancer. She did not have any past history or family history of thromboembolic diseases or risk factors other than hypertension.

On examination, she was dyspnoeic at rest but maintained a saturation of more than 94% without supplemental oxygen. Her heart rate was 110 beats per minute and blood pressure was 100/60 mmHg. Jugular venous pressure was elevated and there were fine bibasal crepitations. TTE was performed 18 h after the onset of chest pain, which revealed hypokinesia of the mid and apical segments of the left ventricle with typical LV apical

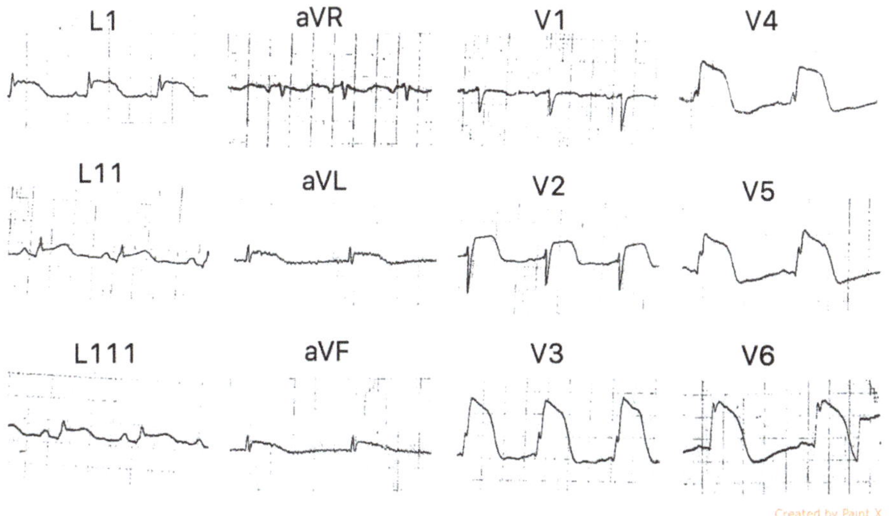

Fig. 1 Electrocardiogram showing ST segment elevation in leads L1, aVL, L11, L111, aVF and V2 to V6

ballooning. Ejection fraction was 40% and a 2.5 cm × 2 cm apical thrombus was detected (Fig. 2)(Additional file 1: Movie S1 and Additional file 2: Movie S2). Because the coronary angiogram performed at the same time showed normal coronary arteries, Takotsubo cardiomyopathy was diagnosed and she was commenced on metoprolol, losartan, atorvastatin, diuretics and aspirin. We continued subcutaneous enoxaparin 1 mg/ kg bd and added warfarin 5 mg daily. Her full blood count (hemoglobin 12 g/dL, white blood cell count 7.79 × $10^{9/}$ L, platelet count 222 × $10^{9/}$ L), renal function tests, liver function tests, thyroid function tests, serum calcium, serum magnesium and coagulation profile were within normal range. The greatest troponin I value was 2.2 ng/ml (normal <0.5 ng/ml). Erythrocyte sedimentation rate was 13 mm in the first hour and C-reactive protein (CRP) was 6.7 mg/L (normal <5 mg/L). Human immunodeficiency virus serology, venereal disease research laboratory and hepatitis serology were also negative. After achieving a therapeutic international normalized ratio of 2–3, enoxaparin was omitted. Her symptoms improved gradually over 1 week. Follow up TTE performed 1 week later showed only mild hypokinesia of the apex of the left ventricle and the thrombus had reduced in size (2.1 cm × 1.8 cm) (Fig. 3). ECG also showed resolving ST elevation (Fig. 4). After 3 weeks, TTE showed normally contracting ventricles and the thrombus had resolved. We discontinued warfarin and continued with the other drugs. She did not experience any thromboembolism.

Discussion

TCM was diagnosed in this patient who had clinical manifestations and ECG abnormalities out of proportion to the cardiac biomarkers with typical apical ballooning evident in TTE and normal coronary angiography [5]. We assumed this event was precipitated by emotional stress due to social problems and the recent upper respiratory tract infection. We assumed that the ventricular thrombus developed due to apical hypokinesia since

the TTE performed 3 months earlier was normal and the thrombus was visualized at the apex as in other cases of TCM. The thrombus also resolved rapidly indicating that it was a newly formed thrombus. The other possible mechanism for thrombus formation in this patient is reduced wall motion due to myocarditis following viral flu she had 1 week back. But this less likely since she did not have symptoms, signs or ECG changes suggestive of cardiac involvement during that admission.

Apical thrombosis complicating TCM was first described in 2003 [6, 7]. Several isolated case reports and 2 case series were published later [4, 8]. A systematic review done in 2008 analyzed 15 patients with left ventricular thrombus formation in TCM. In all 15 cases thrombus was located in the left ventricular apical region and complete thrombus resolution was documented in every patient [9]. Here we summarise 50 cases of takotsubo cardiomyopathy complicated with ventricular thrombosis reported in the literature from 2003 to 2017 (Table 1). Like our patient, the majority of the cases was female (45 out of 49 patients; 92%) and was above 60 years of age (30 out of 49; 61%).

Abnormality in the contraction of the left ventricular apical region resulting in transient apical aneurysm and local hemostasis [4], endocardial injury with local exposure or release of thrombogenic substances [10] and influence of catecholamines on nucleotide-induced platelet aggregation [11, 12] have been postulated as possible mechanisms for the thrombus formation. In TCM, ventricular apical aneurysm always occurs during the acute phase and is often more extensive than in acute myocardial infarction. Plasma catecholamine levels are also much higher in the TCM than in acute coronary syndrome. These might be the causes why out patient developed apical thrombus in the very acute phase.

In our patient, the thrombus was detected using TTE. Ventriculography or cardiac magnetic resonance imaging can also be used to recognize this complication. The cardiac magnetic resonance imaging (MRI) features

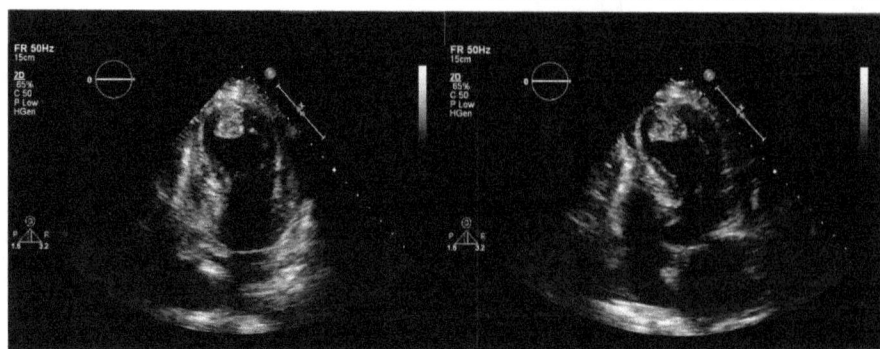

Fig. 2 Transthoracic echocardiogram, performed 18 h after the onset of chest pain, showing hypokinesia of the *left* ventricular apex with apical ballooning. Ejection fraction was 40% and a 2.5 cm × 2 cm apical thrombus was detected

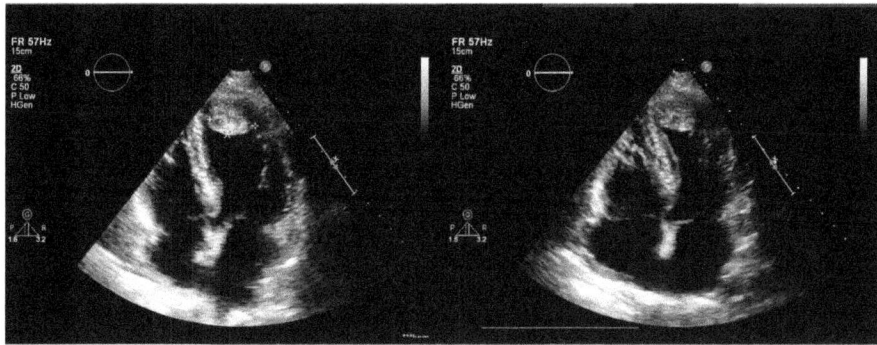

Fig. 3 Follow up transthoracic echocardiogram, done 1 week later, showing only mild hypokinesia of the apex of the *left* ventricle and the thrombus which had reduced in size (2.1 cm × 1.8 cm)

of a thrombus in TCM was first described by Singh, V. et al. [10]. Cardiac MRI [13] and contrast CT [14] have been used to identify ventricular thrombi that are not visualized by echocardiography and provide more information on the myocardium. In our patient, we did not perform cardiac MRI or CT and ventriculography was not performed due to increased risk of thromboembolism.

The significant feature in our case is the rapid development of ventricular thrombus within 24 h, despite administration of streptokinase and heparin. We could only find one other reported case, which described a ventricular thrombus found on TTE performed within 24 h from the onset of symptoms [8]. Kimura, K. et al., had reported a giant apical thrombus which had formed within 2 days [15]. In all but 3 cases the thrombus was identified within 14 days. Lee, P.H. et al., had reported a case of TCM in which a newly developed apical thrombus was noted 5 weeks later in serial TTE which is the longest time period reported in literature [16]. This patient had a multi-septated liver abscess with adjacent hepatic venous thrombosis, a very low ejection

fraction of 18% and had to be treated at the medical intensive care unit with inotropic support. Another case report describes a patient who developed a renal infarct 11 weeks after TCM, with TTE demonstrating a thrombus attached to the left ventricular apical wall [17]. Here serial TTE had not been performed, so the exact time taken for the development of thrombus was not certain. This patient had a bicuspid aortic valve and aortic regurgitation, so the author highlights that a ventricular thrombus should be considered not only as an early but also as a delayed complication of TCM, especially in a patient with organic heart disease. Shim, I.K. et al., reported a case in which an apical thrombus was visualized on TTE performed 3 weeks after TCM [18]. This patient had a 25-year history of systemic lupus erythematosus and the apical ballooning persisted for more than 3 weeks.

We were unable to find any case reports of TCM complicated with thrombus formation despite administration of streptokinase and heparin on admission. In one case report, TTE performed 24 h later revealed a solid thrombus in the akinetic apical region of the left

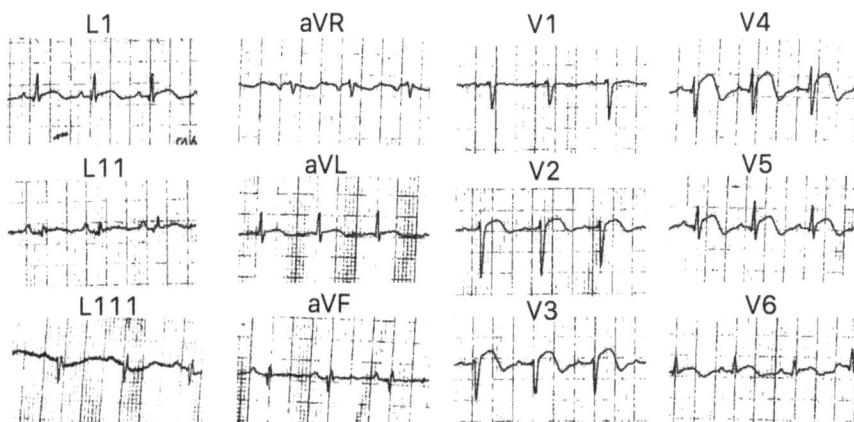

Fig. 4 ECG done 1 week later showing resolving ST elevations

Table 1 Case report review of takotsubo cardiomyopathy complicated with ventricular thrombus formation from 2003 to 2017

Year	Age (Years)	Gender	Day of diagnosis[a]	Site of the thrombus	Treatment[b]	Time for resolution[c]	Ejection Fraction %	Thrombo Embolism[d]	Reference
2003	74	F	4	4 × 4 mm, LV apex	Warfarin	2w		Right hemiparesis	[6]
2003	64	F	2	LV	Anticoagulation	12w	40		[7]
2004	76	F	6		Heparin and warfarin	2w			[35]
2004	57	F	2	LV apex, 2.0 × 1.5 cm	Heparin and warfarin	4w		Right upper limb hemiplegia	[36]
2004	44	F	11 weeks	LV apex	Urokinase, warfarin			Renal infarct	[17]
2006	64	F		LV apex, 13 × 8 mm	Anticoagulant	4w			[37]
2006	76	F		LV apex	Anticoagulant	3w	35		[38]
2007	54	F	2	LV apex	Heparin and warfarin	1w			[15]
2007	74	F	3	LV apex	Heparin and warfarin	12d	33		[39]
2007	70	F	3	LV apex	Anticoagulant	3 m		Sensory aphasia	[40]
2007	74	M	14	20 × 15 mm LV apex	Anticoagulant	7w	30		[10]
2007	74	F		LV apex	Anticoagulant	2 m	40		[41]
2008	69	F	1	LV apex, Two mobile thrombi 5 × 6 mm and 8 × 10 mm	Heparin and phenprocoumon	4w	39		[8]
2008	69	F	8	Mobile thrombus adjacent to the posteromedial papillary muscle	Heparin	9d	30		[8]
2008	43	F	4	LV apex	Heparin	11d	34		[8]
2008	69	F	3	28 × 22 mm anterior and anteroseptal wall, 4 × 4 mm mobile thrombus adjacent to the anterolateral papillary muscle	Heparin	27d	45		[8]
2008	55	F	2	LV apex	Heparin and warfarin	1 m			[19]
2008	53	F		LV apex	Heparin aspirin	2w	32		[42]
2008	74	F		Multiple thrombotic masses	Warfarin	2w	35	Dysphasia, right arm paresis	[26]
2008	43	F	5	LV apex	Heparin and warfarin	8d	<25	Right renal infarct	[43]
2008	64	F		LV apex	Warfarin		45	Broca's aphasia	[44]
2009	28	F	3	LV apex	Heparin and warfarin	3w	25		[20]
2009	57	M		LV apex	Heparin and warfarin	2w	48		[45]
2011	78 87 71 82 55	F F F F F		Mural in 2 cases and protruding in 3 cases	Anticoagulant	4w	45 ± 6%	Cerebral infarction in one patient	[4]
2011	62	F	35	LV apex	Heparin and warfarin	3 m	18		[16]
2011	76	F	8	LV apex, 24 × 25 mm	Heparin and warfarin	1w	18	Multiple brain embolic infarctions	[46]
2011	68	F	3	LV apex, 26 × 29 mm	Heparin and warfarin	12d			[47]

Table 1 Case report review of takotsubo cardiomyopathy complicated with ventricular thrombus formation from 2003 to 2017 *(Continued)*

Year	Age	Sex		Location	Treatment				Ref
2011	69	F	6	LV apex	Anticoagulant	14d			[48]
2012	78	F		LV apex	Anticoagulant	2w	50		[49]
2012	70	F	13	LV apex	Anticoagulant		55		[50]
2012	29	F	2	Mid right ventricular cavity, 16 × 9 8 mm,	Anticoagulant	7d			[22]
2012	48	M	15	Apical inferior wall, 28 × 16 mm	Sx				[25]
2012	78	F	7	LV apex	Heparin	17d			[30]
2013	52	F	3	LV apex, 37 × 21 mm	Heparin and warfarin			Multifocal micro infarctions in the brain, pleen and kidneys	[27]
2013	78	F		Attached to septoapical wall, 30 × 15 mm	Aspirin, heparin		35	Left hemiparesis and dysarthria, large thrombus at the trunk and branches of the superior mesenteric artery	[24]
2013	50	M		LV apex, 3.6 cm × 1.7 cm	Enoxaparin, Clopidogrel and warfarin	7w	45	Dense left sided hemiplegia, left homonymous hemianopia, aphasia	[31]
2013	63	F	3 weeks	LV apex, 1.10 × 2.12 cm	Heparin and warfarin	3 m	43		[18]
2013	58	F	2		Heparin, warfarin and sx				[33]
2015	66	F		LV apex	Heparin, acetyl-salicylic acid and clopidogrel	17d		Ischemic infarctions of the left median cerebral artery	[51]
2015	59	F	13	LV apex	Heparin, Warfarin, sx		<25		[21]
2016	48	F		LV apex	Anticoagulant	3 m		Right femoral artery embolism	[52]
2016	57	F	4	LV apex, 2.3 × 3.3 cm	Warfarin	15d	35		[53]
2016	61	F		LV apex	Heparin and warfarin		35		[14]
2016	55	F		LV apex, 20 × 10 mm	Warfarin	3 m			[54]
2017	48	F		LV apex	Heparin and warfarin		30		[55]
2017	88	F		Biventricular	Heparin		35		[21]
2003	74	F	4	4 × 4 mm, LV apex	Warfarin	2w		Right hemiparesis	[6]
2003	64	F	2	LV	Anticoagulation	12w	40		[7]
2004	76	F	6		Heparin and warfarin	2w			[35]
2004	57	F	2	LV apex, 2.0 × 1.5 cm	Heparin and warfarin	4w		Right upper limb hemiplegia	[36]
2004	44	F	11 weeks	LV apex	Urokinase, warfarin			Renal infarct	[17]
2006	64	F		LV apex, 13 × 8 mm	Anticoagulant	4w			[37]
2006	76	F		LV apex	Anticoagulant	3w	35		[38]
2007	54	F	2	LV apex	Heparin and warfarin	1w			[15]
2007	74	F	3	LV apex	Heparin and warfarin	12d	33		[39]

Table 1 Case report review of takotsubo cardiomyopathy complicated with ventricular thrombus formation from 2003 to 2017 (Continued)

Year	Age	Sex		Location	Treatment	Duration	EF	Complications	Ref
2007	70	F	3	LV apex	Anticoagulant	3 m		Sensory aphasia	[40]
2007	74	M	14	20 × 15 mm LV apex	Anticoagulant	7w	30		[10]
2007	74	F		LV apex	Anticoagulant	2 m	40		[41]
2008	69	F	1	LV apex, Two mobile thrombi 5 × 6 mm and 8 × 10 mm	Heparin and phenprocoumon	4w	39		[8]
2008	69	F	8	Mobile thrombus adjacent to the posteromedial papillary muscle	Heparin	9d	30		[8]
2008	43	F	4	LV apex	Heparin	11d	34		[8]
2008	69	F	3	28 × 22 mm anterior and anteroseptal wall, 4 × 4 mm mobile thrombus adjacent to the anterolateral papillary muscle	Heparin	27d	45		[8]
2008	55	F	2	LV apex	Heparin and warfarin	1 m			[19]
2008	53	F		LV apex	Heparin aspirin	2w	32		[42]
2008	74	F		Multiple thrombotic masses	Warfarin	2w	35	Dysphasia, right arm paresis	[26]
2008	43	F	5	LV apex	Heparin and warfarin	8d	<25	Right renal infarct	[43]
2008	64	F		LV apex	Warfarin		45	Broca's aphasia	[44]
2009	28	F	3	LV apex	Heparin and warfarin	3w	25		[20]
2009	57	M		LV apex	Heparin and warfarin	2w	48		[45]
2011	78 87 71 82 55	F F F F F		Mural in 2 cases and protruding in 3 cases	Anticoagulant	4w	45 ± 6%	Cerebral infarction in one patient	[4]
2011	62	F	35	LV apex	Heparin and warfarin	3 m	18		[16]
2011	76	F	8	LV apex, 24 × 25 mm	Heparin and warfarin	1w	18	Multiple brain embolic infarctions	[46]
2011	68	F	3	LV apex, 26 × 29 mm	Heparin and warfarin	12d			[47]
2011	69	F	6	LV apex	Anticoagulant	14d			[48]
2012	78	F		LV apex	Anticoagulant	2w	50		[49]
2012	70	F	13	LV apex	Anticoagulant		55		[50]
2012	29	F	2	Mid right ventricular cavity, 16 × 9 8 mm,	Anticoagulant	7d			[22]
2012	48	M	15	Apical inferior wall, 28 × 16 mm	Sx				[25]
2012	78	F	7	LV apex	Heparin	17d			[30]
2013	52	F	3	LV apex, 37 × 21 mm	Heparin and warfarin			Multifocal micro infarctions in the brain, spleen and kidneys	[27]

Table 1 Case report review of takotsubo cardiomyopathy complicated with ventricular thrombus formation from 2003 to 2017 (Continued)

2013	78	F		Attached to septoapical wall, 30 × 15 mm	Aspirin, heparin		35	Left hemiparesis and dysarthria, large thrombus at the trunk and branches of the superior mesenteric artery	[24]
2013	50	M		LV apex, 3.6 cm × 1.7 cm	Enoxaparin, Clopidogrel and warfarin	7w	45	Dense left sided hemiplegia, left homonymous hemianopia, aphasia	[31]
2013	63	F	3 weeks	LV apex, 1.10 × 2.12 cm	Heparin and warfarin	3 m	43		[18]
2013	58	F	2		Heparin, warfarin and sx				[33]
2015	66	F		LV apex	Heparin, acetyl-salicylic acid and clopidogrel	17d		Ischemic infarctions of the left median cerebral artery	[51]
2015	59	F	13	LV apex	Heparin, Warfarin, sx		<25		[21]
2016	48	F		LV apex	Anticoagulant	3 m		Right femoral artery embolism	[52]
2016	57	F	4	LV apex, 2.3 × 3.3 cm	Warfarin	15d	35		[53]
2016	61	F		LV apex	Heparin and warfarin		35		[14]
2016	55	F		LV apex, 20 × 10 mm	Warfarin	3 m			[54]
2017	48	F		LV apex	Heparin and warfarin		30		[55]
2017	88	F		Biventricular	Heparin		35		[21]
2003	74	F	4	4 × 4 mm, LV apex	Warfarin	2w		Right hemiparesis	[6]
2003	64	F	2	LV	Anticoagulation	12w	40		[7]
2004	76	F	6		Heparin and warfarin	2w			[34]
2004	57	F	2	LV apex, 2.0 × 1.5 cm	Heparin and warfarin	4w		Right upper limb hemiplegia	[35]
2004	44	F	11 weeks	LV apex	Urokinase, warfarin			Renal infarct	[17]
2006	64	F		LV apex, 13 × 8 mm	Anticoagulant	4w			[36]
2006	76	F		LV apex	Anticoagulant	3w	35		[37]
2007	54	F	2	LV apex	Heparin and warfarin	1w			[15]
2007	74	F	3	LV apex	Heparin and warfarin	12d	33		[38]
2007	70	F	3	LV apex	Anticoagulant	3 m		Sensory aphasia	[39]
2007	74	M	14	20 × 15 mm LV apex	Anticoagulant	7w	30		[10]
2007	74	F		LV apex	Anticoagulant	2 m	40		[40]
2008	69	F	1	LV apex, Two mobile thrombi 5 × 6 mm and 8 × 10 mm	Heparin and phenprocoumon	4w	39		[8]
2008	69	F	8	Mobile thrombus adjacent to the posteromedial papillary muscle	Heparin	9d	30		[8]
2008	43	F	4	LV apex	Heparin	11d	34		[8]

Table 1 Case report review of takotsubo cardiomyopathy complicated with ventricular thrombus formation from 2003 to 2017 *(Continued)*

Year	Age	Sex		Location	Treatment		EF	Complications	Ref
2008	69	F	3	28 × 22 mm anterior and anteroseptal wall, 4 × 4 mm mobile thrombus adjacent to the anterolateral papillary muscle	Heparin	27d	45		[8]
2008	55	F	2	LV apex	Heparin and warfarin	1 m			[19]
2008	53	F		LV apex	Heparin aspirin	2w	32		[41]
2008	74	F		Multiple thrombotic masses	Warfarin	2w	35	Dysphasia, right arm paresis	[24]
2008	43	F	5	LV apex	Heparin and warfarin	8d	<25	Right renal infarct	[42]
2008	64	F		LV apex	Warfarin		45	Broca's aphasia	[43]
2009	28	F	3	LV apex	Heparin and warfarin	3w	25		[44]
2009	57	M		LV apex	Heparin and warfarin	2w	48		[45]
2011	78 87 71 82 55	F F F F F		Mural in 2 cases and protruding in 3 cases	Anticoagulant	4w	45 ± 6%	Cerebral infarction in one patient	[4]
2011	62	F	35	LV apex	Heparin and warfarin	3 m	18		[16]
2011	76	F	8	LV apex, 24 × 25 mm	Heparin and warfarin	1w	18	Multiple brain embolic infarctions	[46]
2011	68	F	3	LV apex, 26 × 29 mm	Heparin and warfarin	12d			[47]
2011	69	F	6	LV apex	Anticoagulant	14d			[48]
2012	78	F		LV apex	Anticoagulant	2w	50		[49]
2012	70	F	13	LV apex	Anticoagulant		55		[50]
2012	29	F	2	Mid right ventricular cavity, 16 × 9 8 mm,	Anticoagulant	7d			[20]
2012	48	M	15	Apical inferior wall, 28 × 16 mm	Sx				[23]
2012	78	F	7	LV apex	Heparin	17d			[28]
2013	52	F	3	LV apex, 37 × 21 mm	Heparin and warfarin			Multifocal micro infarctions in the brain, spleen and kidneys	[25]
2013	78	F		Attached to septoapical wall, 30 × 15 mm	Aspirin, heparin		35	Left hemiparesis and dysarthria, large thrombus at the trunk and branches of the superior mesenteric artery	[22]
2013	50	M		LV apex, 3.6 cm × 1.7 cm	Enoxaparin, Clopidogrel and warfarin	7w	45	Dense left sided hemiplegia, left homonymous hemianopia, aphasia	[29]
2013	63	F	3 weeks	LV apex, 1.10 × 2.12 cm	Heparin and warfarin	3 m	43		[18]
2013	58	F	2		Heparin, warfarin and sx				[31]

Table 1 Case report review of takotsubo cardiomyopathy complicated with ventricular thrombus formation from 2003 to 2017 (Continued)

Year	Age	Sex	Day of diagnosis	Location	Treatment	Time for resolution	EF	Thrombo Embolism	Reference
2015	66	F		LV apex	Heparin, acetyl-salicylic acid and clopidogrel	17d		Ischemic infarctions of the left median cerebral artery	[51]
2015	59	F	13	LV apex	Heparin, Warfarin, sx		<25		[32]
2016	48	F		LV apex	Anticoagulant	3 m		Right femoral artery embolism	[52]
2016	57	F	4	LV apex, 2.3 × 3.3 cm	Warfarin	15d	35		[53]
2016	61	F		LV apex	Heparin and warfarin		35		[14]
2016	55	F		LV apex, 20 × 10 mm	Warfarin	3 m			[54]
2017	48	F		LV apex	Heparin and warfarin		30		[55]
2017	88	F		Biventricular	Heparin		35		[21]

F female, M male,

Day of diagnosis[a] = the date of diagnosis from the onset of symptoms / diagnosis of takotsubo cardiomyopathy, given in number of days, in 2 cases given in weeks

Treatment[b] = anticoagulant = In case reports which has not specified the anticoagulant used, Sx = ventriculotomy and surgical thrombectomy

Time for resolution[c] = d days, w weeks, m months

Thrombo Embolism[d] = Thrombo embolic episodes diagnosed after the detection of ventricular thrombus

ventricle [19] despite an oral dose of aspirin 300 mg and a bolus of intravenous heparin 4000 U given on admission. In another case report, an apical clot was visualized on day 3 and in this patient, aspirin, intravenous heparin, and glycoprotein IIb/IIIa inhibitor was started on admission, but stopped on the same day [20]. Niino, T. et al., reported a case in which TTE revealed an apical thrombus on day 13 and this patient received heparin from day 1 to day 6 [21]. One patient had developed a thrombus while on full dose of low molecular weight heparin [8].

As in most cases described in literature, in our patient a single thrombus was visualized at the apex of the left ventricle. Only one case report described a thrombus in the right ventricular cavity attached to the akinetic right ventricular free wall [22]. A recent case repot describes a 88 years old female with biventricular TCM complicated by biventricular thrombosis [23]. A thrombus attached to the septo-apical wall [24], a thrombus attached to the apical inferior wall by a thin stalk [25], a thrombus attached to an akinetic segment of the anterior and anteroseptal wall, a mobile thrombus adjacent to the anterolateral papillary muscle [8], a mobile thrombus adjacent to the posteromedial papillary muscle [8], two mobile thrombi in the left ventricular apex [8] and multiple thrombotic masses in the left ventricular apex [26] were also described.

The feared complication of a left ventricular thrombus is embolisation and fortunately our patient did not have any embolic events, which was probably prevented by early treatment. Out of the 49 cases we summarized, 8 cases had isolated cerebral thromboemboli, one case had an isolated renal infarct [17], one case had multifocal micro infarctions in the brain, spleen and kidneys [27] and one case had cerebral and superior mesenteric artery thromboembolism [24] (Table 1). The management of TCM with ventricular thrombus is directed to prevent embolic episodes and in most cases heparin and warfarin were used for anticoagulation (Table 1). In one case, urokinase was used for lysis of the thrombus [17]. Since no guidelines are available for management, indirect data can be used from randomized trials that evaluated anticoagulation to prevent left ventricular thrombus formation and embolisation in patients with acute myocardial infarction. For patients with anterior myocardial infarction and left ventricular thrombus or at high risk for left ventricular thrombus (ejection fraction less than 40%, antero- apical wall motion abnormality) American College of Chest Physician's Evidence-Based Clinical Practice Guidelines recommend warfarin (plus antiplatelet for ischemic heart disease) [28]. The duration of warfarin therapy for these patients with acute myocardial infarction is at least for 3 months according to guidelines. However the wall motion abnormalities in TCM are known to improve rapidly and completely compared to acute myocardial infarction, so the optimum duration of anticoagulation in not clear - in most cases thrombus resolved within 1 month (39 out of 49; 80%) and in all cases the thrombus resolved within 3 months. Serial TTE was performed for the majority of cases to confirm thrombus resolution. We could find only one case report describing repeated embolic events despite anticoagulation with subcutaneous enoxaparin and aspirin treatment [24]. Myocardial necrosis and cardiac rupture [29], massive hemorrhagic effusion following ventricular wall rupture [30], large cerebral infarct with mass effect and hemorrhagic transformation [31] can complicate the medical management. Most thrombi described were smooth, conform to the cavity shape and are relatively stable. Thrombectomy is rarely recommended if they are mobile or pedunculated, due to the high risk of embolization [32]. Ventriculotomy and surgical thrombectomy was only indicated in 3 of the reported cases [21, 25, 33]. Based on the available evidence, we commenced enoxaparin with warfarin and the thrombus resolved in 3 weeks following which anticoagulation was omitted.

Use of prophylactic anticoagulation to prevent thrombus formation in TCM is not practiced and no specific clinical, radiological or biochemical marker is available to risk categorize these patients. Haghi, D. et al., have stated that elevated serum CRP levels and thrombocytosis indicate higher risk of developing thrombi [8] and Ouchi, K. et al., have suggested D-dimer levels as a screening test for thrombosis [14]. In our patient, CRP was not significantly elevated and the platelet count was normal. Only a few case reports are available, and in most of them full biochemical analysis was not performed, limiting our ability to formulate risk factors to predict thrombus formation in TCM. No particular features to predict the occurrence of left ventricular thrombosis were identified in the only published systematic review either [9]. The number of echocardiograms performed in a patient, the operator skill and the use of cardiac MRI and CT influence thrombus detection making the determination of the true incidence of left ventricular thrombosis in TCM difficult, again limiting recommendations regarding prophylactic anticoagulation. Since most of the patients with TCM present with chest pain and ST segment elevation [34], the chances of receiving thrombolytic therapy, antiplatelets and anticoagulation on presentation are high, as was the case for our patient. This may reduce the chance of thrombus formation, because the majority of those who developed the complication had not received any form of anticoagulation prior to detection of the thrombus.

Conclusion
Although severe systolic dysfunction is observed in almost all patients with TCM, intraventricular thrombus formation is rarely reported in the literature. Most thrombi were detected during the first 2 weeks, emphasising the importance of follow up echocardiography at least 2 weeks later. The management of a left ventricular thrombus in TCM is controversial and in most cases warfarin and heparin

is used for a short duration. Most of the thrombi resolved within 2 weeks of therapy and serial TTE can be used to monitor response. The role of prophylactic anticoagulants in TCM and risk factors to predict thrombosis should be examined further as current data is not enough to formulate a firm recommendation.

Additional files

Additional file 1: Movie S1. TTE performed 18 h after the onset of chest pain, revealing hypokinesia of the mid and apical segments of the left ventricle with typical LV apical ballooning. Ejection fraction was 40% and a 2.5 cm × 2 cm apical thrombus was detected. (AVI 17890 kb)

Additional file 2: Movie S2. TTE performed 18 h after the onset of chest pain, revealing hypokinesia of the mid and apical segments of the left ventricle with typical LV apical ballooning. Ejection fraction was 40% and a 2.5 cm × 2 cm apical thrombus was detected. (AVI 15305 kb)

Abbreviations
CRP: C-reactive protein; ECG: electrocardiogram; MRI: magnetic resonance imaging; STEMI: ST elevation myocardial infarction; TCM: Takotsubo cardiomyopathy; TTE: transthoracic echocardiogram

Acknowledgements
This case reports were supported by ward doctors in acquisition, analysising and interpretation of data. We are thankful to the patients relatives for the support given in providing data.

Funding
No source of funding.

Authors' contributions
Dr.H.M.M.T.B.H, Dr. L.C.L., Dr. S.V. and Dr. M.W. collected data, followed up the patient and did the literature review and drafted the manuscript. Dr.S.P.P, Dr. S.W and Dr. V.S. corrected the manuscript. All authors read and approved the final manuscript.

Competing interests
The authors declare that they have no competing interests.

Author details
[1]National Hospital, Colombo, Sri Lanka. [2]University of Edinburg, National Hospital, University of Edinburg, Scotland, Sri Lanka.

References
1. Akashi YJ, Goldstein DS, Barbaro G, Ueyama T. Takotsubo cardiomyopathy: a new form of acute, reversible heart failure. Circulation. 2008;118(25):2754–62.
2. Wittstein IS, Thiemann DR, Lima JA, Baughman KL, Schulman SP, Gerstenblith G, et al. Neurohumoral features of myocardial stunning due to sudden emotional stress. N Engl J Med. 2005;352(6):539–48.
3. Paur H, Wright PT, Sikkel MB, Tranter MH, Mansfield C, O'Gara P, et al. High levels of circulating epinephrine trigger apical cardiodepression in a beta2-adrenergic receptor/Gi-dependent manner: a new model of Takotsubo cardiomyopathy. Circulation. 2012;126(6):697–706.

4. Kurisu S, Inoue I, Kawagoe T, Ishihara M, Shimatani Y, Nakama Y, et al. Incidence and treatment of left ventricular apical thrombosis in Tako-tsubo cardiomyopathy. Int J Cardiol. 2011;146(3):e58–60.

5. Prasad A, Lerman A, Rihal CS. Apical ballooning syndrome (Tako-Tsubo or stress cardiomyopathy): a mimic of acute myocardial infarction. Am Heart J. 2008;155(3):408–17.

6. Kurisu S, Inoue I, Kawagoe T, Ishihara M, Shimatani Y, Nishioka K, et al. Left ventricular apical thrombus formation in a patient with suspected tako-tsubo-like left ventricular dysfunction. Circ J. 2003;67(6):556–8.

7. Barrera-Ramirez CF, Jimenez-Mazuecos JM, Alfonso F. Apical thrombus associated with left ventricular apical ballooning. Heart. 2003;89(8):927.

8. Haghi D, Papavassiliu T, Heggemann F, Kaden JJ, Borggrefe M, Suselbeck T. Incidence and clinical significance of left ventricular thrombus in tako-tsubo cardiomyopathy assessed with echocardiography. QJM. 2008;101(5):381–6.

9. de Gregorio C, Grimaldi P, Lentini C. Left ventricular thrombus formation and cardioembolic complications in patients with Takotsubo-like syndrome: a systematic review. Int J Cardiol. 2008;131(1):18–24.

10. Singh V, Mayer T, Salanitri J, Salinger MH. Cardiac MRI documented left ventricular thrombus complicating acute Takotsubo syndrome: an uncommon dilemma. Int J Cardiovasc Imaging. 2007;23(5):591–3.

11. Ardlie NG, Glew G, Schwartz CJ. Influence of catecholamines on nucleotide-induced platelet aggregation. Nature. 1966;212(5060):415–7.

12. Nunez-Gil IJ, Bernardo E, Feltes G, Escaned J, Mejia-Renteria HD, De Agustin JA, et al. Platelet function in Takotsubo cardiomyopathy. J Thromb Thrombolysis. 2015;39(4):452–8.

13. Sharkey SW, Windenburg DC, Lesser JR, Maron MS, Hauser RG, Lesser JN, et al. Natural history and expansive clinical profile of stress (tako-tsubo) cardiomyopathy. J Am Coll Cardiol. 2010;55(4):333–41.

14. Ouchi K, Nakamura F, Ikutomi M, Oshima T, Ishiwata J, Shinohara H, et al. Usefulness of contrast computed tomography to detect left ventricular apical thrombus associated with takotsubo cardiomyopathy. Heart Vessel. 2016;31(5):822–7.

15. Kimura K, Tanabe-Hayashi Y, Noma S, Fukuda K. Images in cardiovascular medicine. Rapid formation of left ventricular giant thrombus with Takotsubo cardiomyopathy. Circulation. 2007;115(23):e620–1.

16. Lee PH, Song JK, Park IK, Sun BJ, Lee SG, Yim JH, et al. Takotsubo cardiomyopathy: a case of persistent apical ballooning complicated by an apical mural thrombus. Korean J Intern Med. 2011;26(4):455–9.

17. Sasaki N, Kinugawa T, Yamawaki M, Furuse Y, Shimoyama M, Ogino K, et al. Transient left ventricular apical ballooning in a patient with bicuspid aortic valve created a left ventricular thrombus leading to acute renal infarction. Circ J. 2004;68(11):1081–3.

18. Shim IK, Kim BJ, Kim H, Lee JW, Cha TJ, Heo JH. A case of persistent apical ballooning complicated by apical thrombus in takotsubo cardiomyopathy of systemic lupus erythematosus patient. J Cardiovasc Ultrasound. 2013;21(3):137–9.

19. Azzarelli S, Galassi AR, Amico F, Giacoppo M, Argentino V, Giordano G, et al. Apical thrombus in a patient with takotsubo cardiomyopathy. J Cardiovasc Med (Hagerstown). 2008;9(8):831–3.

20. Tobar R, Rotzak R, Rozenman Y. Apical thrombus associated with Takotsubo cardiomyopathy in a young woman. Echocardiography. 2009;26(5):575–80.

21. Niino T, Unosawa S. Surgical extirpation of apical left ventricular thrombus in Takotsubo Cardiomyopathy. Case Rep Surg. 2015;2015:387037.

22. Robaei D, Buchholz S, Feneley M. Biventricular stress-induced (Tako-tsubo) cardiomyopathy complicated by right ventricular thrombus. J Echocardiogr. 2012;10(3):104–5.

23. De Gennaro L, Ruggiero M, Musci S, Tota F, De Laura D, Resta M, et al. Biventricular thrombosis in biventricular stress(takotsubo)-cardiomyopathy. J Thromb Thrombolysis. 2017;

24. Porta A, Barrabes JA, Figueras J, Millan X, Sambola A, Boye R, et al. Transient apical ballooning complicated with left ventricular thrombus and repeated embolic events with fatal outcome despite anticoagulant therapy. Int J Cardiol. 2013;165(1):e11–2.

25. Seitz MJ, McLeod MK, O'Keefe MD, Seah PW. A rare cause of Takotsubo cardiomyopathy related left ventricular apical thrombus requiring surgery. Heart Lung Circ. 2012;21(4):245–6.

26. de Gregorio C, Cento D, Di Bella G, Coglitore S. Minor stroke in a Takotsubo-like syndrome: a rare clinical presentation due to transient left ventricular thrombus. Int J Cardiol. 2008;130(2):e78–80.

27. Celik M, Yalcinkaya E, Yuksel UC, Celik T, Iyisoy A. Multiple foci of infarction secondary to giant left ventricular thrombus in a patient with takotsubo cardiomyopathy. Oman Med J. 2013;28(4):294.

28. Vandvik PO, Lincoff AM, Gore JM, Gutterman DD, Sonnenberg FA, Alonso-Coello P, et al. Primary and secondary prevention of cardiovascular disease: antithrombotic therapy and prevention of thrombosis, 9th ed: American College of Chest Physicians Evidence-Based Clinical Practice Guidelines. Chest. 2012;141(2 Suppl):e637S–68S.

29. Kumar S, Kaushik S, Nautiyal A, Choudhary SK, Kayastha BL, Mostow N, et al. Cardiac rupture in takotsubo cardiomyopathy: a systematic review. Clin Cardiol. 2011;34(11):672–6.

30. Yoshida S, Miwa K, Matsubara T, Yasuda T, Inoue M, Teramoto R, et al. Stress-induced takotsubo cardiomyopathy complicated with wall rupture and thrombus formation. Int J Cardiol. 2012;161(1):e18–20.

31. Al-Farsi K, Siddiqui AA, Sharef YW, Al-Belushi AK, Al-Hashim H, Al-Ghailani M, et al. Hemorrhagic cardioembolic stroke secondary to a left ventricular thrombus: a therapeutic dilemma. Oman Med J. 2013;28(1):56–9.

32. Early GL, Ballenger M, Hannah H 3rd, Roberts SR. Simplified method of left ventricular thrombectomy. Ann Thorac Surg. 2001;72(3):953–4.

33. Suzuki R, Kudo T, Kurazumi H, Takahashi M, Shirasawa B, Mikamo A, et al. Transapical extirpation of a left ventricular thrombus in Takotsubo cardiomyopathy. J Cardiothorac Surg. 2013;8:135.

34. Tsuchihashi K, Ueshima K, Uchida T, Oh-mura N, Kimura K, Owa M, et al. Transient left ventricular apical ballooning without coronary artery stenosis: a novel heart syndrome mimicking acute myocardial infarction. Angina pectoris-myocardial infarction investigations in Japan. J Am Coll Cardiol. 2001;38(1):11–8.

35. Yasuga Y, Inoue M, Takeda Y, Kitazume R, Hayashi N, Nakagawa Y, et al. Tako-tsubo-like transient left ventricular dysfunction with apical thrombus formation: a case report. J Cardiol. 2004;43(2):75–80.

36. Matsuoka K, Nakayama S, Okubo S, Fujii E, Uchida F, Nakano T. Transient cerebral ischemic attack induced by transient left ventricular apical ballooning. Eur J Intern Med. 2004;15(6):393–5.

37. Camastra GS, Cacciotti L, Kol A, Ansalone G. Stress cardiomyopathy with apical thrombosis promptly diagnosed with cardiovascular MRI. Cardiology. 2006;105(2):108–9.

38. Iengo R, Marrazzo G, Rumolo S, Accadia M, Di Donato M, Ascione L, et al. An unusual presentation of "tako-tsubo cardiomyopathy". Eur J Echocardiogr. 2007;8(6):491–4.

39. Korosoglou G, Haars A, Kuecherer H, Giannitsis E, Katus HA. Prompt resolution of an apical left ventricular thrombus in a patient with takotsubo cardiomyopathy. Int J Cardiol. 2007;116(3):e88–91.

40. Schmidt M, Herholz C, Block M. Apical thrombus in tako-tsubo cardiomyopathy. Heart. 2007;93(11):1368.

41. Robles P, Jimenez JJ, Alonso M. Left ventricular thrombus associated with left ventricular apical ballooning. Heart. 2007;93(7):861.

42. Mrdovic I, Perunicic J, Asanin M, Matic M, Vasiljevic Z, Ostojic M. Transient left ventricular apical ballooning complicated by a mural thrombus and outflow tract obstruction in a patient with pheochromocytoma. Tex Heart Inst J. 2008;35(4):480–2.

43. Nerella N, Lodha A, Tiu CT, Chandra PA, Rose M. Thromboembolism in takotsubo syndrome: a case report. Int J Cardiol. 2008;124(2):e37–8.

44. Grabowski A, Kilian J, Strank C, Cieslinski G, Meyding-Lamade U. Takotsubo cardiomyopathy–a rare cause of cardioembolic stroke. Cerebrovasc Dis. 2007;24(1):146–8.

45. Yoshida T, Hibino T, Fujimaki T, Oguri M, Kato K, Yajima K, et al. Tako-tsubo cardiomyopathy complicated by apical thrombus formation: a case report. Int J Cardiol. 2009;132(3):e120–2.

46. Shin SN, Yun KH, Ko JS, Rhee SJ, Yoo NJ, Kim NH, et al. Left ventricular thrombus associated with takotsubo cardiomyopathy: a cardioembolic cause of cerebral infarction. J Cardiovasc Ultrasound. 2011;19(3):152–5.

47. Wakabayashi K, Dohi T, Daida H. Takotsubo cardiomyopathy associated with epilepsy complicated with giant thrombus. Int J Cardiol. 2011;148(2):e28–30.

48. Yaguchi M, Yaguchi H, Takahashi N. A case of asymptomatic takotsubo cardiomyopathy with intraventricular thrombus associated with epileptic seizure. Brain Nerve. 2011;63(8):897–900.

49. Correia AS, Moreno N, Goncalves A, Araujo V, Pinho T, Rodrigues RA, et al. Cardiac thrombus and conduction disorder in takotsubo cardiomyopathy. Rev Port Cardiol. 2012;31(7–8):513–6.

50. Michels G, Pfister R. De novo left ventricular thrombus during tako-tsubo cardiomyopathy. Dtsch Med Wochenschr. 2012;137(47):2423–6.

51. Finsterer J, Stollberger C, Pulgram T. Paraneoplastic takotsubo syndrome with ventricular thrombus and stroke. Herz. 2015;40(4):632–4.

52. Gulsin G, Serna S, Morris C, Taher A, Loke I. Takotsubo cardiomyopathy with left ventricular thrombus presenting as critical limb ischaemia. Oxf Med Case Reports. 2016;2016(8):omw051.
53. Icli A, Akilli H, Kayrak M, Aribas A, Ozdemir K. Short-term warfarin treatment for apical thrombus in a patient with Takotsubo cardiomyopathy. Cardiovasc J Afr. 2016;27(3):e12–e4.
54. Wong GR, Roberts-Thomson R, Parvar SL, Nelson AJ. Large apical thrombus due to Takotsubo cardiomyopathy. BMJ Case Rep. 2016;2016
55. Ahmed AE, Serafi A, Sunni NS, Younes H, Hassan W. Recurrent takotsubo with prolonged QT and torsade de pointes and left ventricular thrombus. J Saudi Heart Assoc. 2017;29(1):44–52.

28

Left ventricular remodeling in hypertrophic cardiomyopathy patients with atrial fibrillation

Hongwei Tian, Jingang Cui, Chengzhi Yang, Fenghuan Hu, Jiansong Yuan, Shengwen Liu, Weixian Yang, Xiaowei Jiang and Shubin Qiao[*] (iD)

Abstract

Background: Atrial fibrillation (AF) is the most common complication in hypertrophic cardiomyopathy (HCM). The mechanisms of AF is associated with left atrial (LA) structural remodeling in HCM patients. However, the impact of left ventricular (LV) remodeling on the presence of AF in HCM patients has not been evaluated yet. We sought to investigate effect of LV remodeling on the presence of AF assessed by cardiovascular magnetic resonance (CMR) in HCM patients.

Methods: A total of 394 HCM patients were enrolled into this study, including HOCM patients ($n = 293$) and NOHCM patients ($n = 101$). Patients were divided into HCM with AF (50) and HCM without AF ($n = 344$). Data were collected from hospital records.

Results: LA diameter and LV remodeling index (LVRI) were significantly higher in HCM patients with AF than that of HCM patients without AF (46.6 ± 7.4 mm versus 39.9 ± 8.0 mm, $p < 0.001$, and 1.46 ± 0.6 versus 1.2 ± 0.4, $p = 0.002$, respectively). HCM patients with AF were older than HCM patients without AF (53.6 ± 11.7 years versus 47.7 ± 13.6 years, $p = 0.002$). Additionally, LVRI positively correlated to LA size ($r = 0.12$, $p = 0.02$). In a multivariable logistic regression analysis, when adjusting for age and LV end diastolic mass index, LVRI and LA size remained an independent determinant of AF in HCM patients ($OR = 4.7$, $p = 0.001$ and $OR = 1.13$, $P < 0.001$).

Conclusion: HCM patients with AF showed significantly more LA diameter, LVRI and age than HCM patients without AF. LVRI and LA size were strong independent predictor of AF in HCM, suggesting LV remodeling may contribute to the occurrence of AF in HCM patients.

Keywords: Atrial fibrillation, Hypertrophic cardiomyopathy, Left ventricular remodeling

Background

Hypertrophic cardiomyopathy (HCM) is a complex and relatively common form of genetic heart disease characterized by left ventricular (LV) hypertrophy and the most frequent cause of sudden death in the young [1]. Histologically, HCM is characterized by myocyte disarray, scarring and microvascular dysfunction [2].

Atrial fibrillation (AF) is the most common arrhythmia in HCM and was associated with an increased risk for morbidity and mortality [3, 4]. The mechanisms of AF are complex and associated with structural and electrical remodeling in the atria and ventricular myocardium [5, 6]. In HCM patients, increased LA size, late gadolinium-enhancement (LGE) and advanced age have been shown to be independent predictors of the presence of AF [7, 2, 8]. However, the impact of LV remodeling on the presence of AF in HCM patients has not been evaluated yet. Thus, we used cardiovascular magnetic resonance (CMR) to evaluate effect of left ventricular remodeling index (LVRI) on the presence of AF in HCM patients.

---

* Correspondence: qsbfw@sina.com
State Key Laboratory of Cardiovascular Disease, Fuwai Hospital, National Center for Cardiovascular Diseases, Chinese Academy of Medical Sciences and Peking Union Medical College, Beijing 100037, China

Methods

Study population

The protocol study was approved by Fuwai Hospital ethics committee. The informed consents were obtained from all participants. We retrospectively analyzed data from 440 HCM patients who had maximum LV wall thickness ≥ 15 mm (or ≥ 13 mm with an unequivocal family history of HCM) in the absence of other cardiac or systemic causes of left ventricular hypertrophy [9, 10] between November 2012 and August 2016. Evaluation of patients included complete medical history, blood examination, physical examination, 24-h ambulatory electrocardiographic monitoring, transthoracic echocardiography, invasive coronary angiography, 12-lead electrocardiography and cardiovascular magnetic resonance imaging (MRI). Patients were excluded if they had (1) coronary artery disease (coronary artery stenosis > 50%), (2) renal dysfunction, (3) heart failure, (4) cardiac valve disease, (5) permanent mechanical device implantation. Forty-six patients were excluded owing to concomitant coronary artery disease ($n = 44$) and cardiac valve disease ($n = 2$) (Fig. 1). Finally, a total of 394 patients were enrolled into this study, including HOCM patients ($n = 293$) and NOHCM patients ($n = 101$). Patients were divided into HCM with AF (50) and HCM without AF ($n = 344$).

Echocardiography

Standard transthoracic M-mode, 2-dimensional, and pulse-wave and continuous-wave Doppler images were obtained with an iE33 Color Doppler Ultrasound System (Philips Healthcare, Andover, Massachusetts). All measurements were analyzed following the guidelines of the American Society of Echocardiography. The left ventricular outflow tract (LVOT) peak gradient was estimated using the simplified Bernoulli eq. HCM with obstruction was defined as an LVOT peak gradient ≥30 mmHg at rest or provoked LVOT peak gradient > 50 mmHg. Patients were divided into non-obstructive (NOHCM) or obstructive (HOCM) based on left ventricular outflow tract obstruction [11].

Cardiovascular MRI

CMR was performed using a 1.5-T speed clinical scanner (Magnetom Avanto; Siemens Medical Solutions, Erlangen, Germany). All MR image was analysed by a single experienced observer who was blinded to the all HCM patients. Endocardial contours of the LV myocardium were manually traced at end-diastole and end-systole on each LV short-axis cine image. LV end-diastolic volume (LVEDV), stroke volume, LV end-systolic volume (LVESV), LV

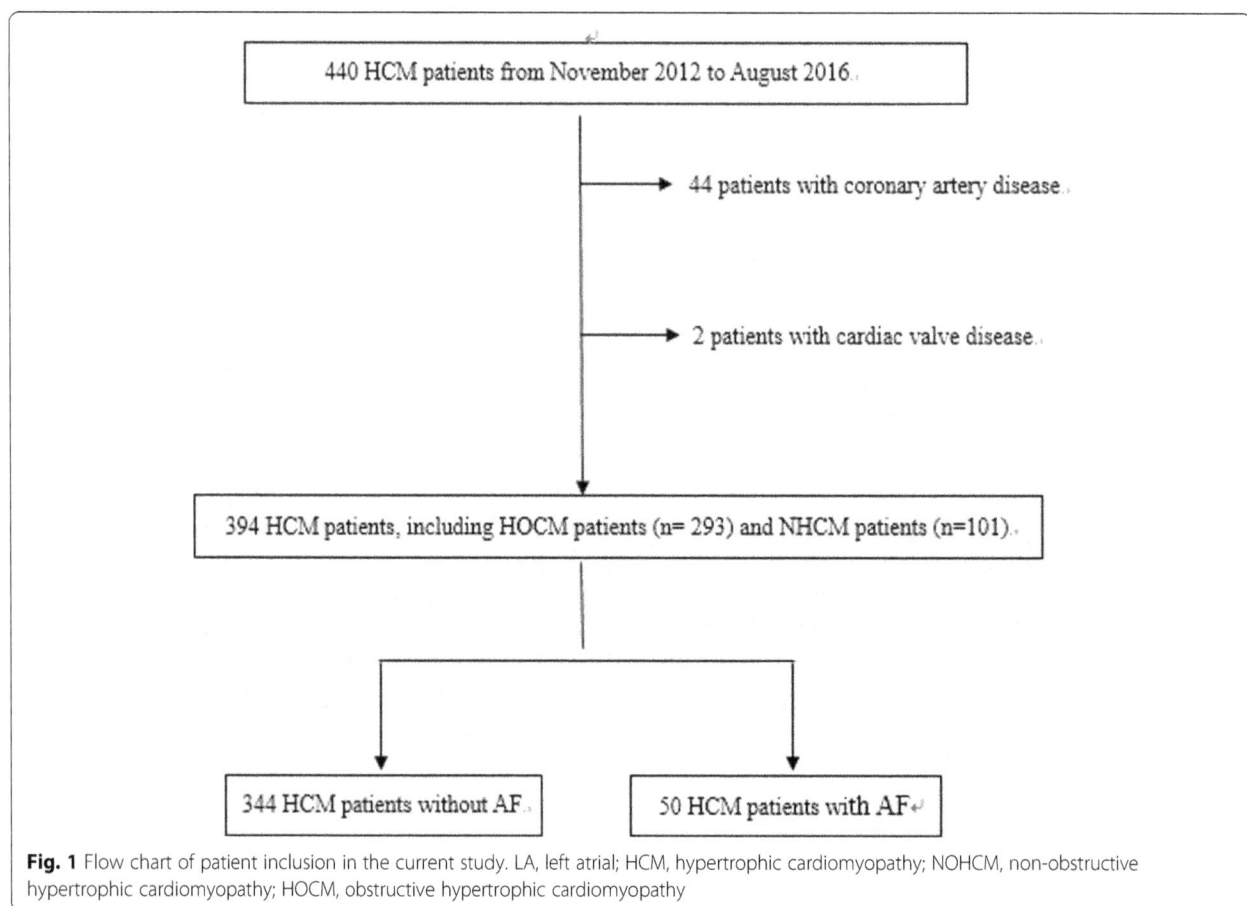

Fig. 1 Flow chart of patient inclusion in the current study. LA, left atrial; HCM, hypertrophic cardiomyopathy; NOHCM, non-obstructive hypertrophic cardiomyopathy; HOCM, obstructive hypertrophic cardiomyopathy

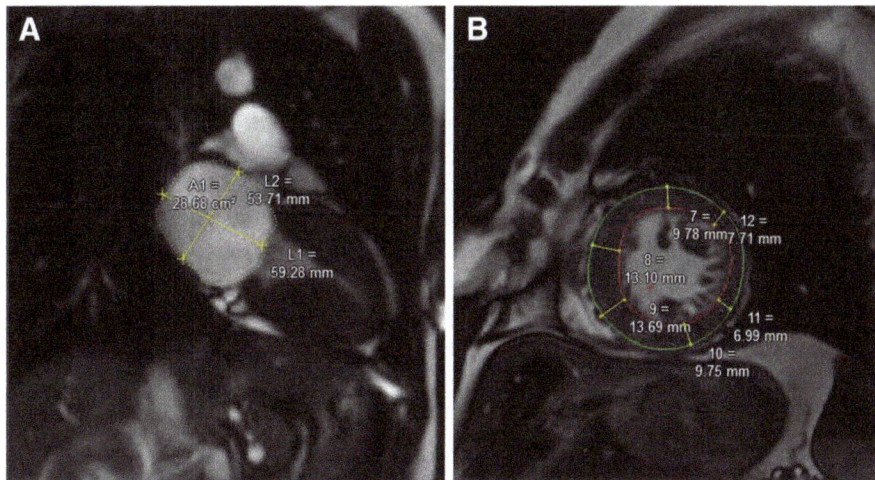

Fig. 2 CMR images showed LA size (**a**) (yellow line) and contours of endocardial and epicardial (**b**) (red circle and green circle). CMR, cardiovascular magnetic resonance; LA, left atrial

ejection fraction (EF), and cardiac output were then calculated in a standard fashion. The LV end-diastolic diameter (EDD) was measured from short axis at LV end-diastolic phase and left atrial diameter (LAD) (Fig. 2a) was measured from transverse axis at LV end-systolic phase [11]. Left ventricular mass (LVM) was obtained on the basis of end-diastolic endocardial and epicardial contours (Fig. 2b) and calculated as the product of myocardial volume and specific density of myocardial tissue (1.05 g/ml). LVM and LV EDV were indexed to body surface area. Left ventricular remodeling index (LVRI = LVM/LV EDV) was calculated used the methods described previously [12].

Atrial fibrillation

The diagnosis of AF was based on 12-lead electrocardiography or 24 h dynamic electrocardiogram recordings, or by an established history of paroxysmal or chronic AF [13].

Table 1 Patient Demographics and Baseline Characteristics

Variable	All Patients (n = 394)	Patients with AF (n = 50)	Patients without AF (n = 344)	P value
Age, y	48.5 ± 13.5	53.6 ± 11.7	47.7 ± 13.6	0.002
Male, n (%)	247 (62.7%)	37 (74%)	210 (61%)	0.08
Body surface area, m^2	1.8 ± 0.2	1.8 ± 0.3	1.8 ± 0.2	0.41
NYHA class	2.4 ± 0.9	2.5 ± 0.9	2.4 ± 0.9	0.45
Heart rate, beats/min	70.5 ± 10.3	68.6 ± 9.9	70.8 ± 10.4	0.15
SBP (mmHg)	118.7 ± 17.2	120.0 ± 19.0	118.8 ± 15.7	0.63
DBP (mmHg)	73.0 ± 10.3	74.5 ± 10.9	72.7 ± 9.9	0.28
Syncope, n (%)	97 (24.6%)	13 (26%)	84 (24.4%)	0.81
Dyspnea, n (%)	319 (81%)	42 (84%)	277 (80.5%)	0.56
Hypertension, n (%)	116 (29.4%)	18 (36%)	98 (28.5%)	0.28
Diabetes mellitus, n (%)	13 (3.3%)	4 (8%)	9 (2.6%)	0.05
Family history of HCM, n (%)	56 (14.2%)	7 (14%)	49 (14.2%)	0.96
Family history of SCD, n (%)	24 (6.1%)	1 (2%)	23 (6.7%)	0.33
Medications, n (%)				
β-Blockers	261 (66.2%)	36 (72%)	225 (65.4%)	0.36
Echocardiography				
Systolic anterior motion	293 (74.4%)	36 (72%)	257 (74.7%)	0.68
LVOTPG at rest (mmHg)	74.9 ± 37.1	68.4 ± 46.9	75.9 ± 35.4	0.34

HCM hypertrophic cardiomyopathy, *LV* left ventricular, *LVOTG* LV outflow tract gradient, *NS* not significance; Values are expressed as either mean ± SD or number (percentage)

Table 2 CMR assessment

Variable	Patients with AF	Patients without AF	P value
LA dimension, mm	46.6 ± 7.4	39.9 ± 8.0	< 0.001
LVEDD, mm	47.0 ± 5.1	46.5 ± 5.3	0.48
LV ejection fraction, %	63.4 ± 12.3	67.2 ± 9.8	0.015
Septal wall thickness, mm	26.6 ± 4.5	24.7 ± 5.5	0.26
LV end diastolic volume index, ml/m^2	69.6 ± 21.9	70.7 ± 16.7	0.72
LV ESVI	26.3 ± 14.5	23.7 ± 11.4	0.22
CI	3.0 ± 1.0	3.2 ± 0.8	0.14
LV end diastolic mass index, g/m^2	95.8 ± 36.7	85.7 ± 34.8	0.07
LVRI	1.46 ± 0.6	1.2 ± 0.4	0.002

Data are presented as ± standard deviation. Volumes are indexed to body surface area. *EDD* end diastolic dimension, *LA* left atrial, *LV* left ventricular, *ESVI* end-systolic volume index, *CI* Cardiac index

Statistical analysis

Statistical calculations were performed using SPSS 20.0 (SPSS Inc.; Chicago, IL, USA). In the case of a $p < 0.05$, the result was considered statistically significant. Data are expressed as mean ± SD for normally distributed continuous variables. Differences between means were measured by Student's t-tests. Noncontinuous data were compared by chi-square tests as appropriate. Pearson correlation was used to evaluate the correlation between LA size and LVRI. Multivariate analysis was performed with logistic regression analysis using block entry of the following variables: LVRI, LA size, LV end diastolic mass index, and age to evaluate if these variables were independent predictors of AF, provided to have a $p < 0.10$ in univariate analysis.

Results

Patients characteristics

In our study, AF was documented in 50 HCM patients (12.7%). Baseline characteristics are presented in Table 1. No significant differences were observed for gender, systolic blood pressure (SBP), diastolic blood pressure (DBP), heart rate, NYHA class, body surface area (BSA), LVOT peak gradient. HCM patients with AF were older than HCM patients without AF (53.6 ± 11.7 years versus 47.7 ± 13.6 years, $p = 0.002$). The proportion of syncope, dyspnea, family history of HCM, family history of SCD, diabetes mellitus, hypertension, systolic anterior motion and use of medications did not differ significantly between HCM patients with AF and without AF groups.

LA and LV parameters, LV end diastolic mass index and LVRI were all comparable between HCM patients with AF and without AF, Table 2. Left atrial diameter and LVRI were significantly higher in HCM patients with AF than that of HCM patients without AF (46.6 ± 7.4 mm versus 39.9 ± 8.0 mm, $p < 0.001$, and 1.46 ± 0.6 versus 1.2 ± 0.4, $p = 0.002$). Additionally, pearson correlation analysis showed LVRI positively correlated to LA size ($r = 0.12$, $p = 0.02$) in all HCM patients, Fig. 3.

In HOCM patients, LA dimension ($p = 0.025$), LV ejection fraction ($p < 0.001$), septal wall thickness ($p < 0.001$), LV end diastolic mass index ($p < 0.001$) and LVRI ($p < 0.001$) were significantly larger and LV EDD ($p < 0.001$) was lower compared to NOHCM patients. However, there was no significant differences between HOCM patients and NOHCM patients regarding the occurrence of AF (12.6% vs. 12.9%, $p = 0.95$), see Table 3.

In a multivariable logistic regression analysis, when adjusting for age and LV end diastolic mass index, LVRI and LA size remained an independent determinant of AF in HCM patients (OR = 4.7, $p = 0.001$ and OR = 1.13, $P < 0.001$), see Table 4.

Discussion

The present study demonstrates that HCM patients with AF had higher LA diameter, age and LVRI than HCM patients without AF. LA size mildly correlated to LVRI in all HCM patients. When adjusting for age and LV end

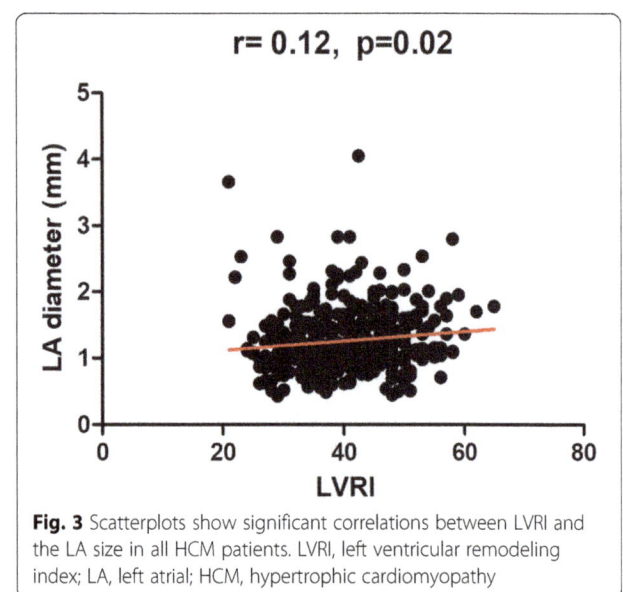

Fig. 3 Scatterplots show significant correlations between LVRI and the LA size in all HCM patients. LVRI, left ventricular remodeling index; LA, left atrial; HCM, hypertrophic cardiomyopathy

Table 3 Comparison of left ventricular and left atrial dimensions between HOCM and NOHCM patients

Variable	HOCM	NOHCM	P value
AF, %	12.6%	12.9%	0.95
LA dimension, mm	40.4 ± 8.5	38.4 ± 7.7	0.025
LVEDD, mm	46.0 ± 5.2	48.3 ± 5.0	< 0.001
LV ejection fraction, %	68.5 ± 9.2	61.7 ± 11.2	< 0.001
Septal wall thickness, mm	23.6 ± 5.4	21.0 ± 6.3	< 0.001
LV end diastolic volume index, ml/m^2	71.4 ± 18.6	68.2 ± 13.2	0.12
LV ESVI, ml/m^2	23.1 ± 11.7	26.8 ± 11.9	0.008
CI, ml/m^2	3.3 ± 0.9	2.8 ± 0.7	< 0.001
LV end diastolic mass index, g/m^2	91.4 ± 35.5	74.4 ± 31.0	< 0.001
LVRI	1.3 ± 0.5	1.1 ± 0.5	< 0.001

AF atrial fibrillation, *LA* left atrial, *EDD* end diastolic dimension, *LV* left ventricular, *ESVI* end-systolic volume index, *CI* Cardiac index, *LVRI* left ventricular remodeling index

diastolic mass index, LVRI and LA size remained an independent determinant of AF in HCM patients.

AF is a commonly reported complication in HCM that affects quality of life and increases risk for morbidity and mortality. It has been previously revealed that the diagnosis of HCM precedes the presence of AF in the majority of HCM patients [3] which strongly suggests that the structural and physiological changes related to the development of AF. In HCM patients, diastolic dysfunction, advanced age, myocardial ischemia, myocardial fibrosis, LA diameter and congestive heart failure symptoms have been shown to be associated with the development of AF [7, 14]. However, the impact of LV remodeling on the presence of AF in HCM patients has not been evaluated yet. The aim of the present study was to investigate whether LV remodeling is related to the occurrence of AF in HCM patients.

LA dimension is one of the most important determinants of AF occurrence in HCM patients. In our study, we showed that LA diameter and age was significantly higher in HCM patients with AF than that of HCM patients without AF, these findings confirm previous study [2, 13, 15]. In the present study, we also showed LVRI positively correlated to LA size, suggesting that LV remodeling may contribute to the enlargement of LA. LA enlargement is a multifactorial process in HCM,

including LA overload, mitral regurgitation, intrinsic myocardial stiffness, LV diastolic dysfunction and rhythm disturbances [14, 16, 17].

The LVRI which was calculated as the ratio of LV mass and end-diastolic volume can evaluate the degree of LV remodeling [6]. In our study, HCM patients with AF had higher LV mass index and LVRI. In a multivariable logistic regression analysis, LVRI and LA size remained an independent determinant of AF in HCM patients. These observations indicate that LA size and progressive LV remodeling may contribute to the occurrence of AF in HCM patient. The main underlying structural abnormalities in HCM include myocardial cell disarray, coronary microvasculature dysfunction and remodeling changes [18, 19]. LV myocardial remodeling that occur as a compensatory mechanism and can involve changes to the fibroblasts, myocytes and interstitium. LV remodeling and increased LV mass impaired diastolic function due to increased myocardial stiffness and decreased chamber compliance [17]. Moreover, LV diastolic dysfunction can lead to LA enlargement and associated rhythm disturbances [20]. Patients with AF frequently have the left atrial appendage remodeling in which there is dilation, stretching, and reduction in pectinate muscle volume [21]. Prior studies have showed that LA diameter and P wave dispersion values are the most significant predictors for AF occurrence in patients with HCM [22]. All these findings suggested that the AF was a result of electrical remodeling and myocardial remodeling [23].

Limitations
There may be some limitations in our study. Firstly, we did not evaluate the impact of late gadolinium enhanced (LGE) on the presence of AF in HCM patients owning to the absence of LGE examination. Secondly, in this study, patients with hypertension were not excluded.

Conclusions
HCM patients with AF showed significantly more LA diameter, LVRI and age than HCM patients without AF. LVRI and LA size were strong independent predictor of AF in HCM, suggesting that the LA enlargement and progressive LV remodeling may contribute to the occurrence of AF in HCM patients.

Table 4 Predictors of AF in HCM group by univariate and multivariable logistic regression

Variable	Univariate analysis			Multivariable logistic regression		
	P value	Crude OR	95% CI	P value	Adjusted OR	95% CI
Age	0.004	1.0	1.0~ 1.1	0.01	1.0	1.0~ 1.1
LA dimension, mm	< 0.001	1.1	1.1~ 1.2	< 0.001	1.13	1.1~ 1.2
LV end diastolic mass index, g/m^2	0.06	1.0	1.0~ 1.02	0.07	0.99	0.97~ 1.0
LVRI	0.003	2.3	1.3~ 4.0	0.001	4.7	1.9~ 11.8

LA left atrial, *LV* left ventricular, *LVRI* left ventricular remodeling index

Abbreviations

AF: Atrial fibrillation; CMR: Cardiovascular magnetic resonance; DBP: Diastolic blood pressure; EDD: End-diastolic diameter; EF: Ejection fraction; HCM: Hypertrophic cardiomyopathy; HOCM: Obstructive hypertrophic cardiomyopathy; LA: left atrial; LAD: Left atrial diameter; LGE: Late gadolinium-enhancement; LV: Left ventricular; LVEDV: LV end-diastolic volume; LVESV: LV end-systolic volume; LVM: Left ventricular mass; LVOT: Left ventricular outflow tract; LVRI: LV remodeling index; NOHCM: Non-obstructive hypertrophic cardiomyopathy; SBP: systolic blood pressure

Acknowledgements

The authors thank the study patients for participating and the study personnel for their invaluable contribution. The authors also thank All staffs at the department of nuclear magnetic resonance for performing and assisting with the cardiovascular MRI analysis.

Funding

This study was supported by grants from the National Natural Science Foundation of China (nos. 81370327).

Authors' contributions

HWT, SBQ, CZY, and JGC contributed to the design of the study. HWT, JSY and FHH contributed to the analysis, while all authors (HWT, JGC, CZY, FHH, JSY, SWL, WXY, XWJ, SBQ) contributed to the interpretation of data. HWT drafted the manuscript and SWL, WXY, and XWJ contributed significantly to the preparation. All the authors critically revised the manuscript and gave final approval and agree to be accountable for all aspects of the work, ensuring both its integrity and accuracy.

Competing interests

The authors declare that they have no competing interests.

References

1. Maron BJ. Hypertrophic cardiomyopathy: a systematic review. Jama. 2002; 287(10):1308–20.
2. Papavassiliu T, Germans T, Flüchter S, Doesch C, Suriyakamar A, Haghi D, et al. CMR findings in patients with hypertrophic cardiomyopathy and atrial fibrillation. J Cardiovasc Magn Reson. 2009;11(1):1–9.
3. Olivotto I, Cecchi F, Casey SA, Dolara A, Traverse JH, Maron BJ. Impact of atrial fibrillation on the clinical course of hypertrophic cardiomyopathy. Circulation. 2001;104(21):2517–24.
4. Doi Y, Kitaoka H. Hypertrophic cardiomyopathy in the elderly: significance of atrial fibrillation. J Cardiol. 2001;37(Suppl 1):133.
5. Dzeshka MS, Lip GYH, Snezhitskiy V, Shantsila E. Cardiac fibrosis in patients with atrial fibrillation: mechanisms and clinical implications. J Am Coll Cardiol. 2015;66(8):943–59.
6. De-Castro S, Caselli SM, Pelliccia A, Cavarretta E, Maddukuri P, Cartoni D, et al. Left ventricular remodelling index (LVRI) in various pathophysiological conditions: a real-time three-dimensional echocardiographic study. Heart. 2007; 93(2):205–9.
7. Olivotto I, Cecchi F, Casey SA, Dolara A, Traverse JH, Maron BJ. Impact of atrial fibrillation on the clinical course of hypertrophic cardiomyopathy. Circulation. 2002;11(3):58.
8. Yamaji K, Fujimoto S, Yutani C, Ikeda Y, Mizuno R, Hashimoto T, et al. Does the progression of myocardial fibrosis lead to atrial fibrillation in patients with hypertrophic cardiomyopathy? Cardiovasc Pathol. 2001;10(6):297.
9. Maron BJ, Towbin JA, Thiene G, Antzelevitch C, Corrado D, Arnett D, et al. Contemporary definitions and classification of the cardiomyopathies: an American Heart Association scientific statement from the council on clinical cardiology, heart failure and transplantation committee; quality of care and outcomes research and functional genomics and translational biology interdisciplinary working groups; and council on epidemiology and prevention. Circulation. 2006;113(14):1807–16.
10. Elliott P, Andersson B, Arbustini E, Bilinska Z, Cecchi F, Charron P, et al. Classification of the cardiomyopathies: a position statement from the european society of cardiology working group on myocardial and pericardial diseases. Eur Heart J. 2008;29(2):270–6.
11. Schulzmenger J, Abdelaty H, Busjahn A, Wassmuth R, Pilz B, Dietz R, et al. Left ventricular outflow tract planimetry by cardiovascular magnetic resonance differentiates obstructive from non-obstructive hypertrophic cardiomyopathy. J Cardiovasc Magn Reson. 2006;8(5):741–6.
12. Schulzmenger J, Abdelaty H, Rudolph A, Elgeti T, Messroghli D, Utz W, et al. Gender-specific differences in left ventricular remodelling and fibrosis in hypertrophic cardiomyopathy: insights from cardiovascular magnetic resonance. Eur J Heart Fail. 2008;10(9):850–4.
13. Siontis KC, Geske JB, Ong K, Nishimura RA, Ommen SR, Gersh BJ. Atrial fibrillation in hypertrophic cardiomyopathy: prevalence, clinical correlations, and mortality in a large high-risk population. J Am Heart Assoc. 2014;3(3):e001002.
14. Manuguerra R, Callegari S, Corradi D. Inherited structural heart diseases with potential atrial fibrillation occurrence. J Cardiovasc Electrophysiol. 2015;27(2):242–52.
15. Losi MA, Betocchi S, Aversa M, Lombardi R, Miranda M, D'Alessandro G, et al. Determinants of atrial fibrillation development in patients with hypertrophic cardiomyopathy. Am J Cardiol. 2004;94(7):895–900.
16. Yang H, Woo A, Monakier D, Jamorski M, Fedwick K, Wigle ED, et al. Enlarged left atrial volume in hypertrophic cardiomyopathy: a marker for disease severity. J Am Soc Echocardiogr. 2005;18(10):1074–82.
17. Barbero U, Destefanis P. An Indian-look right into restrictive cardiomyopathies. Indian Heart J. 2015;67(6):512–3.
18. Poliac LC, Barron ME, Maron BJ. Hypertrophic cardiomyopathy | anesthesiology | ASA publications. Anesthesiology. 2006;104(1):183.
19. Camici PG, Olivotto I, Rimoldi OE. The coronary circulation and blood flow in left ventricular hypertrophy. J Mol Cell Cardiol. 2012;52(4):857–64.
20. Hensley N, Dietrich J, Nyhan D, Mitter N, Yee MS, Brady M. Hypertrophic cardiomyopathy: a review. Anesth Analg. 2015;120(3):554–69.
21. Barbero U, Ho SY. Anatomy of the atria: A road map to the left atrial appendage. Herzschrittmacherther Elektrophysiol. 2017;28(4):347–54.
22. Ozdemir O, Soylu M, Demir AD, Topaloglu S, Alyan O, Turhan H, et al. P-wave durations as a predictor for atrial fibrillation development in patients with hypertrophic cardiomyopathy. Int J Cardiol. 2004;94(2–3):163–6.
23. Liu T, Li G. Potential mechanisms between atrial dilatation and atrial fibrillation. Am Heart J. 2006;151(2):e1.

29

Basal wall hypercontraction of Takotsubo cardiomyopathy in a patient who had been diagnosed with dilated cardiomyopathy

Noboru Ichihara, Shuichi Fujita, Yumiko Kanzaki, Tomohiro Fujisaka, Michishige Ozeki and Nobukazu Ishizaka* ⓘ

Abstract

Background: Takotsubo cardiomyopathy is characterized by the basal hypercontractility and apical ballooning of the left ventriculum and T-wave inversion in the electrocardiogram. It has been suggested that Takotsubo cardiomyopathy might underlie the pathogenesis of persistent cardiac dysfunction; however, few reports are present demonstrating the advent of Takotsubo cardiomyopathy in patients with idiopathic cardiomyopathy.

Case presentation: A 64-year-old women was admitted due to dyspnea on effort and lower extremity edema. She had been diagnosed with idiopathic dilated cardiomyopathy 2.5 years before owing to the reduced left ventricular ejection fraction (24%), normal coronary artery, and interstitial fibrosis of the myocardial samples. On admission, her electrocardiogram showed giant negative T wave in II, III, aVF, and precordial leads. Echocardiography showed dyskinesis of the left ventricular apex and hypercontraction of the basal wall, which had not been observed in the previous examinations. Coronary angiography showed normal coronary arteries, and apical ballooning and basal hypercontractility was confirmed by left ventriculography. On day 15 of admission, contraction of apical wall was recovered, and basal hypercontraction was disappeared.

Conclusion: The present case is the first report demonstrating appearance the transient basal wall hypercontraction along with the advent of Takotsubo cardiomyopathy in a patient diagnosed with dilated cardiomyopathy. Whether such findings are indicative of fair prognosis and have the utility of understanding the pathogenesis of dilated cardiomyopathy needs further investigation.

Keywords: Takotsubo cardiomyopathy, Idiopathic cardiomyopathy, Hypercontraction, Pathogenesis, Percutaneous coronary intervention, Emotional stress

Background

Takotsubo cardiomyopathy is characterized by transient left ventricular apical ballooning, which typically occurs in older women after emotional or physical stress [1]. The pathophysiology of Takotsubo cardiomyopathy remains obscure, but it may occur after emotional or physical stress, so-called "triggering events". In order to diagnose Takotsubo cardiomyopathy, several disorders that might show reversible abnormal cardiac contraction should be excluded, including obstructive coronary artery disease [2], subarachnoid hemorrhage, pheochromocytoma crisis, intra-cranial or subarachnoid bleeding myocarditis, tachycardia-induced cardiomyopathy, and hypertrophic cardiomyopathy [3–6]. On the other hand, the possibility exists that some of these conditions might present together with Takotsubo cardiomyopathy and underlie it as a triggering event [7, 8]. There have been few reports, until now, about Takotsubo cardiomyopathy in the dilated cardiomyopathic heart. We herein present a case of basal cardiac wall hypercontraction during the acute-phase of Takotsubo cardiomyopathy that occurred in a patient with idiopathic dilated cardiomyopathy.

* Correspondence: ishizaka@osaka-med.ac.jp
Department of Cardiology, Osaka Medical College, Takatsuki-shi
Daigaku-machi 2-7, Osaka 569-8686, Japan

Case presentation

A 64-year-old woman who complained of worsening nocturnal dyspnea was admitted to our hospital. Two and half years previously, the patient had felt exertional chest pain and lower extremity edema and had been admitted to our hospital. She did not have a history of hypertension, diabetes, or smoking. On her previous admission, chest X-ray showed an enlarged cardiac silhouette with a cardiothoracic ratio of 68.7% and right side pleural effusion. Electrocardiogram showed T-wave inversion in leads II, III, aVF, and precordial leads (Fig. 1a). Echocardiography showed that left ventricular wall motion was diffusely reduced with the left ventricular ejection fraction of 24% (Fig. 1b, c). The end-diastolic left ventricular dimension was 53 mm. Coronary artery angiography showed no physiologically significant stenosis and left ventriculography showed diffuse hypokinesis of the left ventricle (Fig. 1d, e). Histological examination of endomyocardial biopsy samples showed interstitial fibrosis, but neither amyloid deposition nor granulomatous degeneration was observed. Echocardiography 1.5 years later also showed the reduced global left ventricular contractility (Fig. 1f, g).

The chief complaint of the patient on the current admission was exertional dyspnea and edema of lower extremities. On admission, her body temperature was 35.8°C, blood pressure was 104/79 mmHg, and pulse rate was 100 bpm. Electrocardiography showed T wave inversion on leads I, II, aVF, and precordial leads, which was more prominent than that observed previously (Fig. 2a). Echocardiography showed dyskinesis of the apical (Fig. 2b, c, arrows) and hypercontraction of the basal walls (Fig. 2b, c). Emergency coronary angiography showed, again, no significant stenosis in the coronary arteries (Fig. 2d, e) and apical ballooning and basal hypercontraction were demonstrated by left ventriculography (Fig. 1f, g). Laboratory examinations showed elevated levels of serum creatine kinase, its MB fraction, and plasma B-type natriuretic peptide (Table 1). In addition to the treatment with diuretic drugs, the patient was treated with anticoagulant drugs because of the thrombus formation in the left ventricular apex – intravenous administration of heparin for 12 days followed by the oral administration of warfarin. Administration of beta blocker, bisoprolol, was also started. On day 15, follow-up electrocardiogram showed no apparent changes in the giant T-wave inversion (Fig. 3a); however, echocardiography showed the disappearance of hypercontraction of the left ventricular basal wall (Fig. 3b, c, arrowheads) in addition to recovery of the contraction of the thickened apical wall (arrows). The patient was diagnosed with Takotsubo cardiomyopathy [9]. Finding of electrocardiogram, T-wave inversion, normalized at 3 months after the discharge and it remained normal at 8 months after the discharge.

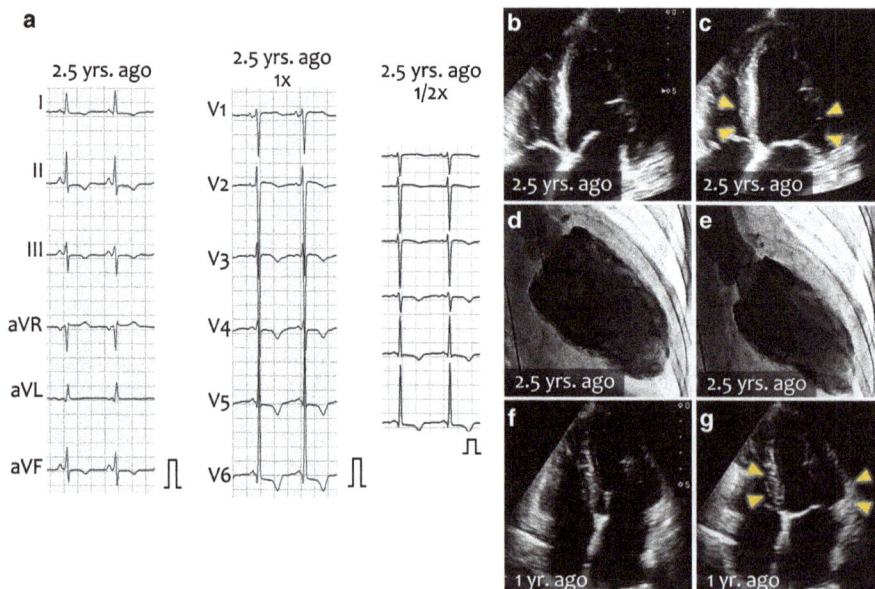

Fig. 1 Electrocardiogram and echocardiographic images prior to the current admission. **a** Electrocardiogram 2.5 years before the current admission. T-wave inversion was observed in II, III, aVF and precordial leads. **b, c** Echocardiography 2.5 years before the current admission at end diastole (**b**) and end systole (**c**). Left ventricular wall motion was diffusely decreased including the base of the left ventricle (arrowheads).**d, e** Left ventriculogram at end diastole (**d**) and at end systole (**e**). **f, g** Echocardiography 2.5 years before the current admission at end diastole (**f**) and end systole (**g**). Wall motion of left ventricle, including the base (arrowheads) remained impaired. The calibration of the electrocardiogram indicates 1 mV

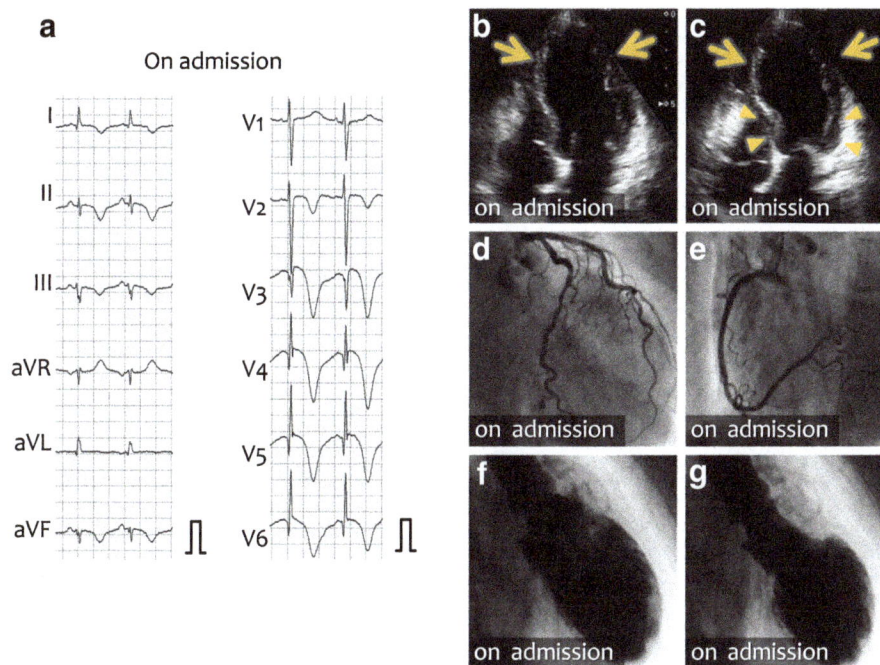

Fig. 2 Electrocardiogram and echocardiographic and radiologic images on the current admission. **a** Electrocardiogram on the current admission. T-wave inversion became more prominent. **b, c** Echocardiography on the current admission at end diastole (**a**) and end systole (**f**). Dyskinetic wall motion was observed at the eft ventricular apex (arrows), but the base of left ventriculum showed hypercontraction. **d, e** Coronary angiography showed normal left (**d**) and right (**e**) coronary arteries. **f, g** Left ventriculogram at end diastole (**f**) and at end systole (**g**). Basal hypercontraction and apical ballooning were demonstrated

Discussion

In the present case, we demonstrated the occurrence of Takotsubo cardiomyopathy in a patient who had been diagnosed with dilated cardiomyopathy. Of note, in the acute phase, the left ventricular basal wall showed hypercontraction together with the advent of apical ballooning,

Table 1 Laboratory data on the current admission

Blood cell count	
White blood cell count, $\times 10^3/\mu L$	11.59
Red blood cell count, $\times 10^6/\mu L$	4.93
Hemoglobin, g/dL	14.8
Platelet count, $\times 10^3/\mu L$	304
Biochemistry	
Total protein, mg/dL	8.1
serum creatinine, mg/dL	0.81
Creatine kinase, U/L	773
Creatine kinase MB, U/L	76
C-reactive protein, mg/dL	1.22
Na, mEq/L	144
K, mEq/L	4.3
Cl, mEq/L	106
BNP, pg/mL	940.8

BNP indicates brain natriuretic peptide

although these findings were transient and disappeared within 2 weeks. These findings indicated that basal wall hypercontraction can occur in patients diagnosed with dilated cardiomyopathy.

Whether there were any relationships between previously diagnosed idiopathic dilated cardiomyopathy and Takotsubo cardiomyopathy remains unclear; however, there are some possibilities. Although wall motion abnormality is, in general, transient in Takotsubo cardiomyopathy [10], several previous studies suggested that Takotsubo cardiomyopathy might be emerging as a chronic form [11], causing congestive heart failure and acute coronary syndrome-like symptoms. It is increasingly recognized that Takotsubo cardiomyopathy may not always be benign [12], and may cause left ventricular fibrosis [13] leading to appearance as a non-ischemic cardiomyopathy [14]. In addition, presence of Takotsubo cardiomyopathy may not be able to be recognized or diagnosed when it is not associated with anginal chest pain [15].

Considering that our patient had T-wave inversion in her electrocardiogram 2.5 years before the current admission, and the chief complaint of the current admission was not chest pain, typical for Takotsubo cardiomyopathy, there is a possibility that dilated cardiomyopathy diagnosed 2.5 years before the current admission might have been attributed to the cardiac

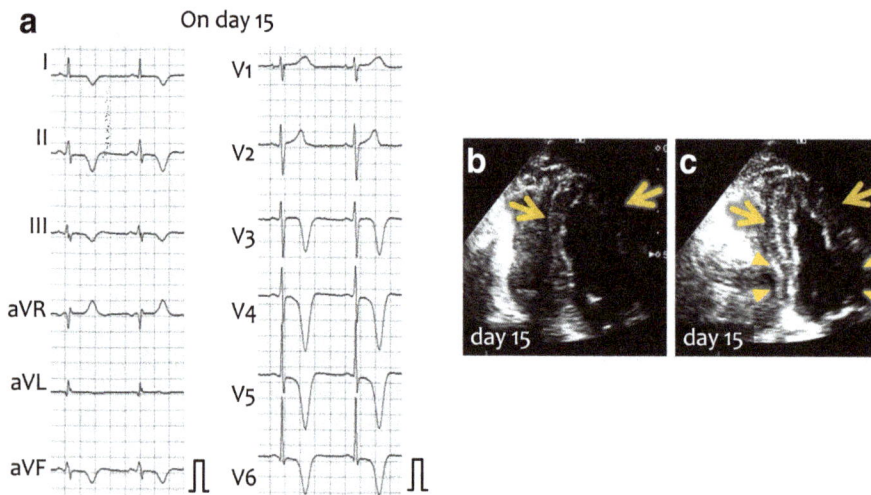

Fig. 3 Electrocardiogram and echocardiographic images at day 15. **a** Electrocardiogram at day 15. Giant negative T waves were still present. **b, c** Echocardiography at day 15 at end diastole (**b**) and end systole (**c**). Basal hypercontraction disappeared, and thickening of the apical wall was emerging

remodeling by chronic and recurrent Takotsubo cardiomyopathy.

It has been demonstrated that contractile reserve assessed by the administration of catecholamine predicts long-term prognosis in patients with dilated cardiomyopathy [16–18]. Therefore, whatever the etiology of cardiac dysfunction of our patient is, improved left basal contraction during the advent of Takotsubo cardiomyopathy, a potential *intrinsic* catecholamine-mediated cardiomyopathy, might indicate the fair prognosis of our patient, although circulating catecholamine levels are not always increased in Takotsubo cardiomyopathy [19].

Conclusion

We showed a case who had been diagnosed with dilated cardiomyopathy who demonstrated left ventricular basal hypercontraction at the advent of Takotsubo cardiomyopathy on the latest admission. Such findings might provide important information on the possibility of chronic or recurrent Takotsubo cardiomyopathy as the underlying cause of dilated cardiomyopathy in some patients.

Acknowledgments
None.

Funding
The authors declare that there are no relationships with the company relating to employment, consultancy, patents, products in development or marketed products.

Authors' contributions
NI (Ichihara), collected data, analyzed, and interpreted data. SF and YK, extracted the data and provided the clinical information. TF and MO, helped to interpret the data and draft the manuscript. NI (ishizaka) made substantial contributions to acquisition and interpretation of data and prepared the drafted the manuscript. All authors read and approved the final manuscript.

Competing interests
The authors declare that they have no competing interests.

References
1. Ono R, Falcao LM. Takotsubo cardiomyopathy systematic review: Pathophysiologic process, clinical presentation and diagnostic approach to Takotsubo cardiomyopathy. Int J Cardiol. 2016;209:196–205.
2. Lee SR, Lee SE, Rhee TM, Park JJ, Cho H, Lee HY, Choi DJ, BH O. Discrimination of stress (Takotsubo) cardiomyopathy from acute coronary syndrome with clinical risk factors and coronary evaluation in real-world clinical practice. Int J Cardiol. 2017.
3. Abe Y, Kondo M. Apical ballooning of the left ventricle: a distinct entity? Heart. 2003;89(9):974–6.
4. Bybee KA, Kara T, Prasad A, Lerman A, Barsness GW, Wright RS, Rihal CS. Systematic review: transient left ventricular apical ballooning: a syndrome that mimics ST-segment elevation myocardial infarction. Ann Intern Med. 2004;141(11):858–65.
5. Redfors B, Shao Y, Lyon AR, Omerovic E. Diagnostic criteria for takotsubo syndrome: a call for consensus. Int J Cardiol. 2014;176(1):274–6.
6. Wittstein IS. Stress cardiomyopathy: a syndrome of catecholamine-mediated myocardial stunning? Cell Mol Neurobiol. 2012;32(5):847–57.
7. YH S. Myocarditis and takotsubo syndrome: are they mutually exclusive? Int J Cardiol. 2014;177(1):149–51.
8. Abreu G, Rocha S, Bettencourt N, Azevedo P, Vieira C, Rodrigues C, Arantes C, Braga C, Martins J, Marques J. An unusual trigger causing Takotsubo syndrome. Int J Cardiol. 2016;223:118–20.
9. Prasad A, Lerman A, Rihal CS. Apical ballooning syndrome (Tako-Tsubo or stress cardiomyopathy): a mimic of acute myocardial infarction. Am Heart J. 2008;155(3):408–17.

10. Akashi YJ, Musha H, Kida K, Itoh K, Inoue K, Kawasaki K, Hashimoto N, Miyake F. Reversible ventricular dysfunction takotsubo cardiomyopathy. Eur J Heart Fail. 2005;7(7):1171–6.

11. Madias JE. Is there a "chronic Takotsubo syndrome"? Could "smart-phone"based technology be of aid? Int J Cardiol. 2015;186:297–8.

12. Morley-Smith AC, Lyon AR. Challenges of chronic cardiac problems in survivors of Takotsubo syndrome. Heart Fail Clin. 2016;12(4):551–7.

13. Iacucci I, Carbone I, Cannavale G, Conti B, Iampieri I, Rosati R, Sardella G, Frustaci A, Fedele F, Catalano C, et al. Myocardial oedema as the sole marker of acute injury in Takotsubo cardiomyopathy: a cardiovascular magnetic resonance (CMR) study. Radiol Med. 2013;118(8):1309–23.

14. Madias JE. Is there a link between Takotsubo syndrome and some cases of nonischemic cardiomyopathy? A proposal of an animal model. Int J Cardiol. 2014;172(1):e212–3.

15. Aoki Y, Kodera S, Shakya S, Ishiwaki H, Ikeda M, Kanda J. Isolated deep T-wave inversion on an electrocardiogram with normal wall motion. Clin Case Rep. 2015;3(7):594–7.

16. Matsumura Y, Takata J, Kitaoka H, Hamada T, Okawa M, Kubo T, Doi Y. Low-dose dobutamine stress echocardiography predicts the improvement of left ventricular systolic function and long-term prognosis in patients with idiopathic dilated cardiomyopathy. J Med Ultrason (2001). 2006;33(1):17–22.

17. Stipac AV, Otasevic P, Popovic ZB, Cvorovic V, Putnikovic B, Stankovic I, Neskovic AN. Prognostic significance of contractile reserve assessed by dobutamine-induced changes of Tei index in patients with idiopathic dilated cardiomyopathy. Eur J Echocardiogr. 2010;11(3):264–70.

18. Lee JH, Yang DH, Choi WS, Kim KH, Park SH, Bae MH, Park HS, Cho Y, Chae SC, Jun JE. Prediction of improvement in cardiac function by high dose dobutamine stress echocardiography in patients with recent onset idiopathic dilated cardiomyopathy. Int J Cardiol. 2013;167(4):1649–50.

19. YH S, Henareh L. Plasma catecholamine levels in patients with takotsubo syndrome: implications for the pathogenesis of the disease. Int J Cardiol. 2015;181:35–8.

30

Right precordial-directed electrocardiographical markers identify arrhythmogenic right ventricular cardiomyopathy in the absence of conventional depolarization or repolarization abnormalities

Daniel Cortez[1,2]* ⓘ, Anneli Svensson[3], Jonas Carlson[1], Sharon Graw[4], Nandita Sharma[2], Francesca Brun[4,5], Anita Spezzacatene[4,5], Luisa Mestroni[4,5] and Pyotr G. Platonov[1,6]

Abstract

Background: Arrhythmogenic right ventricular dysplasia/cardiomyopathy (ARVD/C) carries a risk of sudden death. We aimed to assess whether vectorcardiographic (VCG) parameters directed toward the right heart and a measured angle of the S-wave would help differentiate ARVD/C with otherwise normal electrocardiograms from controls.

Methods: Task Force 2010 definite ARVD/C criteria were met for all patients. Those who did not fulfill Task Force depolarization or repolarization criteria (−ECG) were compared with age and gender-matched control subjects. Electrocardiogram measures of a 3-dimentional spatial QRS-T angle, a right-precordial-directed orthogonal QRS-T (RPD) angle, a root mean square of the right sided depolarizing forces (RtRMS-QRS), QRS duration (QRSd) and the corrected QT interval (QTc), and a measured angle including the upslope and downslope of the S-wave (S-wave angle) were assessed.

Results: Definite ARVD/C was present in 155 patients by 2010 Task Force criteria (41.7 ± 17.6 years, 65.2% male). -ECG ARVD/C patients (66 patients) were compared to 66 control patients (41.7 ± 17.6 years, 65.2% male). All parameters tested except the QRSd and QTc significantly differentiated -ECG ARVD/C from control patients ($p < 0.004$ to $p < 0.001$). The RPD angle and RtRMS-QRS best differentiated the groups. Combined, the 2 novel criteria gave 81.8% sensitivity, 90.9% specificity and odds ratio of 45.0 (95% confidence interval 15.8 to 128.2).

Conclusion: ARVD/C disease process may lead to development of subtle ECG abnormalities that can be distinguishable using right-sided VCG or measured angle markers better than the spatial QRS-T angle, the QRSd or QTc, in the absence of Taskforce ECG criteria.

Keywords: Arrhythmogenic right ventricular cardiomyopathy, Vectorcardiography, ECG, Cascade screening

* Correspondence: dr.danielcortez@gmail.com
[1]Department of Cardiology, Clinical Sciences, Lund University, Lund, Sweden
[2]Electrophysiology/Cardiology, Penn State Milton S. Hershey Medical Center, Hershey, USA
Full list of author information is available at the end of the article

Background

Arrhythmogenic right ventricular dysplasia/cardiomyopathy (ARVD/C) is an inherited cardiomyopathy characterized by fibro-fatty replacement of predominately the right ventricle, which predisposes patients to life-threatening ventricular arrhythmias and usually slowly progressive ventricular dysfunction [1]. The disease is inherited as an autosomal dominant trait with incomplete penetrance and highly variable expressivity [1]. Diagnosis is made by combining multiple sources of diagnostic information as prescribed by the Task Force criteria, which were updated in 2010 to increase diagnostic sensitivity while maintaining specificity [2].

First-degree relatives often have incomplete expression of the disease [3]. Clinical cascade screening of family members in genotype-negative ARVD/C is complicated by the lack of early specific signs of disease that would identify those individuals prone to development of disease. Electrocardiographic (ECG) changes may develop before histologic evidence of myocyte loss or clinical evidence of RV dysfunction [4, 5]. However, ECG depolarization and repolarization changes, based on current criteria, are typically only apparent in around half of family members who eventually progress to meet Definite ARVD/C by 2010 criteria [5].

The spatial QRS-T angle, a vectorcardiographic parameter easily derivable from the 12-lead ECG [6], has been shown to improve detection of left sided cardiomyopathy, particularly hypertrophic cardiomyopathy [7], as well as the prediction of susceptibility to ventricular tachycardia and cardiac death both in general populations [8–10] and in patients with known cardiac pathology [11–13]. Given this mainly right-sided heart disease, we hypothesize that right-precordial-directed vectorcardiographic parameters, particularly a right precordial-directed-orthogonal QRS-T angle (RPD angle), right-sided depolarization magnitude (right root mean square of the QRS, RtRMS-QRS) (Fig. 1) from a baseline ECG would improve detection of ARVD/C patients who have no depolarization or repolarization abnormalities otherwise but who still meet criteria for definite ARVD/C by 2010 taskforce criteria (by criteria other than ECG).

Methods
Population

A cross-sectional study of patients with ARVC/D from an international cohort from the University of Colorado (Denver, CO, USA), Skåne University Hospital (Lund, Sweden), Linköping University Hospital (Sweden) and the University of Trieste (Italy) undergoing routine follow-up, classified as definite ARVD/C by the 2010 Task Force criteria was performed [2]. Normal variant ECGs from patients, who did not have signs of bundle branch block and not fitting 12-lead ECG major or minor depolarization or repolarization criteria by 2010 Task Force guidelines (electrocardiographically concealed

ARVD/C) were compared with ECGs recorded from 1:1 age- and gender-matched control subjects who were screened in cardiology clinic at the University of Colorado (Denver, CO) or at Skåne University Hospital (Lund, Sweden) for murmurs or chest pain without family history of ARVD/C and through ultrasound and clinical observations were deemed normal. None of the control subjects had other underlying cardiac disease (no cardiomyopathy or other notable cardiac disease) nor did they have obvious obstructive or restrictive lung disease or thromboembolisms. All ECG's were taken from the first time the patient had presented to the particular institution and no patients were on antiarrhythmic treatment at the time of their ECG. The study was approved by the Institutional Review Boards at each of the institutions noted above.

Electrocardiogram

The resting ECG closest to time of diagnostic echocardiogram or magnetic resonance imaging studies from ARVD/C patients at a speed of 25 mm/s and with voltages of 10 mm/mV were assessed (GE, WI, USA or Phillips Healthcare, MA, USA). Digital recordings were changed to PDF files and assessed at up to 150% magnification and used for vectorcardiographic derivations. Approximations of the Kors' quasi-orthogonal spatial peaks QRS-T angle (normally based on V6 defined as the X-axis, lead II as the Y-axis and $-0.5*V2$ as the Z-axis) were used with direction particularly toward the R-wave in V1 (as the Z-axis QRS vector magnitude) and S-wave in V5 (as the X-axis QRS vector magnitude) while ignoring magnitudes of the S-wave in V1 and the R-wave in V5 (as an attempt to have right-precordial-directed vector magnitude and angle). Lead II measures maximum deviation from baseline (whether R or S) was used as the Y-axis QRS vector magnitude, similar to Kors' quasi-orthogonal method [6]. Right-precordial-directed orthogonal QRS-T angles (RPD angle, degrees, Fig. 2), right-precordial-directed vector magnitudes (RtRMS-QRS, mV, Fig. 1), and spatial peaks QRS-T angles (SPQRS-T angle, degrees) were measured in ARVD/C and compared to the same parameters from control patients. The Bazett corrected QT interval (QTc) and the QRS duration (QRSd) were measured in milliseconds (ms).

The spatial QRS-T angle was calculated based on the visual transform estimation based on using selected leads and multipliers of those leads to approximate an orthogonal system. This is based on the Kors' visual estimations regression-related method, which has been described previously [6].

The RPD angle is similar in calculation to the Kors' quasi-orthogonal angle, but is a right-side restrictive measure meaning only the QRS maximum deviation in the orthogonal planes according to the following principles:

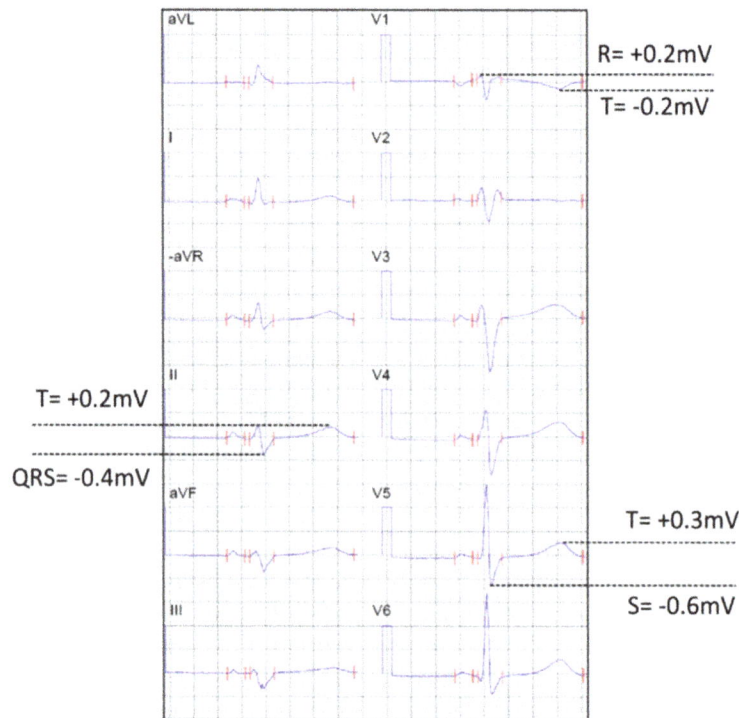

Fig. 1 Calculation of the right spatial peaks QRS-T angle (RtSPQRS-T angle) and the right root mean square QRS (RtRMSQRS). 0.1 mV × 40 ms = 1 little box. SV5 = Swave maximum deviation from baseline (negative number). QRSmaxII: QRS maximum deviation from baseline (positive or negative number) RV1: Rwave maximum deviation from baseline (positive number). RtRMS-QRS= $\sqrt{SV5^2 + QRSmaxII^2 + (-0.5 * RV1)^2}$ = $\sqrt{-0.6mV^2 + (-0.4mV)^2 + (-0.5 * 0.2mV)^2}$ = 0.73 mV. RtRMST=$\sqrt{TV5^2 + TII^2 + (-0.5 * TV1)^2}$ = $\sqrt{0.3mV^2 + 0.2mV^2 + (-0.5 * -0.2mV)^2}$ = 0.37 mV. RPD- angle= $\cos^{-1}([(SV5*TV5) + (QRSmaxII*TII) - 0.5(RV1*TV1)]/RtRMSQRS*RtRMST)$ =$\cos^{-1}([(-0.6mV*0.3mV) + (-0.4mV*0.2mV) - 0.5(0.2mV * -0.2mV)]/0.73 mV*0.37 mV)$ = 172.4 degrees

- X-axis: the S-wave deviation only in V5 (ignoring the R-wave in V5, even if it has a greater deviation from baseline than the S-wave);
- Y-axis: the R or S maximum deviation from lead II;
- Z-axis: the negative one half of the deviation of the R in lead V1.

These measures are then applied in the equation (Fig. 1 legend) and inverse cosine is taken between the QRS deviations and the T-wave deviations (positive or negative in leads V6 (X-axis), II (Y-axis) and negative one half of the deviation in V1 (Z-axis)). Please see Fig. 1 for further detail.

The RtRMS-QRS is the vector magnitude of the QRS complex based on right-precordial-directed measures (please see equation noted above and Fig. 1).

V5 also more consistently demonstrated an S-wave than V6, thus the S-wave in V5 was used.

All parameters were assessed by the first author if not otherwise noted above, while 10% of the sample was assessed by the 5th author to calculate inter-observer variability (per below).

Statistics

Parametric measures are given as mean ± standard deviation, while non-parameteric measures are given as median (1st quartile to 3rd quartile) and were used to assess statistical significance between the two groups. A p-value of 0.05 or less was considered significant. Receiver operating characteristic curves were used to assess optimum cut-off values for sensitivity and specificity measures. Odds ratios were used. All data were de-identified. Intra-class correlation coefficients were used to determine inter-/intra-observer variability by the 1st and 5th authors' measurements of the RPD angle, and the RtRMS-QRS.

Results

Population

Of a total of 155 patients with the diagnosis of definite ARVD/C by 2010 Task Force criteria, 66 patients did not have depolarization or repolarization changes consistent with either major or minor criteria (ECG-negative patients) who were compared with 1:1 age- and gender matched control patients. Tables 1 and 2 summarize

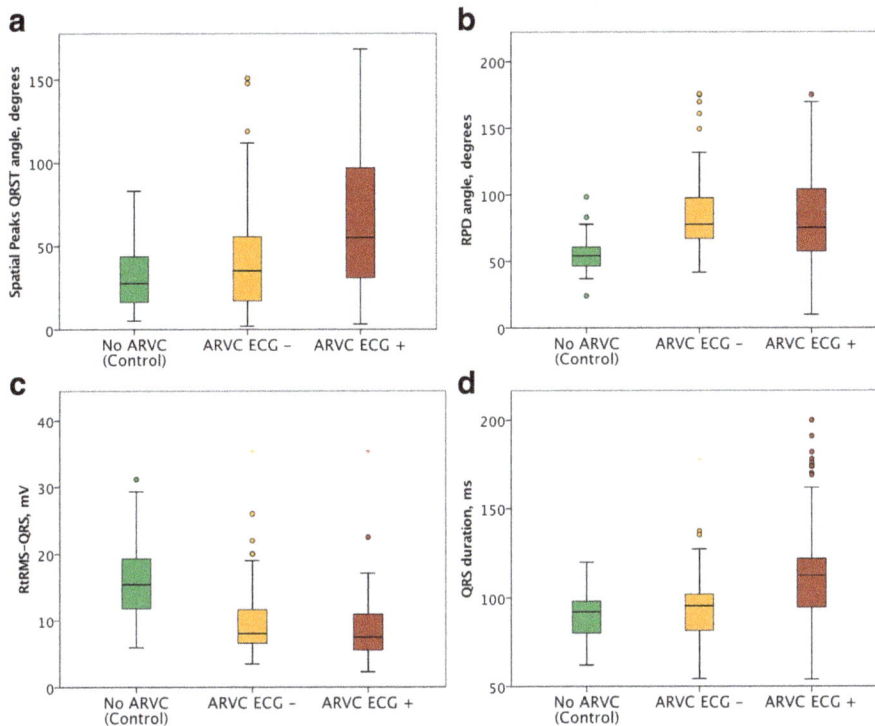

Fig. 2 a-d: Box plots comparing parameter values for controls, ECG-negative and ECG-positive comparisons of the **a**: Spatial peaks QRS-T angle (median with 1st to 3rd quartiles), **b**: RPD angle (mean with 2 standard deviations), **c**: RtRMS-QRS (mean with 2 standard deviations), **d**: QRS duration (mean with 2 standard deviations)

patient demographic data. Apart from the ECG-related differences between ECG-positive and ECG-negative ARVD/C patients, on which group definitions were based, no other diagnostic criteria appeared to demonstrate significant difference between the groups (Table 1). Borderline significant difference was observed in regard to the greater prevalence of patients fulfilling minor arrhythmia criterion in ECG-positive ARVD/C patients.

However, we observed significant differences in regard to the major MRI volume criteria, which was twice as common in ARVD/C patients who met ECG criteria (ECG-positive ARVD/C) than in those who did not meet 12-lead ECG criteria (ECG-negative ARVD/C). Figure 2 shows how the patients were sorted in various categories to determine the overall ability to detect ECG-negative ARVD/C patients. Figure 2a-d shows comparisons of various parameters for controls, ECG-negative and ECG-positive patients.

QTc and QRSd

Five of our ECG-negative ARVD/C patient had right bundle branch blocks. While QRSd did not significantly differentiate ECG-negative ARVD/C patients from controls (Table 2), the QTc was significantly longer in ECG-negative ARVD/C than in control subjects (Table 3), with resultant optimum sensitivity, specificity, positive

and negative predictive values shown in Table 4 with an odds ratio of 5.3 for QTc (95% confidence interval 0.6 to 46.6). The QRSd and the QTc significantly differentiated the ECG-positive versus ECG-negative ARVD/C patients (p-values of <0.001 and 0.002, respectively).

Spatial peaks QRS-T angles

Both the SPQRS-T angle and the RPD angle demonstrated significant differences between ECG-negative ARVD/C patients and control subjects (p-value < 0.001, Table 3). The RPD angle showed much better sensitivity and specificity than the spatial QRS-T angle (Table 4) and with an odds ratio 34 times higher than that for the SPQRS-T angle at 41.3 l95% CI 13.1 to 130.2).

The SPQRS-T angle demonstrated stepwise increase from the lowest value in the control group to ECG-negative ARVD/C and the highest value observed in the ECG-positive ARVD/C patients.

Right root mean square QRS voltage

The right root mean square QRS (RtRMS-QRS) progressively and significantly decreased stepwise from the highest mean value observed in the control group to the lowest among the ECG-positive ARVD/C. In regard to discrimination between control subjects and ECG-negative ARVD/C patients, the ROC curve gave an

Table 1 All ARVD/C, ARVD/C with (+ECG) and without (−ECG) 2010 ECG taskforce criteria

	ARVC Total (N = 155)	ECG-positive ARVC (N = 89)	ECG-negative ARVC (N = 66)	p-value ECG-positive vs ECG-negative
Age	42.1 ± 17.3	42.0 ± 17.4	41.7 ± 17.6	0.861
Sex (% male)	106 (68.4%)	63 (70.8%)	43 (65.2%)	0.488
Proband (%)	111 (71.6%)	71 (79.8%)	30 (45.5%)	0.012
I. Imaging	155 (100%)	89 (100%)	66 (100%)	1.000
major, %	111 (71.6%)	68 (76.4%)	43 (65.2%)	0.082
minor, %	89 (57.4%)	60 (67.4%)	29 (43.9%)	0.005
II. Tissue characterization of the wall, biopsies performed (% of patients)	70 (45.2%)	39 (43.8%)	31 (47.0%)	0.745
major, %	53 (75.7%)	31 (79.1%)	22 (71.0%)	0.576
minor, %	63 (90.0%)	36 (92.3%)	27 (87.1%)	0.454
III. Repolarization abnormality				
major, %	54 (34.8%)	54 (60.7%)	0 (0.0%)	<0.001
minor, %	20 (12.9%)	20 (22.5%)	0 (0.0%)	<0.001
IV. Depolarization abnormality				
major, %	13 (8.4%)	13 (14.6%)	0 (0.0%)	<0.001
minor, %	17 (11.0%)	17 (19.1%)	0 (0.0%)	<0.001
V. Arrhythmia				
major, %	44 (28.4%)	26 (29.2%)	18 (27.3%)	0.858
minor, %	64 (41.3%)	42 (47.2%)	22 (33.3%)	0.1000
VI. Family history				
major, %	84 (54.2%)	48 (53.9%)	35 (53.0%)	1.000
VII. Genotype positive	48 (31.0%)	29 (32.6%)	19 (28.8%)	0.726
PLN (% genotype positive)	1 (2.1%)	0 (0.0%)	1 (5.3%)	0.396
TTN (% genotype positive)	11 (22.9%)	8 (27.6%)	3 (15.8%)	0.488
PKP2 (% genotype positive)	23 (47.9%)	17 (58.6%)	6 (31.2%)	0.083
DSC2 (% genotype positive)	2 (4.2%)	1 (3.5%)	1 (5.3%)	1.000
DSG2 (% genotype positive)	12 (25.0%)	6 (20.7%)	6 (31.5%)	0.501
DSG3 (% genotype positive)	2 (4.2%)	1 (3.5%)	1 (5.30%)	1.000
DSP (% genotype positive)	8 (16.7%)	6 (20.7%)	2 (10.56%)	0.4510

optimum cut-off value of 0.81 mV giving an odds ratio of 13.0 (4.6 to 36.4). Please see Tables 3 and 4.

Combined right-precordial directed parameters
Based on combined right-precordial-directed-sided parameters including the RPD angle and RtRMS-QRS, at the above noted cut-off values, the sensitivity, specificity and odds ratios were 90.9%, 83.3%, and 45.0 (95% CI 15.8 to 128.2), respectively. Figure 2a-d shows depolarization parameter box plots.

ECG-negative proband versus ECG-negative non-proband
Thirty patients without abnormalities on the 12-lead ECG were probands (45.5%). At the cut-off values above (70.2 degrees for RPD angle and 0.81 mV for the RtRMS-QRS, respectively), the sensitivity for probands

was 86.7% and for non-probands 72.5% for identification of those without 12-lead ECG abnormalities otherwise, while of course maintaining specificity 92.4% and 94.0% respectively.

ECG-based 2010 taskforce criteria and their relationship to the right-precordial ECG parameters
When the whole ARVD/C cohort was assessed (N = 155), the RtRMS-QRS significantly differentiated those with TAD (upslope of the S-wave ≥55 ms, minor depolarization criterion) versus those ARVD/C patients with upslope of the S-wave <55 ms (p = 0.006).

Patients with and without epsilon waves did not demonstrate significant difference in regard to the novel right-precordial parameters (Table 5). Patients with different extent of repolarization abnormalities, such as no

Table 2 Detailed electrocardiographical and imaging characteristics of ECG-positive and ECG-negative ARVC/D patients including Epsilon waves, upslope S-wave, Signal Average ECG measurements (SAECG) including fractional QRS duration (fqrsd), low amplitude signal under 40 microV in the latter part of QRS (LAS40) and root mean square amplitude in the last 40milliseconds (RMS40), repolarization abnormalities and echocardiogram/magnetic resonance imaging (MRI) including right ventricular end-diastolic volumes (RVEDV)

	ARVD/C (n = 155)	ARVD/C ECG-positive (N = 84)	ARVD/C ECG-negative (N = 66)	P-value ECG positive/ negative
ECG: Depolarization				
- Epsilon waves	13 (8.4%)	13 (15.5%)	0 (0.0%)	<0.001
- upslope S-wave ≥55 ms V1,V2 or V3	17 (11.0%)	17 (20.2%)	0 (0.0%)	<0.001
Bundle branch blocks	22 (14.1%)	17 (20.2%)	0 (0.0%)	0.035
SAECG performed (% total)	63 (40.7%)	32 (38.1%)	31 (41.7%)	0.515
- fQRSd ≥114 ms (% of SAECG)	33 (52.4%)	17 (53.1%)	16 (51.6%)	1.000
- LAS40 ≥ 38 ms (% of SAECG)	31 (49.2%)	18 (56.3%)	13 (41.9%)	0.317
- RMS40 ≤ 20 µV (% of SAECG)	28 (44.4%)	13 (40.6%)	15 (48.4%)	0.616
ECG: Repolarization				
- T-wave inversions V1-V3 > 14 years no RBBB	54 (34.8%)	54 (64.3%)	0 (0.0%)	<0.001
- T-wave inversions V1-V4 with RBBB	12 (7.7%)	12 (14.3%)	0 (0.0%)	<0.001
- T-wave inversions V1 and V2 or in V4,V5,V6	8 (5.2%)	8 (9.5%)	0 (0.0%)	0.008
Imaging				
Echocardiograms performed (% total)	155 (100.0%)	84 (100.0%)	66 (100.0%)	1.000
- Regional akinesia/dyskinesia/aneurysm (% echo)	111 (71.6%)	65 (77.4%)	43 (65.2%)	0.108
MRI's performed (% total)	124 (80.0%)	72 (85.7%)	52 (73.2%)	0.070
- Regional akinesia/dyskinesia/aneurysm (% MRI)	89 (71.8%)	58 (80.6%)	31 (59.6%)	0.272
- RVEDV ≥110 ml/m² (M), 100 ml/m² (F) (%MRI)	65 (52.4%)	49 (68.1%)	16 (30.8%)	<0.001
- RVEDV ≥100 ml/m² but <110 ml/m² (M), ≥90 ml/m² but <100 ml/m² (F) (%MRI)	24 (19.4%)	10 (11.9%)	14 (26.9%)	0.106

T-wave inversion/T-wave inversion in V1 (repolarization criterion is not present), T-wave inversion in V1 and V2 only (minor repolarization criterion) or T-wave inversions in V1-V3 or beyond (major repolarization criterion) were not differentiated by the right-precordial parameters (Table 5). The spatial QRS-T angle was lower for those with only T-wave inversions in V1 and V2, versus those with more precordial T-wave inversions or those without T-wave inversions in the precordial leads (Table 5).

Left ventricular involvement and clinical parameters
Twelve total ARVD/C patients had left-sided disease (7.7%). Eleven had decreased left ventricular ejection

Table 3 Vector and protractor measured angles and their respective p-values for the QRS duration (QRSd, milliseconds), corrected QT interval (QTc, milliseconds), the right precordial directed angle (RPD angle), and right root mean square QRS (RtRMS-QRS)respectively for different subsets of patients including controls, arrhythmogenic right ventricular dysplasia/cardiomyopathy patients who meet 12-lead 2010 Taskforce criteria (ECG-positive), who don't meet 12-lead 2010 Taskforce criteria (ECG-negative), who are ECG-negative without bundle branch blocks (BBB) and who are ECG-negative who have signal average ECG's do not have any late potentials (SAECG-). P-values as compared to controls

Parameter	QRSd (ms),[p-value]	QTc (ms),[p-value]	SPQRS-T angle	RPD angle	RtRMS-QRS
Controls (N = 66)	91.5 (85.5 to 99.0)	405.0 (387.5 to 430.2)	24.1 (13.5 to 42.1)	54.4 (48.9 to 61.5)	1.54 (1.17 to 1.90)
ARVD/C ECG-positive (N = 89)	104.0 (94.0 to 122.0), [<0.001]*	425.0 (403.0 to 449.0), [0.022]*	43.8 (23.6 to 72.9), [0.228]	74.8 (58.4 to 94.7), [0.971]	0.81 (0.63 to 1.13), [0.371]
ARVD/C ECG- and no BBB (N = 66)	98.0 (86.0 to 104.0), [0.052]s	412.0 (399.0 to 430.0), [0.061]	33.6 (16.7 to 54.2), [0.004]	76.2 (62.3 to 92.9), [<0.001]	0.81 (0.64 to 1.15), [<0.001]
ARVD/C ECG-, no BBB, SAECG-negative (N = 20)	93.0 (85.5 to 100.0), [0.947]	420.5 (397.5 to 430.0), [0.057]	40.9 (22.3 to 55.7), [0.081]	71.2 (60.4 to 84.7) [<0.001]	0.77 (0.67 to 1.18), [<0.001]

*indicated significant p-value < 0.050

Table 4 Derived-vectorcardiographic angles and their respective sensitivities, specificities, positive and negative predictive values (PPV, NPV, respectively) and odds ratios (95% confidence intervals) for optimal cut-off values based on ROC curve analysis for the corrected QT interval (QTc), spatial peaks QRS-T angle (SPQRS-T angle), the right precordial directed angle (RPD angle angle), right root mean square QRS (RtRMS-QRS), and for both right parameters (RPD angle angle and RtRMS-QRS) at the above cut-off values) for ECG-negative ARVD/C versus controls

Parameter	Optimum cut-off	AUC	p-value	Sensitivity (%)	Specificity (%)	PPV (%)	NPV (%)	Odds ratio
QRSd	99.0 ms	0.64	0.026	48.5	83.3	74.4	61.8	4.7 (2.1 to 10.6)
QTc	451.0 ms	0.56	0.289	12.1	100.0	100.0	53.2	19.3 (1.1 to 342.1)
SPQRS-T angle	50.8°	0.68	<0.001	30.0	94.0	53.6	50.9	1.2 (0.5 to 2.7)
RPD angle	70.2°	0.86	<0.001	72.7	94.0	91.7	80.5	41.3 (13.1 to 130.2)
RtRMS-QRS	0.81 mV	0.85	<0.001	51.5	92.4	92.3	77.5	13.0 (4.6 to 36.4)
Both right parameters	N/A	N/A	N/A	81.8	90.9	90.0	83.3	45.0 (15.8 to 128.2)

fraction (median 52.5%, IQR 50.5 to 54.0%) and three had LVEDVi >100 ml/m^2 (median 30.8 ml/m^2, IQR 26.5 to 97.0 ml/m^2). Three patients were ECG-negative and one had no late potentials. There was only a significant difference in the QRSd with those without LV changes at median 100 ms (IQR 90-113 ms) versus those with left sided changes at a median of 97 ms (IQR 91.5 to 101 ms). The median values for ARVD/C patients with left-sided changes for the QTc, SPQRS-T angle, RPD angle and RtRMS-QRS were 417 ms (IQR 401 to 457 ms), 23.0 degrees (IQR 15.6 to 51.5 degrees), 79.4 degrees (IQR 70.0 to 99.8 degrees), and 0.91 mV (IQR 0.54 to 1.21 mV), respectively.

Intra-observer and inter-observer variability
Intra-class correlation coefficients for the intra-/inter-observer variability for the RPD angle were 0.93 and 0.92, for the RtRMS-QRS were 0.94 and 0.92. For the SPQRS-T angle, intra-/inter-observer variability has previously been described [6, 14, 15].

Variability between automated analyses and 1st author calculations gave intra-class correlation coefficients of 0.971 and 0.917 for RtRMS-QRS and RPD angle.

Magnetic resonance imaging correlates
MRI indexed volumes and ejection fractions were compared to the VCG/ECG parameters above. The highest

R-squared value for a VCG or ECG parameter was 0.24 for the SPQRS-T angle correlating to left ventricular ejection fraction (EF). Otherwise the RPD angle and RtRMS-QRS correlated poorly to RV indexed volume (indexed RVEDV) with R-squared values at 0.15 and 0.07, respectively and with RV EF R-squared values of 0.06 and 0.19, respectively, all without significant p-values. QRSd also correlated poorly with indexed RVEDV and RVEF with R-squared values of 0.10 and 0.11, respectively without significant p-values.

Discussion
Main findings
We aimed to assess whether patients with definite ARVD/C diagnosed using the 2010 revised Task Force criteria exhibit subtle electrocardiographic abnormalities, which do not fit in the frame of the depolarization and repolarization criteria outlined in the Task Force 2010 document. By comparing with a cohort of healthy controls we found that ostensibly normal ECG pattern in patients with ECG-negative ARVD/C contain signs of abnormal ventricular depolarization and repolarization that can be quantified using novel right precordial-adjusted VCG markers. RPD angle, SPQRS-T angle, and the RtRMS-QRS demonstrated significant ability to differentiate patients with electrocardiographically concealed ARVD/C from healthy controls. In addition,

Table 5 Novel right-precordial and vectorcardiographic values compared to ARVD/C patients and 2010 Taskforce criteria values currently used

	SPQRS-T angle (degrees)	RPD angle (degrees)	RtRMS-QRS (millivolts)
Epsilon-wave +, n = 13	54.4 ± 31.3	100.5 ± 42.5	1.0 ± 0.8
Epsilon-wave -, n = 142	54.6 ± 42.0	81.2 ± 31.2	0.9 ± 0.4
TAD > = 55 ms, n = 17	67.0 ± 41.1	92.9 ± 40.7	0.7 ± 0.3[a]
TAD < 55 ms, n = 138	53.1 ± 41.1	81.7 ± 31.4	0.9 ± 0.5[a]
No T-wave inversion/only in V1, n = 26	56.7 ± 31.0	83.8 ± 33.8	1.0 ± 0.6
T-wave inversion V1-V2, n = 56	35.0 ± 28.0[a]	87.5 ± 31.8	0.9 ± 0.4
T-wave inversion V1-V3 or beyond, n = 73	67.7 ± 46.8	78.1 ± 32.4	0.8 ± 0.4

[a]indicates significantly different novel parameter values per 2010 Taskforce ECG parameter differentiation mentioned

SPQRS-T angle exhibited stepwise increase and RtRMS-QRS a decrease when control cohort was compared with ECG-negative and ECG-positive ARVD/C patients thus suggesting novel markers potential for quantification of electrocardiographic ARVD/C phenotype. These may aid in early detection in clinical cascade screening.

QRSd and QTc

The QRSd was not a specific marker for -ECG ARVC/D, which is not surprising, given the patients don't meet 2010 taskforce criteria including epsilon waves or delayed S-wave upstroke. It does significantly differentiate ECG-positive ARVD/C from ECG-negative ARVD/C. The QTc did significantly differentiate patients with ECG-negative ARVD/C with minimal diagnostic assistance. The QTc also prolongs significantly as the ARVD/C patients develop Taskforce 2010 ECG criteria, which may or may not assist in diagnosis.

Spatial angles

Although conventional VCG markers have shown use in left sided heart disease [7–11], they have shown limited use in right heart disease [13]. For instance, in hypertrophic cardiomyopathy, the spatial QRS-T angle improves diagnostic ability for detection of hypertrophic cardiomyopathy over conventional 12-lead ECG parameters, however only detected part of our ECG-negative ARVD/C cohort [7]. This same angle, however showed limited prognostic ability in other right-ventricle disease patients, namely those with Tetralology of Fallot [13, 14]. The RPD angle had the highest identification ability out of all parameters tested and gave the highest odds ratio for identification of ECG-negative ARVD/C. Although the SPQRS-T angle significantly differentiates controls from ECG-negative ARVD/C, it did not prove as clinically useful with less sensitivity and less specificity than the RPD angle. Although some cases of ARVD/C include left sided disease (12 patients in our cohort), more often than not a right-sided only phenotype is present [2]. Thus, even though the SPQRS-T angle has prognostic and diagnostic use [7–11], and specifically for a generally left sided cardiomyopathy [7], it is not surprising that a right-sided specific marker is more helpful in identification of disease in those without other depolarization/repolarization abnormalities in ARVD/C as suggested by our findings. This also seemed to be particularly a good marker for those family members detected by cascade screening, who likely represent an early ARVC/D phenotype. This may be a useful marker for screening and can be programmed in most ECG software.

Right root mean square

The RtRMS-QRS or right precordial-directed QRS vector magnitude is simply a measure of depolarization dispersion in the right ventricle which should become smaller as more fibrosis occurs. The lower the RtRMS-QRS, the more dispersion of depolarization in the right ventricle would likely occur. The RtRMS-QRS had significant identification ability in those with ECG-negative ARVD/C compared to control patients with a high specificity. This is useful as it is a simple parameter to calculate (Fig. 1). Similar to other right side-specific voltage parameters, it has low sensitivity for detection of right heart disease in this study, however as a non-invasive and cost-effective test, this simple method still detected over one half of patients who were not initially detected by ECG [15]. Given the fibro-fatty infiltration of right ventricular myocardium often observed in ARVD/C, it seems logical that dispersion of depolarization (ie. lower RtRMS-QRS) would be affected [1]. Again, this would also particularly be helpful in identification of those with early ARVC/D disease, as it was able to detect those non-proband family members who represent an early stage of ARVC/D and meet 1 of their major criteria by family association alone.

Combined right-sided parameters

Combined, the diagnostic value of these parameters demonstrated superior identification power than each parameter alone. Combined, without compromising specificity, these parameters identified 65/71 (91.6%) of patients who would not have otherwise been identified with ECG screening. A high odds ratio was determined. These right-sided specific parameters, although not perfectly sensitive, combined have an additive identification ability without compromising specificity for patients who might otherwise fit 2010 taskforce criteria for definite ARVD/C based on genetic testing or further imaging [2].

Novel right-precordial parameters and the degree of ARVD/C phenotype manifestation

In the case of the S-wave angle and RtRMS-QRS, there appears to be a significant step-wise progression from control patients to ECG-negative and further on to the ECG-positive ARVD/C patients, which suggests that these novel VCG/ECG markers may be considered as electrocardiographic equivalent of the disease substrate in ARVC/D. RtRMS-QRS appears to be related to the conventional electrocardiographic disease markers such as terminal activation delay in the right precordial leads, however they perform well in differentiating patients with ARVC/D from controls also in the "normal" TAD range. This demonstrates the ability of the novel VCG/ECG markers to detect ARVC/D manifesting with subtle depolarization abnormalities only and indicate their potential in identification of affected family members, which requires additional studies.

The RPD angle did not have a step-wise progression, but was similar in number between those ARVD/C patients with and those without other depolarization or repolarization abnormalities. Also, this parameter did not differentiate the degree of T-wave inversion (Table 5), thus must be more affected by depolarization versus repolarization abnormalities. Even though not a significant difference, the RPD angle (as well as the other right-precordial parameters) demonstrated trends with Epsilon wave differentiation, which seem to indicate dependence on dispersion of depolarization.

Regardless, all three parameters detect ARVD/C patients with electrographically concealed changes. Further studies are warranted to define these changes over time as well as genotype differences.

Limitations

The retrospective nature of this study gives inherent limitations. The study control patients were from the USA and from Sweden and did not include those from Italy, specifically, which may bias our control results to some extent. Furthermore, any type of estimation from an ECG of a parameter, if not automated carries some inherent error, although our correlation coefficients were reasonable for intra–/inter-observer variability.

Conclusion

Patients with ECG-negative ARVD/C bear subtle ECG abnormalities that can be detected using right-sided measures including the RPD angle and the RtRMS-QRS. In combination these parameters can identify almost all patients with ECG-negative ARVD/C without compromising specificity. Future studies are warranted to identify changes in these parameters over time as well as to identify their utility in clinical cascade screening. If independently reproduced, these parameters should be considered for addition to current ARVD/C guidelines and may help to cost-effectively screen for ARVD/C in family members or those at risk.

Abbreviations

ARVC/D: Arrhythmogenic right ventricular cardiomyopathy/dysplasia; BBB: Bundle branch blocks; DSC2: Desmocollin 2; DSG2: Desmoglein 2; DSG3: Desmoglein 3; DSP: Desmoplakin; ECG: Electrocardiogram; F: Female; fQRSd: Filtered QRS duration; ICD: internal cardiac defibrillator; LAS40: Low amplitude duration < 40 mV; M: Male; Mri: Magnetic resonance imaging; Ms.: millisecond; mV: millivolt; NPV: Negative predictive value; OR: Odds ratio; PKP2: Plakophilin 2; PLN: Phospholamban; PPV: Positive predictive value; QRSd: QRS duration; QTc: Corrected QT interval; RMS40: Root mean square voltage last 40 milliseconds of the QRS; ROC: receiver operating characteristic curve; RPD angle: Right precordial-directed angle; RtRMS-QRS: Right root mean square QRS (millivolts); RVEDV: Right ventricular end-diastolic volume; SAECG: Signal average electrocardiogram; SPQRS-T angle: Spatial peaks QRS-T angle; TTN: Titin

Acknowledgements

Not otherwise applicable.

Funding

This work was supported by the Swedish National Health Service, Donation funds at Skåne University Hospital, Lund, Sweden, the Swedish Heart-Lung Foundation (20140734), and the Region Skåne.

Authors' contributions

DC made substantial contributions to data conception, design, analysis and interpretation; he wrote the manuscript. AS was responsible a good portion of the data collection, and was thoroughly involved in drafting the manuscript. JC was responsible for the data, analysis and interpretation; he was involved in drafting the manuscript. SG made substantial contributions to data collection, and revision of the manuscript. NS was responsible for inter-observer variability, conception and design of the project and manuscript revision. FB made substantial contributions to the data collection and manuscript revision. AS made substantial contributions to the data collection and manuscript revision. LM made substantial contributions to the conception, design, data acquisition and manuscript revision PP made substantial contributions to conception, design, data acquisition, analysis and interpretation; he was involved in drafting and revising the manuscript; agreed to be accountable for all aspects of work in ensuring that any questions related to accuracy or integrity are appropriately investigated and resolved. All authors read and approved the final manuscript.

Competing interests

The authors declare that they have no competing interests.

Author details

[1]Department of Cardiology, Clinical Sciences, Lund University, Lund, Sweden. [2]Electrophysiology/Cardiology, Penn State Milton S. Hershey Medical Center, Hershey, USA. [3]Department of Cardiology and Department of Medical and Health Sciences, Linkoping University, Linkoping, Sweden. [4]Cardiovascular Institute and Adult Medical Genetics Program, University of Colorado Denver AMC, Aurora, CO, USA. [5]Cardiovascular Department, Ospedali Riuniti and University of Trieste, Trieste, Italy. [6]Arrhythmia Clinic, Skåne University Hospital, Lund, Sweden.

References

1. Basso C, Corrado D, FI M, Nava A, Thiene G. Arrhythmogenic right ventricular cardiomyopathy. Lancet. 2009;373:1289–300.
2. FI M, McKenna WJ, Sherrill D, Basso C, Bauce B, Bluemke DA, Calkins H, Corrado D, Cox MG, Daubert JP, Fontaine G, Gear K, Hauer R, Nava A, Picard MH, Protonotarios N, Saffitz JE, Sanborn DM, Steinberg JS, Tandri H, Thiene G, Towbin JA, Tsatsopoulou A, Wichter T, Zareba W. Diagnosis of arrhythmogenic right ventricular cardiomyopathy/dysplasia: proposed modification of the task force criteria. Circulation. 2010;121:1533–41.
3. Hamid MS, Norman M, Quraishi A, .Firoozi S, Thaman R, Gimeno JR, Sachdev B, Rowland E, Elliott PM, McKenna WJ: Prospective evaluation of relatives for familial arrhythmogenic right ventricular cardiomyopathy/dysplasia reveals a need to broaden diagnostic criteria. J Am Coll Cardiol 2002; 40: 1445-1450.
4. Kaplan SR, Gard JJ, Protonotarios N, Tsatsopoulou A, Spiliopoulou C, Anastasakis A, Squarcioni CP, McKenna WJ, Thiene G, Basso C, Brousse N, Fontaine G, Saffitz JE. Remodeling of myocyte gap junctions in arrhythmogenic right ventricular cardiomyopathy due to deletion in plakoglobin. Heart Rhythm. 2004;1:3–11.
5. Te Riele AS, James CA, Rastegar N, Bhonsale A, Murray B, Tichnell C, Judge DP, Bluemke DA, Zimmerman SL, Kamel IR, Calkins H, Tandri H. Yield of serial evaluation in at-risk family members of patients with ARVD/C. J Am Coll Cardiol. 2014;64:293–301.
6. Cortez D, Sharma N, Devers C, Devers E, Schlegel TT. Visual transform applications for estimating the spatial QRS-T angle from the conventional 12-lead ECG: Kors is still most frank. J Electrocardiol. 2014;47:12–9.
7. Poplock Potter SL, Holmqvist F, Platonov PG, Steding K, Arheden H, Pahlm O, Starc V, McKenna WJ, Schlegel TT. Detection of hypertrophic Cardiomyopathy is improved when using advanced rather than strictly conventional 12-lead electrocardiogram. J Electrocardiol. 2010;43:713–8.

8. Kardys I, Kors JA, van der Meer IM, Hofman A, van der Kuip DA, Witteman JC. Spatial QRS-T angle predicts cardiac death in a general population. Eur Heart J. 2003;24:1357–64.

9. Kors JA, Kardys I, van der Meer IM, van Herpen G, Hofman A, van der Kuip DA, Witteman JC. Spatial QRS-T angle as a risk indicator of cardiac death in an elderly population. J Electrocardiol. 2003;36(Suppl):113–4.

10. Yamazaki T, Froelicher VF, Myers J, Chun S. Wang pl: spatial QRS-T angle predicts cardiac death in a clinical population. Heart Rhythm. 2005;2:73–78.16.

11. Borleffs CJ, Scherptong RW, Man SC, van Welsenes GH, Bax JJ, van Erven L, Swenne CA, Schalij MJ. Predicting ventricular arrhythmias in patients with ischemic heart disease: clinical application of the ECG-derived QRS-T angle. Circ Arrhythm Electrophysiol. 2009;2:548–54.

12. Cortez D, Graw S, Mestroni L. Hypertrophic cardiomyopathy, the spatial peaks QRS-t angle identifies those with sustained ventricular arrhythmias. Clin Cardiol. 2016;39:459–63.

13. Cortez D, Ruckdeschel E, McCanta AC, Collins K, Sauer W, Kay J, Nguyen D. Vectorcardiographic predictors of ventricular arrhythmia inducibility in patients with tetralogy of Fallot. J Electrocardiol. 2015;48:141–4.

14. Cortez D, Barham W, Ruckdeschel E, Sharma N, McCanta AC, von Alvensleben J, Sauer WH, Collins KK, Kay J, Patel S, Ngueyen DT. Noninvasive predictors of ventricular arrhythmias in patients with tetralogy of Fallot undergoing pulmonary valve replacement. JACC Clin Electrophysiol. 2017;3:162–170.

15. Whitman IR, Patel VV, Soliman EZ, Bluemke DA, Praestgaard A, Jain A, Herrington D, Lima JA, Kawut SM. Validity of the surface electrogram criteria for right ventricular hypertrophy: the MESA-RV study (multi-ethnic study of atherosclerosis-right ventricle). J Am Coll Cardiol. 2014;63:672–8.

Permissions

List of Contributors

Julia Daher Carneiro Marsiglia, Flávia Laghi Credidio, Théo Gremen Mimary de Oliveira, Rafael Ferreira Reis, José Eduardo Krieger and Alexandre Costa Pereira
Laboratory of Genetics and Molecular Cardiology, Heart Institute (InCor), University of São Paulo, São Paulo, Brazil

Murillo de Oliveira Antunes, Charles Mady and Edmundo Arteaga-Fernandez
Clinical Unit of Cardiomyopathies, Heart Institute (InCor), University of São Paulo, São Paulo, Brazil

Aloir Queiroz de Araujo
Federal University of Espírito Santo, Vitória, Brazil

Rodrigo Pinto Pedrosa
Chagas Disease and Heart Failure Outpatient Service, PROCAPE-University of Pernambuco/UPE, Recife, Brazil

João Marcos Bemfica Barbosa-Ferreira
Federal University of Amazonas, Manaus, Brazil

Kamilu Musa Karaye
Department of Medicine, Bayero University and Aminu Kano Teaching Hospital, 3 New Hospital Road, Kano, Nigeria

Kamilu Musa Karaye, Krister Lindmark and Michael Henein
Department of Public Health and Clinical Medicine, Umea University, SE-901 87 Umea, Sweden

Krister Lindmark and Michael Henein
Department of Cardiology, Umea Heart Centre, SE-901 87 Umea, Sweden

Daiva Bironaite and Algirdas Venalis
Dept. of Stem Cell Biology, State Research Institute, Center for Innovative Medicine, Zygimantu 9, LT01102 Vilnius, Lithuania

Dainius Daunoravicius, Sigitas Cibiras, Edvardas Zurauskas and Virginija Grabauskiene
Department of Pathology, Forensic Medicine and Pharmacology, Vilnius University, Faculty of Medicine, Vilnius, Lithuania

Julius Bogomolovas and Siegfried Labeit
Department of Integrative Pathophysiology, Universitäts medizin Mannheim, Mannheim, Germany

Dalius Vitkus
Department of Physiology, Biochemistry, Microbiology and Laboratory Medicine, Vilnius University, Faculty of Medicine, Vilnius, Lithuania

Ieva Zasytyte, Kestutis Rucinskas and Virginija Grabauskiene
Vilnius University, Faculty of Medicine, Clinic of Cardiovascular Diseases, Vilnius, Lithuania

Wei Yang, Yuan Li, Fawei He and Haixiang Wu
Department of Ultrasonics, The Second Hospital of Sichuan, No. 55, People's South Road, Wuhou District, 610041 Chengdu, Sichuan, China

Jun Guan, Wen-Qi Liu and Hong-Yan Dai
Department of Cardiology, Qingdao Municipal Hospital, Qingdao, Shandong, China

Wen-Qi Liu, Yue Shi and Xue-Ying Tan
Qingdao University Medical College, Qingdao, Shandong, China

Ming-Qing Xing
Department of Clinical laboratory, Qingdao Municipal Hospital,
Qingdao, Shandong, China.

Wen-Qi Liu and Xue-Ying Tan
Key Laboratory of cellular transplantation, Chinese Ministry of Public Health, Qingdao Municipal Hospital, Qingdao, Shandong, China

Chang-Qing Jiang
Department of pathology department, Qingdao Municipal Hospital, Qingdao, Shandong, China

Jochen Hefner and Herbert Csef
Section of Psychosomatic Medicine and Psychotherapy, Department of
Internal Medicine II, Julius-Maximilian-University of Wuerzburg, Oberduerrbacher Str. 6, D- 97080 Wuerzburg, Germany

Stefan Frantz
Unit of Cardiology, Department of Internal Medicine I, Julius-Maximilian-University of Wuerzburg, Wuerzburg, Germany
Comprehensive Heart Failure Center, Julius-Maximilian-University of Wuerzburg, Wuerzburg, Germany

Nina Glatter and Bodo Warrings
Department of Psychiatry, Psychosomatics and Psychotherapy, Julius-Maximilian-University of Wuerzburg, Wuerzburg, Germany

Thomas Emil Christensen, Lia E. Bang and Lene Holmvang
Department of Cardiology, Copenhagen University Hospital, Rigshospitalet, Copenhagen, Denmark

Thomas Emil Christensen, Philip Hasbak and Andreas Kjaer
Department of Clinical Physiology, Nuclear Medicine & PET and Cluster for Molecular Imaging, Copenhagen University Hospital, Rigshospitalet and University of Copenhagen, Copenhagen, Denmark

Per Bech
Psychiatric Research Unit, Psychiatric Center North Zealand, Copenhagen University Hospital, Hillerød, Denmark

Søren Dinesen Østergaard
Department of Clinical Medicine, Aarhus University Hospital, Aarhus, Denmark
Department P - Research, Aarhus University Hospital, Risskov, Denmark

Cong Liu, Chang-Yang Xing, Jing Ma, Yun-You Duan and Li-Jun Yuan
Department of Ultrasound Diagnostics, Tangdu Hospital, Fourth Military Medical University, #569 Xinsi RoadBaqiao District, Xi'an 710038, China

Xiao-Zhao Lu and Ming-Zhi Shen
Department of Biochemistry and Molecular Biology, Fourth Military Medical University, Xi'an, China

Xiaoping Li and Wei Fang
Department of Cardiology, Sichuan Academy of Medical Sciences and Sichuan Provincial People's Hospital, Hospital of the University of Electronic Science and Technology of China, Chengdu, Sichuan 610072, China

Xiaoping Li, Guodong Niu and Wei Hua
Cardiac Arrhythmia Center, State Key Laboratory of Cardiovascular Disease, Cardiovascular Institute and Fuwai Hospital, National Center for Cardiovascular Diseases, Chinese Academy of Medical Sciences and Peking Union Medical College, Beijing 100037, People's Republic of China

Rong Luo
Temperature and Inflammation Research Center, Key Laboratory of Colleges and Universities in Sichuan Province, Chengdu Medical College, Chengdu 610500, People's Republic of China

Xiaolei Xu
Division of Cardiovascular Diseases, Mayo Clinic College of Medicine, Rochester, MN 55905, USA

Yixian Xu
Department of Cardiology, Lanzhou University Second Hospital, Lanzhou, Gansu 730030, People's Republic of China

Michael Fu
Department of Medicine, Sahlgrenska University hospital/Östra hospital, Gothenburg, Sweden

Xiushan Wu
The Center of Heart Development, Key Lab of MOE for Development Biology and Protein Chemistry, College of Life Science, Hunan Normal University, Changsha 410081, People's Republic of China

Zhongshu Liang, Sunnar Leo, Helin Wen, Mao Ouyang, Weihong Jiang and Kan Yang
Department of Cardiology, Third Xiangya Hospital, Central South University, Changsha, Hunan 410013, People's Republic China

Ole De Backer, Sofie Gevaert and Peter Gheeraert
Department of Cardiology, Ghent University Hospital, De Pintelaan 185, B-9000 Ghent, Belgium

Ole De Backer, Philippe Debonnaire, Sofie Gevaert, Luc Missault and Luc Muyldermans
Department of Cardiology, AZ Sint-Jan Hospital, Bruges, Belgium

Kyoichiro Yazaki, Yoichi Ajiro, Fumiaki Mori, Masahiro Watanabe, Kei Tsukamoto, Takashi Saito, Keiko Mizobuchi and Kazunori Iwade
Department of Cardiology, National Hospital Organization Yokohama Medical Center, 3-60-2 Harajuku, Totsuka-ku, Yokohama-shi, Kanagawa 245-8575, Japan

Toru Kubo, Yuichi Baba, Takayoshi Hirota, Katsutoshi Tanioka, Naohito Yamasaki, Takashi Furuno and Hiroaki Kitaoka
Department of Cardiology, Neurology and Aging Science, Kochi Medical School, Oko-cho, Nankoku-shi 783-8505Kochi, Japan

Shigeo Yamanaka and Tetsuro Sugiura
Department of Laboratory Medicine, Kochi Medical School, Kochi, Japan

Tatsuo Iiyama and Naoko Kumagai
Clinical Trial Center, Kochi Medical School, Kochi, Japan

Marcelo Dantas Tavares de Melo, José Arimateia Batista de Araújo Filho, Jose Rodrigues Parga Filho, Camila Rocon de Lima, Charles Mady, Roberto Kalil-Filho and Vera Maria Cury Salemi
Heart Institute (InCor) do Hospital das Clínicas da Faculdade de Medicina da Universidade de São Paulo, São Paulo, Brazil

Justin Berk, Raymond Wade, Hatice Duygu Baser and Joaquin Lado
Department of Internal Medicine, Texas Tech University Health Sciences Center, School of Medicine, 3601 4th St Stop 9410, Lubbock, TX 79416, USA

Stepan Havranek, Tomas Palecek, Tomas Kovarnik, Miroslav Psenicka and Ales Linhart
2nd Department of Medicine – Department of Cardiovascular Medicine, First Faculty of Medicine, Charles University and General University Hospital in Prague, U Nemocnice 2, Prague 128 08, Czech Republic

Ivana Vitkova
Institute of Pathology, First Faculty of Medicine, Charles University and General University Hospital in Prague, Studnickova 2, 128 00 Prague, Czech Republic

Dan Wichterle
Department of Cardiology, Institute for Clinical and Experimental Medicine, Videnska 1958/9, Prague 140 21, Czech Republic

Peter Magnusson
Cardiology Research Unit, Department of Medicine, Karolinska Institutet, Karolinska University Hospital/Solna, SE-171 76 Stockholm, Sweden

Peter Magnusson, Jessica Jonsson and Lennart Fredriksson
Centre for Research and Development, Uppsala University/Region Gävleborg, SE-80187 Gävle, Sweden

Stellan Mörner
Department of Public Health and Clinical Medicine, Umeå University, SE-90187 Umeå, Sweden

Nobila Valentin Yaméogo, André Koudnoaga Samadoulougou, Koudougou Jonas Kologo, Georges Rosario Christian Millogo, Anna Thiam and Patrice Zansonré
Department of Cardiology, Yalgado Ouedraogo University Hospital, Ouagadougou, Burkina Faso

Larissa Justine Kagambèga
Medical Sciences Department, University of Ouagadougou, Ouagadougou, Burkina Faso

Charles Guenancia
Department of Cardiology, University Hospital, 14 rue Paul Gaffarel, 21079 Dijon CEDEX, France PEC2, UFR Sciences de Santé, University Bourgogne Franche-Comté, Dijon, France

Gustav Mattsson, Hoshmand Tawfiq and Peter Magnusson
Centre for Research and Development, Uppsala University/Region Gävleborg, SE-801 87 Gävle, Sweden

Abdullah Baroudi
Department of Medicine, Kiruna sjukhus, Region Norrbotten, SE-981 28 Kiruna, Sweden

Abdullah Baroudi and Peter Magnusson
Cardiology Research Unit, Department of Medicine, Karolinska Institutet, SE-171 76 Stockholm, Sweden

Jun Huang, Zi-Ning Yan, Yi-Fei Rui, Li Fan, Chang Liu and Jie Li
Department of Echocardiography, the Affiliated Changzhou No.2 People's Hospital of Nanjing Medical University, Changzhou, China

Nadine Abanador-Kamper, Judith Wolfertz, Marc Vorpahl and Melchior Seyfarth
Department of Cardiology, Helios University Hospital Wuppertal, University Witten/Herdecke, Germany
Center for Clinical Medicine Witten/Herdecke University Faculty of Health, Wuppertal, Germany

Lars Kamper and Patrick Haage
Department of Diagnostic and Interventional Radiology, Helios University Hospital Wuppertal, University Witten/Herdecke, Germany
Center for Clinical Medicine Witten/Herdecke University Faculty of Health, Wuppertal, Germany

Jun Huang, Zi-Ning Yan, Li Fan, Yi-Fei Rui and Xiang-Ting Song
Department of Echocardiography, ChangZhou No.2 People's Hospital Affiliated to NanJing Medical University, ChangZhou 213003, China

Tetsuya Yamamoto, Tsuneaki Kenzaka, Masanori Matsumoto, Ryo Nishio, Satoru Kawasaki and Hozuka Akita
Department of Internal Medicine, Hyogo Prefectural Kaibara Hospital, 5208-1, Kaibara, Kaibara-cho, Tanba, Hyogo 669-3395, Japan

Tsuneaki Kenzaka and Ryo Nishio
Division of Community Medicine and Career Development, Kobe University Graduate School of Medicine, 2-1-5, Arata-cho, Hyogo-ku, Kobe, Hyogo 652-0032, Japan

Uzair Ansari, Ibrahim El-Battrawy, Christian Fastner, Michael Behnes, Katherine Sattler, Aydin Huseynov, Stefan Baumann, Erol Tülümen, Martin Borggrefe and Ibrahim Akin
First Department of Medicine, University Medical Center Mannheim, University of Heidelberg, Mannheim, Germany

Ibrahim El-Battrawy, Martin Borggrefe and Ibrahim Akin
DZHK (German Center for Cardiovascular Research) partner site Mannheim, Mannheim, Germany

Uzair Ansari
First Department of Medicine, University Medical Center Mannheim, Theodor-Kutzer-Ufer 1-3, 68167 Mannheim, Germany

Tarun Pant and Zeljko J. Bosnjak
Department of Medicine, Medical College of Wisconsin, 8701 Watertown Plank Road, Milwaukee, WI 53226, USA

Zhi-Dong Ge
Department of Ophthalmology, Stanford School of Medicine, 1651 Page Mill Road, Stanford, CA 94304, USA

Juan Fang
Department of Pediatrics, Medical College of Wisconsin, 8701 Watertown Plank Road, Milwaukee, WI 53226, USA

Xiaowen Bai
Department of Cell Biology, Neurology & Anatomy, Medical College of Wisconsin, 8701 Watertown Plank Road, Milwaukee, WI 53226, USA

Xiaowen Bai, Zeljko J. Bosnjak and Mingyu Liang
Department of Physiology, Medical College of Wisconsin, 8701 Watertown Plank Road, Milwaukee, WI 53226, USA

Tarun Pant and Anuradha Dhanasekaran
Centre for Biotechnology, Anna University, Chennai, Tamil Nadu, India

Chen-Yu C. Guo
Lewis Katz School of Medicine, Temple University, 3500 N. Broad Street, Philadelphia, PA 19140, USA

Nan-Sung Chou
Department of Surgery, Madou Sin-Lau Hospital, 20 Lingzilin, Tainan 72152, Taiwan

H. M. M. T. B. Herath, S. P. Pahalagamage, S. Vinothan, Sampath Withanawasam, Vajira Senarathne and Milinda Withana
National Hospital, Colombo, Sri Lanka

Laura C. Lindsay
University of Edinburg, National Hospital, University of Edinburg, Scotland, Sri Lanka

Hongwei Tian, Jingang Cui, Chengzhi Yang, Fenghuan Hu, Jiansong Yuan, Shengwen Liu, Weixian Yang, Xiaowei Jiang and Shubin Qiao
State Key Laboratory of Cardiovascular Disease, Fuwai Hospital, National Center for Cardiovascular Diseases, Chinese Academy of Medical Sciences and Peking Union Medical College, Beijing 100037, China

Noboru Ichihara, Shuichi Fujita, Yumiko Kanzaki, Tomohiro Fujisaka, Michishige Ozeki and Nobukazu Ishizaka
Department of Cardiology, Osaka Medical College, Takatsuki-shi Daigaku-machi 2-7, Osaka 569-8686, Japan

Daniel Cortez, Jonas Carlson and Pyotr G. Platonov
Department of Cardiology, Clinical Sciences, Lund University, Lund, Sweden

Daniel Cortez
Electrophysiology/Cardiology, Penn State Milton S. Hershey Medical Center, Hershey, USA

Anneli Svensson
Department of Cardiology and Department of Medical and Health Sciences, Linkoping University, Linkoping, Sweden

Sharon Graw, Francesca Brun, Anita Spezzacatene and Luisa Mestroni
Cardiovascular Institute and Adult Medical Genetics Program, University of Colorado Denver AMC, Aurora, CO, USA

Francesca Brun, Anita Spezzacatene and Luisa Mestroni
Cardiovascular Department, Ospedali Riuniti and University of Trieste, Trieste, Italy

Pyotr G. Platonov
Arrhythmia Clinic, Skåne University Hospital, Lund, Sweden

Index

Non-ischemic Syndrome, 170
Non-sustained Ventricular Tachycardia, 3-4, 122
Non-thyroidal Illness Syndrome, 107-108, 111-112
Noncompaction Cardiomyopathy, 103, 106, 138-139

O
Oral Anticoagulation, 103, 149, 152-153
Outflow Tract Obstruction, 36, 50, 82, 89, 98-99, 155, 206
Oxidative Phosphorylation, 29, 33, 36, 78

P
Pancreatitis, 164, 168-169
Parvovirus B19, 164, 169
Periostin, 38-45
Peripartum Cardiomyopathy, 7, 13-14, 68, 129-131, 134
Plaque Rupture, 47, 83, 150
Pulmonary Artery Systolic Pressure, 8, 13, 68, 70

R
Radiofrequency Ablation, 90-91, 93, 95
Right Ventricular Systolic Dysfunction, 7, 13-14

S
Sarcomere Protein Gene, 96-97
Septum Wall, 140, 144, 146, 157, 160

Spontaneous Scar, 90-94
Streptokinase, 192-193, 195
Streptozocin, 58-59, 64, 75, 77, 181
Subendocardial, 82, 154-162
Syncope, 1, 119, 122, 207-208
Systemic Inflammatory Response Syndrome, 107-108, 111
Systolic Anterior Motion, 82-83, 85, 88, 207-208
Systolic Radial Strain, 140-141, 144-146

T
T-lymphocytes, 15-16, 20, 23, 25
Takotsubo Cardiomyopathy, 50, 52, 57, 82, 84, 87-89, 170, 176-177, 188, 190-194, 196-201, 203-204, 211-215
Trichrome Staining, 42, 58, 60, 62-63
Triptolide, 74-80

V
Vasospasm, 82
Vectorcardiography, 216
Ventricular Conduction Block, 66, 70